MW00845922

HEALING

CHILDREN'S ATTENTION & BEHAVIOR

PROFESSIONAL EDITION

HEALING
CHILDREN'S ATTENTION
& BEHAVIOR DISORDERS

Complementary Nutritional
& Psychological Treatments

DR ABRAM HOFFER, MD, FRCP(C)

CCNM
PRESS

Copyright © The Estate of Abram Hoffer, 2011.
All rights reserved.

The publisher does not advocate the use of any particular treatment program,
but believes that the information presented in this book should be available to
the pubic. The nutritional, medical, and health information presented in this
book is based on the research, training, and personal experiences of the author,
and is true and complete to the best of the author's knowledge. However, this
book is intended only as an informative guide to those wishing to know more
about good health. It is not intended to replace or countermand the advice given
by the reader's physician. Because there is always some risk involved, the author
and the publisher are not responsible for any adverse effects or consequences
from any of the suggestions made in this book. And because each person and
each situation is unique, the author and the publisher urge the reader to consult
with a qualified professional before using any procedure where there is a question
as to its appropriateness.

Previously published in a trade paperback edition as *Dr Hoffer's ABC of Natural
Nutrition for Children* (Quarry Health Books, 1999) and later revised as *Healing
Children's Attention & Behavior Disorders* (CCNM Press, 2004).

Cataloging in publication data is available.

ISBN-10 1-897025-41-6
ISBN-13 978-1-897025-41-3

Edited by Bob Hilderley.
Design by Sari Naworynski.

Printed and bound in Canada.

Published by CCNM Press Inc., 1255 Sheppard Avenue East,
Toronto, Ontario M2K 1E2 Canada.
ccnmpress@ccnm.edu

CONTENTS

ACKNOWLEDGEMENTS

I thank Bob Hilderley for editing this book. Incorporating my clinical data, presented in my sparse technical style of writing, Mr Hilderley has edited, reshaped, and restructured my manuscript.

I also thank my son, L. John Hoffer MD PhD, Associate Professor of Medicine, McGill University, Lady Davis Institute for Medical Research, who, while in his third year of medical school, spent two summer months interviewing the children whose cases are described in this book. I have included his views about these patients, but the conclusions about them are my own.

My experience with disturbed children is truly presented in this volume. If the program described here is followed by physicians and by patients and their families, there is no doubt that the vast majority of the children so treated will recover, and without the need for medication.

Abram Hoffer

The Troubled Child and the Battered Parent

One evening, early in 1962, my friend George called to say he was very worried about his youngest son, Ben. Nine years old, Ben had become a behavioral problem with a learning disability. Today he would be diagnosed as suffering from ADD (Attention Deficit Disorder) or one of its many variants. Progress at school was so slow his teachers began to prepare his parents to have him go to a school for slow learners, perhaps even to a school for the mentally retarded. But before anyone was aware that Ben had such a problem, he had tested 120 on an I.Q. (intelligence quotient) test. To his father, a public administrator, and his mother, a teacher, this was not only perplexing but very disturbing. I asked George to bring Ben to my office on the fifth floor of the University Hospital, now Royal University Hospital, in Saskatoon. At the time, I was Director of Psychiatric Research, Psychiatric Services Branch, Department of Public Health, Saskatchewan, and Associate Professor of Psychiatry at the Medical School.

I was not very keen on seeing Ben since I had little experience in treating children. The few children I had seen in the previous ten years were all considered either slow learners or had various degrees of severe retardation and no treatment was available for them. The 1960 view of these children was that they were primarily failures of the educational system and required special pedagogic skills and programs in order to deal with the problem. None of these special educational efforts was very effective. This was why the hospitals for the retarded were not called hospitals but rather training schools. We had one in Moose Jaw and a second one was created later on in Prince Albert after the building was closed as a special hospital for treating patients with tuberculosis. These hospitals (training schools) had more teachers and psychologists than physicians on their staff compared to mental hospitals housing schizophrenics and "real" mentally sick patients. To perpetuate this idea some American hospitals for these children called themselves "campuses."

The modern type hyperactive learning disordered child was extremely rare in 1960, however. This was also the view of celebrated pediatrician and children's health advocate Dr Benjamin Spock. I met Dr Spock just before we were both to appear on a TV program in Toronto in the mid 1960s and I asked him whether he had seen many "hyperactive" children when he was still practicing. He asked me to describe what I meant by hyperactive and later said that he could not recall having seen any children with this problem. But George was so disturbed I set aside my worry about making a proper assessment of Ben.

Ben came into my office with his father. He was a good looking boy, appeared healthy, with none of the physical stigmata of the seriously retarded children seen in old psychiatric textbooks. He did not know why he had been brought to see me, and he denied having any problems or symptoms. His father gave me his developmental history. He was walking by 14 months and speaking by 20. Both parents considered him an ideal child until he entered Grade 2 when he was 7 years old. By the end of 1960, his mother noticed a change in behavior. He became more anxious, could not fall asleep at night, and if he did sleep, woke up frequently during the night. School became harder for Ben. When the family moved to a different part of the city and he was moved to a different school, he had even more problems. His teachers were worried about his erratic performance at school and told his parents he was in a "shell." Reading and spelling were very poor. He finished Grade 3 with a D average in spite of extensive tutoring and drilling at home by his mother.

In July 1961 he was examined by a mental health clinic specializing in treating children. Ben's mother told them he had a very poor memory, reversed letters, and had no knowledge of phonics. His eyes skipped back and forth so much she tried to keep him focussed by using a ruler under the lines. His teachers reported he was not working up to his best ability, spent a lot of time day-dreaming, wasting time, and therefore falling behind. His marks were very low. He did not complete his assignments and did not bother to write his exams, nor could he be motivated. At home Ben was negative to his father, missed a lot of school, and often would come home after school hours not having gone to school that day. The clinic blamed (1) the move to a new school and (2) sibling rivalry with his brother, a year and a half older. They recommended remedial reading, which proved to be ineffective.

After my examination, I was puzzled. Nothing appeared which could explain the deterioration of this child to his present state. I arranged to analyze his urine for the "mauve factor." This was a substance which my research group had discovered in the urine of a majority of schizophrenic patients we treated, but it was also found in a smaller number of patients with other diagnoses. Over the previous few years, I had found that any patient with this substance in their urine more closely resembled schizophrenia than they did other diagnostic groups and that they responded very well to large doses of vitamin B-3 (niacin or niacinamide). We called it the mauve factor and later identified it as kryptopyrrole (KP).

The next day we found large quantities of KP in Ben's urine. I started Ben on niacinamide 1 gram three times each day after meals. His parents continued this regimen for several months.

George called me again that fall and told me that Ben was normal. He had been given remedial reading for two months by the clinic, who then pronounced him well, but he had shown no progress whatever before starting on the vitamin. He had spent the summer happily getting caught up with his reading.

One of his teachers prepared a report on Ben which she sent to me in 1973. George had advised her that Ben had done so badly in previous classes that he was called "stupid" in school and had responded by not answering any questions during class. But to her surprise she found him active in group discussions and volunteering answers. Here is what she wrote. "The first thing that his parents noticed in Ben's improvement after he showed an improvement in his health was his desire to go to school. Ben started to do his assignments, but at first he found the excuse of hunting for his books and pencils in his desk to delay him in starting his assignments promptly." The teacher started keeping his books on her desk for some time, but midway through the term Ben took the initiative to get his books out promptly and began his assignments. Previous to vitamin therapy, Ben had no desire to take down all the notes given in the allotted time. When anything was dictated, Ben would have hard time keeping up. Then he would become very tense and, so to speak, 'fold up'. This would happen in some exams, especially in Spelling and Arithmetic, which he was slow doing, and then he would run out of time.

These problems soon began to disappear. Many other improvements were noted physically, socially, emotionally and educationally. Ben at the beginning of the term would pride himself with the fact his mother was also a teacher. Later on in the term, Ben also started to mention his father and brother. "Ben is no longer shy," his teacher reported. "He is a sparkling personality; not afraid to speak up. He has started to take an interest in sports, in which he excels and which should be encouraged. He now gets along well with the children at school and at camp. He will assume leadership and organization duties. Ben now can read with eye-reversal not noticeable in reading and seldom in writing. Ben would go up on the stage to sing, say a speech, and read the morning scripture to the whole student body and the staff. All of the these things he did well with little nervousness and tension noticeable. Ben, also, reads books without being told and enjoys reading them."

In 1966 Ben had completed Grade 7 with a low A average. In Grade 9 he went to a track meet, participated in extra curricular activities, and worked as stage manager for a school play. He was so busy he wound up his scholastic year with a C average. Nevertheless, his parents were delighted with his state of normality.

In 1970 his mother wanted me to see him again. Ben had not taken niacinamide for two years, and she was worried that he might relapse. Ben had forgotten he had ever seen me and did not understand why he should take vitamin pills. I explained the situation to him, and he agreed he would start again and keep taking vitamin B-3 until age 18. Later Ben married.

He is raising a family and has a responsible permanent job. He meets my criteria for recovery – he is free of symptoms and signs of illness, he gets on well with his family and with the community, he is employed and pays taxes.

Although Ben was one of the first children I tested for mauve factor (KP) and advised to take large doses of niacinamide, he is an excellent example of what can be done for these children with so-called learning disabilities and behavioral disorders if they are examined, diagnosed, and treated with the correct "orthomolecular" or nutritional approach. Ben's treatment and response to a vitamin in megadoses is a prototype of what can be achieved through diet and nutrient supplements, not only for "ill" children like Ben, but also for "healthy" children. Since then I have diagnosed and treated over 1,500 children under the age of 14 suffering some learning disability, behavioral disorder, or chronic disease with a regimen of a sugar-free natural diet and optimum doses of vitamins, minerals, amino acids, and essential fatty acids.

Ben's recovery led to my first family study of the mauve factor (KP) and introduced a physician, the father of this family, to the use of megavitamin therapy. From being the usual medical skeptic he became a dedicated proponent of orthomolecular or nutritional therapy. A friend of Ben's mother had been worried about her 12-year-old only son "Mike," who had been a behavioral problem for several years. Mike's mother called me to seek an appointment and informed me her husband was a doctor. He would make the referral. I could not see Mike for several weeks and advised his mother to start him immediately on 2 grams of niacinamide daily.

I finally examined him 28 May 1963. He had been normal until kindergarten, where it was found he was very slow. He passed into Grade 2 with a C standing, but in Grade 3 slipped to a D average. He was shy, nervous, easily discouraged but cheerful and friendly. When nervous, he had a marked speech impediment. Early in 1959 he went to the same mental health clinic for children that had treated Ben. With therapy his reading ability improved from a Grade 1 to a Grade 2 level. This was considered striking by his worker. He was then given speech therapy for one year and gained 4 months of reading skill over that year. In June of 1960 he was in Grade 4 with a C average. The clinic and his school were still unhappy with his progress and remedial reading was intensified. By May 1961 he was reading fairly well, but his speech was slow and labored and he could not enunciate clearly. He tired easily, daydreamed a lot, and needed tranquilizers to relax him.

By May 1963, when I first saw him, he still needed special teaching. He could not locate the source of sound and had even been considered deaf. His mother remarked on his strong body odor, more pronounced when he was active. I have found this odor characteristic of many schizophrenic patients, especially noticeable when one smells their head, but gone when they are well. This odor troubled him and irritated his family. Between May 1959 and May 1961, after a lot of special attention and teaching at school and at the mental health clinic, his reading ability was increased from Grade 1 to Grade 5.4 level. He was then discharged from the clinic. However, his reading skills began to deteriorate, falling to 4.6 two years later.

Then after one month on the vitamin B-3 regimen, his score surged up to a 6.3 level and no longer fluctuated. In 1967 he told me he had passed out of Grade 10 with an 82 percent average. He found school interesting and enjoyable. He had only a vague recollection of what he had been like two years before as if he had gone through a dream. However, he still had moments of unreality and occasionally believed that people were looking at him too much. Apart from that he was well. I saw him for the last time in 1969 when I increased his niacinamide to 6 grams per day in Grade 12.

Unfortunately, he stopped taking vitamin B-3 in 1971, and by mid 1973 he was living on unemployment benefits and sold pot. By Christmas 1973 his behavior was odd and the next year his behavior became stranger. A public statue appeared alive to him and he was able to talk to it and received messages. He tried to interview a radio announcer and was picked up by the police and taken to the psychiatric ward. He asked the psychiatrist to start him back on niacinamide. His family had given this doctor Mike's history and his rapid response to the vitamin, but the doctor ignored the families wishes. The psychiatrist concluded this was just another delusion and gave him only electroconvulsive therapy having diagnosed him paranoid schizophrenic.

Mike's mother asked me to see her second child "William," born in 1954. She had not realized there was anything wrong until she saw the striking change in Mike. William's behavior had also deteriorated in Grade 2, with him becoming resentful, disobedient, and passive. He could not concentrate, could not judge the passage of time, and refused to play with other children. He had the same body odor as had Mike. I decided I would start him on the vitamin program before I saw him so that I could not be accused of helping him because of my therapeutic personality. The critics of megavitamin therapy had become very vocal. They included almost all the psychiatrists in Canada. The ones who saw my patients admitted that they had recovered but they ascribed this to my personality since they "knew" that vitamins could not possibly play a role. I therefore decided to see what niacinamide would do to a young patient whom I had never seen. Surely they could not credit my personality for this without assuming some type of extra sensory effect. I asked his mother to bring a sample of urine in for testing and then I would advise his father how much vitamin to give him.

William also had KP in his urine. I advised his father to start him on 500 mg after each meal. One week later he was much better and by April 1964 he was normal. I saw him for the first time in September 1967 because his mother wanted a doctor to explain to him why he was taking vitamins. He was well and no longer had KP in his urine. In 1973 he completed Grade 12 and was traveling as a tourist in Europe.

His mother also brought in a urine specimen from her daughter "Gail," born in 1952. She, too, had the peculiar odor, worse under stress, and her school performance had also deteriorated from an A student in Grade 3 to a D Grade average in Grade 6. She was also positive for KP. I started her on niacinamide 500 mg after each meal. In April 1964 she was normal. I saw her for the first time in September 1967. She then told me that before she had started on the vitamin she had suffered periodic episodes of depression. In 1973 she was in third-year university and was well.

Her mother now became worried about an older son, "Bob," born in 1946. He was irritable, hard to get along with, and doing so badly it appeared he would fail Grade 12. He was afraid to make friends, was suspicious of anyone who tried to be friendly with him, and suffered marked swings of mood into depression. He did not have the special body odor. His mother started him on niacinamide 500 mg after each meal. On 1 April 1964 he was better. By May 1965 he was attending university and was well. He then wanted to test himself to see whether he still needed the vitamin. Two months after he stopped, his problems returned. This time he was positive for KP and was placed back on the vitamin, 2 grams after each meal. He took it irregularly, waiting until he had symptoms. In February 1967 he complained of chronic fatigue, worse in the morning. I then placed him on a sugar-free, high protein diet. In March 1968 he was nearly well and negative for KP. In June 1967 he was depressed after he gone off the vitamin again. I started him on niacin, 2 grams, and ascorbic acid, 1 gram, after each meal, adding valium 10 mg at bedtime and neuleptil 5 mg in the morning. One month later he was well and I decreased the niacin to 4 grams daily and the vitamin C to 1.5 grams daily. In October 1972 he was married but the couple were having marital problem. The following year, still on his vitamins, he was normal.

The fifth child in the family, "David," born in 1949, had been normal and was negative for KP when tested in 1963. In February his behavior deteriorated and he was positive. On niacinamide 500 mg after each meal, he was normal in two days. By the end of 1973 he was still normal and in third-year dentistry.

"Felicity," the sixth child, normal and urine negative, began to suffer nightmares and restlessness in 1967. On niacinamide 500 mg after each meal she was normal in a few days. By the end of 1973 she was well as long as she stayed on the vitamin. "Heather," the youngest child, was also normal and negative but in May 1965 she also began to deteriorate in school. I saw her in January 1967 when she failed two classes at university after having passed out of Grade 12 with a high A average. She complained of chronic fatigue. I asked her to eliminate sugar and take niacinamide 1 gram after each meal. One week later she was well. In March 1968 she stopped her vitamins. In June 1970 she was pregnant and went back on. At last contact in 1973 she was well.

Late in 1963 their mother told me that after seeing the response of her children to niacinamide she had started to take it herself. She had been depressed most of her married life. Within a few weeks she became normal. She said this was such a marvelous feeling that she would never go off the vitamins and risk a return of her depression. She, too, had tested positive for the mauve factor.

Although the father of the family tested negative for the mauve factor, this experience with his family changed his medical practice. He became the first physician in Saskatchewan outside of our research group to use vitamin B-3 therapy. By the time he died several years later he had treated over 300 patients and was very enthusiastic about the results of this nutrient treatment. There have been far too few doctors show such enthusiasm for treating children orthomolecularly or nutritionally.

Between 15 percent and 20 percent of children entering school in North American suffer, like Ben and Mike, from one of the many varieties of learning disabilities or behavioral disorders. Many children suffering from these illnesses have been described as "hyperactive." A study in Australia found 18 percent of boys and 5 percent of girls were hyperactive. For a New Zealand group, 22 percent of the boys and 9 percent of the girls were hyperactive. One study in the United States found 9 percent of boys and 4 percent of girls scored hyperactive on behavioral tests. In a German study, 12 percent of boys and 5 percent of girls were in this group. In Britain the figures were 14.5 percent and 5.5 percent. All the evidence points to a figure of about 10 percent for boys and around 3 percent for girls. For good reason, society is very concerned with this problem.

To service this health and education problem – to care for and teach such a large portion of our population – a major "troubled-child" industry has grown since the 1960s when such problems first emerged *en masse*. This health and education industry includes the professional workers who diagnose, treat, and care for these children, such as psychiatrists, general practitioners, psychologists, social workers, special education teachers, and counselors; special facilities where the ill children are treated, housed, and rehabilitated; drug companies who provide medications such as ritalin and physicians who prescribe the drugs; educators who write and publishers who distribute textbooks for special education; clinics devoted to studying this problem and journals dedicated to reporting research studies; and societies for the emotionally disturbed, for the learning disabled, and for infantile autism, among many others.

Despite these efforts, the number of children suffering from learning disabilities and behavioral disorders continues to grow, while families directly involved are no less displeased, irritated, and often injured by current treatments, than the child. The system has not only failed many children but also battered many parents.

In 1970, The National Commission on Emotional & Learning Disorders included a report from the province of Manitoba which concluded that this situation is "all the more tragic when the survey proved categorically not only that existing health, social, and educational services are so stereotyped and rigid as to reject any possibility for change, but that inappropriate training institutions, competition between services, and failure to use adequate personnel resulted in a total fragmentation of the service, in turn totally fragmenting the child." In a subsequent 1974 report on this problem in the province of British Columbia, the health services were described as "the most inefficient, ineffective, out-dated, and discriminatory of all our existing social and medical programs." Reviewing these early reports from the 1960s and 1970s on learning disabled children and children with behavioral problems, Dr R. Glen Green concluded, "this statement could apply to any province or state if we measure effective treatment as a return to health of the patient, making him a productive member of society. There are thousands of intelligent thoughtful people using hundreds of different ideas and methods, most with equivocal results." There is little to suggest that this state of treatment for these children has changed over the years.

At the time, Dr Green proposed a fundamental nutritional approach to this diagnosing and treating this problem through diet. "If there is a common factor in the production of learning disabilities, we should work first at finding out what it is and then get on to specifics. It has been said that from time immemorial diet has been the cure for almost every illness yet it has seldom proven successful in the treatment of any disease or syndrome. Diet is most assuredly a common factor to every person who eats. It may well be the cause of most of our emotional, learning, and physical problems. In the light of recent developments, this statement will prove to be very prophetic – if the diet is properly used." Dr Green has been an advocate of the nutritional approach to medicine I developed with Dr Humphry Osmond during the 1950s while treating schizophrenics with vitamin B-3 (niacin or niacinamide) and vitamin C (ascorbic acid), an approach Nobel Prize Winner Dr Linus Pauling called "orthomolecular" when he adopted our cause and championed this practice of nutritional medicine.

Nutritional (Orthomolecular) Medicine

The idea to use vitamin B-3 and vitamin C for treating children arose out of the "adrenochrome hypothesis" Dr Osmond and I developed after he joined our research group in Saskatchewan in 1951. Before coming to Canada he and his friend Dr J. Smythies had suggested that in the schizophrenic body there might be a substance similar to adrenalin in structure and having the properties of mescalin. Adrenalin is one of the well-known stress mediators made in the body in the adrenal gland and in other nervous tissues, while mescalin is a hallucinogen extracted from peyote buttons, a cactus plant. I found this idea intriguing, and during the fall of 1951 we explored it further.

As the physician-biochemist of the team, I examined the chemical formula of all the known hallucinogens, hoping something might emerge which could lead us to the substance we thought was present in the body. Chemicals with similar structures tend to have similar properties. I looked up the chemical structure of every known hallucinogen we had previously defined not to include compounds which altered the state of consciousness. LSD (d-lysergic acid diethylamide), harmine, and ibogaine were indoles. Mescalin could easily become an indole by the side ring connecting to the benzene ring. We suspected that pink adrenalin, deteriorated adrenalin in solution, also had hallucinogenic properties, but we did not know what that substance was. The similarity in structure suggested that the schizophrenic toxin might be an indole coming from adrenalin, not simply a substance with a structural similarity to adrenalin. At our first meeting of the Saskatchewan Committee on Schizo-phrenia Research early in 1952, Dr D.E. Hutcheon, Professor of Pharmacology, College of Medicine, University of Saskatchewan, told us that the pink adrenalin was adrenochrome. He had studied this compound for his doctoral dissertation in England.

Our guiding hypothesis became the reaction:

$$\text{ADRENALIN} \longrightarrow \text{ADRENOCHROME}$$

To establish this hypothesis we would have to demonstrate (1) that adrenochrome is indeed made in the body; (2) that it is an hallucinogen; and (3) that preventing its formation would be therapeutic for schizophrenia.

A full account of the development of this hypothesis is available in our book *The Hallucinogens*. All these conditions were met. As we were interested in finding a better treatment for schizophrenia, we decided to use this hypothesis as our guide.

There were two ways of shutting down the formation of adrenochrome. We could divert the adrenalin to other compounds rather than allowing it to go to adrenochrome. If we could prevent the addition of methyl groups to noradrenalin, then less adrenalin would be available for forming adrenochrome. To do so we decided to try vitamin B-3. I knew something about vitamins, having studied them while doing the research on vitamins in cereal products during my Ph.D. education at the University of Minnesota. Four natural methyl acceptors are now known – thiamin (vitamin B-1), riboflavin (vitamin B-2), niacin (vitamin B-3), and ubiquinone (coenzyme Q_{10}). Coenzyme Q_{10} was not known then and the vitamins B-1 and B-2 were not as clearly related to psychosis as vitamin B-3 was. Vitamin B-3 was readily available and it was the safest and easiest to administer.

Both forms of vitamin B-3, niacin and niacinamide, are methyl acceptors – that is, they pick up methyl groups. We thought that this vitamin might decrease the formation of adrenalin by making less noradrenalin available. The process of adding and removing methyl groups from molecules is called transmethylation. In 1952 transmethylation had not been established as a normal reaction in the body. We also knew that vitamin B-3 was the anti pellagra vitamin, that it had been used in large doses for treating some organic confusional conditions and some patients with depression, and that it was safe to use even in large doses. In the body, vitamin B-3 is converted into nicotinamide adenine dinucleotide, which is present in both oxidized (NAD) and reduced forms (NADH). But this coenzyme is involved in over 200 reactions in the body involving oxidation reduction in the respiratory chain.

Dr Osmond and I spent a lot of time in defining what would be the ideal treatment. Our first requirement was that the treatment could be given for many years with safety. We realized that the only two treatments then in use, electroconvulsive (ECT) and insulin therapy, even if they were effective for a short time, could not be expected to cure any patients since schizophrenia is a chronic disease much as is diabetes. One does not treat diabetes by giving patients insulin in hospital and then expect them to stay well after discharge without insulin, yet this is what was expected of the schizophrenic patients. We knew that we would have to give large or mega-doses if we were to quench the production of adrenalin from noradrenalin by inhibiting transmethylation. We also thought that if smaller doses had been effective, this would have been reported in the medical literature.

The pellagrologists doing their clinical research between 1935 and 1945 were not squeamish about using what they considered to be large doses of vitamin B-3 to treat pellagra. The largest daily dose was 1.5 grams. Later I discovered that Dr William Kaufman had used up to 4 grams daily for treating patients with arthritis. The 1.5 gram doses had been given to small series of depressed patients and many of them had gotten well.

At the time, vitamins were defined as substances which were needed in very small amounts in order to prevent the development of a vitamin deficiency disease. In the absence of thiamin, patients would get beri beri, in the absence of vitamin B-3, pellagra, and in the absence of vitamin C, scurvy. Conversely, it meant that in the absence of these deficiency diseases these vitamins were not necessary. Mr Ben May, an American philanthropist who funded the Ben May Research Institute for Cancer, later told me that in the 1930s in the southern mental hospitals of the United States vitamin B-3 was given to many of the patients. If they recovered on the smaller doses, they were immediately re-diagnosed as cases of pellagra. If they did not respond to these gram doses, they retained their diagnosis of schizophrenia. This effectively quenched any interest in pursuing vitamin B-3 therapy further.

We did not know in 1952 that chronic patients required much large doses for much longer periods of time. I now know that for some patients up to 10 years of treatment is needed before one sees the maximum benefit from this vitamin and it must be combined with attention to nutrition and the use of other nutrients. We concluded that vitamin B-3, either niacin or niacinamide, individually or combined, could be safely used in 3 or more gram doses for many years. It could be taken by mouth, was readily available in these doses, and was relatively inexpensive. We later found that both forms were acceptable to most patients depending upon the orientation of the physicians. If the physicians did not like them, neither would their patients. That is why skeptics who looked at these vitamins superficially reported many side effects with a high drop out rate, while doctors knowledgeable about them reported fewer side effects and much lower drop out rates.

Vitamin B-3 does decrease the formation of adrenochrome in the brain. The oxidation of adrenalin to adrenochrome takes place in two steps. In the first step, the adrenalin loses one electron to form what has been called oxidized adrenalin. It is a very reactive molecule. In the presence of NAD and NADH, it recaptures one electron once more to form adrenalin and this reaction keeps on going back and forth. But if there is not sufficient NAD and NADH, the oxidized adrenalin loses another electron to become adrenochrome. This can no longer be changed back to adrenalin. Thus, in the absence of vitamin B-3, one of the precursors of NAD, more adrenochrome is formed. The same reactions occur with the other catechol amines. Noradrenalin will be changed to noradrenochrome and dopamine to dopachrome. But at the same time by decreasing the further oxidation of adrenalin to adrenochrome, it also increases the amount of adrenalin which can be used for other physiological purposes.

For example, it is now believed that Parkinsonism is caused by a deficiency of l-dopa. This is why this compound is given to these patients. What has not been taken into account is what happens to the dopamine once it has been given. I have no doubt it is converted to dopachrome and thus it has two activities. It increases the amount of l-dopa in the brain, which helps relieve these patients of some of the symptoms of their disease, but by increasing the amount of dopachrome, it will make many of them psychotic depending on the amount which is given and may, according to some medical authorities, hasten their death. Thus this drug, which is so helpful at the time, decreases life span. However, a recent report supports the finding that vitamin B-3 and coenzyme Q_{10} spare dopamine. J.B. Shulz and colleagues found that in animals made to have Parkinsonism by the administration of MPTP, giving them these two natural substances protected the animals against the dopamine depletion the toxic drug produces. Q_{10} and vitamin B-3 make up what is called complex A in the respiratory chain of respiratory enzymes. I have given two Parkinsonism patients these two vitamins and it has been very effective in helping them.

Preventing the oxidation of adrenalin to adrenochrome by using vitamin C (ascorbic acid) would also be therapeutic, according to our hypothesis. Vitamin C is nature's most powerful water soluble antioxidant. In 1952 we had little information on how adrenalin was oxidized to adrenochrome, nor how vitamin C would modify this reaction. By deliberately using vitamin C as an antioxidant, we were the first medical group to employ antioxidants. For many years this work was totally ignored, but over the past five years the term antioxidant has become fashionable. The two other popular vitamin antioxidants are vitamin E and beta carotene. Coenzyme Q_{10} is becoming much more popular and has many interesting and valuable properties. Only vitamin C was then available, however, and we decided to study its clinical properties as well. We decided to combine vitamin B-3 and vitamin C as our main therapeutic nutrients.

We did combine both of these vitamins in our pilot trials and in our open clinical studies almost every patient receiving vitamin B-3 also was given ascorbic acid. But we could not study both when we began the double blind experiments in Saskatchewan. We had started two double blind controlled experiments to study the therapeutic effect of a yeast nucleotide preparation, at the request of the Department of National Health, Ottawa. This was the first double blind prospective controlled experiment done by any psychiatrists. But we were told that we could not study two variables in the same study as it would make it too complicated and would require much larger series of patients. We therefore had to decide which vitamin we would study, and for the reasons described here, decided to omit ascorbic acid from these controlled trials.

Before beginning our double blind experiments, we had to learn how to use vitamin B-3. We started a small series of pilot studies on acute and a few chronic patients at the Munro Wing, General Hospital, Regina and at the Saskatchewan Hospital at Weyburn where Dr Osmond was superintendent. We concentrated on the early cases since we did not think the chronic patients were the best subjects to study. Any disease is best treated early before there are irreparable physical and psychological damaging changes. After a six-month evaluation of vitamin B-3 in nicotinic acid form, we learned the optimum dose range, the minor side effect (we did not run into any major side effects), and the kind of results we might expect. We also learned it could be combined with any other treatment. The main one then was ECT. By spring of 1952 we reported to the Saskatchewan Committee on Schizophrenia Research that every one of eight acute patents given this vitamin either recovered or were very much better. With this incentive we began our double blind controlled experiments at the Munro Wing, our third but the world's first in psychiatry.

Thirty patients admitted to the Munro Wing and diagnosed schizophrenic by their treating psychiatrist were divided randomly into three groups. One group received placebo, a second group niacinamide, and the third group niacin. The psychiatrist in charge of each patient could also use other treatments, including drugs, psychotherapy, and ECT. The only drugs used were barbituates used to sedate patients. None of these allowed treatments were really effective in treating these patients but something had to be used to control psychotic behavior. In a blind experiment no one is supposed to know which compounds are being given; the nurses, social workers, doctors, and patients would not be allowed to know. That is why it was double blind. However, it is impossible to double blind niacin because it causes a dramatic flush especially at the onset of treatment. We, therefore, added the third group on niacinamide because it does not cause any flushing. We had told the clinical group that we were comparing niacin against placebo. They would therefore assume that every patient turning red would have been getting niacin and that every patient not turning red would be on placebo. In fact half the patients not turning red were on niacinamide. This was a hidden control.

Patients were given 3 grams each day after meals for a month. They were then followed for two years and evaluated before the treatment code was broken. One third of the placebo group were well compared to two thirds of the two vitamin groups. We had improved the 35 percent natural recovery rate to a two year 75 percent recovery rate. Three more double blind experiments yielded similar results. These experiments were very exciting to us and to our patients, but the rest of the psychiatric world remained singularly unimpressed. The main reason was the introduction of tranquilizers into psychiatry in the mid 1950s. These drugs rapidly controlled psychotic behavior whether it was in the acute or chronic patients. There was a revolution in the way patients were treated and it became possible to use these drugs to quiet noisy wards. A psychiatrist tested the therapeutic effect of the tranquilizers on chronic patients by measuring the noise level with a noise meter. Psychiatrists – aided, persuaded, and abetted by the drug companies which held patents on these powerful drugs –

were persuaded that at last we had the answer to the treatment of these patients. These companies are still spending huge sums of money in their search for the ever elusive new miracle tranquilizer, currently such drugs as prozac and ritalin, and their psychiatric colleagues are waiting anxiously for it to be developed.

There was no patent on vitamin B-3 and it is still ignored by drug companies except for those few who manufacture it in bulk. Since then it has been shown over and over that while these drugs are helpful in cooling down symptoms, patients do not recover fully. In fact, I have shown that it is impossible to get well if the only treatment is tranquilizers: the tranquilizer recovery rate is about the same as the natural one third recovery rate. The full story of our research is told in my book *Vitamin B-3 & Schizophrenia: Discovery, Recovery, Controversy.*

In 1967 I resigned from my job as Director of Psychiatric Research, Psychiatric Services Branch, Department of Public Health, and Associate Professor (Research) in Psychiatry, College of Medicine, University of Saskatchewan, at Saskatoon and started a private practice in Saskatoon. I was not receiving adequate support from either of my two employers because they were embarrassed by our claims that vitamins could help schizophrenics. Pressure was increasingly placed upon me to fall in line with our critics, but I did not want to spend my days examining ever more tranquilizers. As a private practitioner I would be free to do what I considered best for my patients and would have access to many more patients. Since each patient would have to be referred by a general practitioner or, in rare cases, by another specialist, seeing their patients get well would eventually persuade them there was something to the nutritional medicine and treatment.

Although I had encouraged Dr Silverman, the foremost pediatrician in North Dakota, to use megavitamin therapy with children during our research years and treated an odd child like Ben and "Mike," I had not intended to treat children in my private practice. However, a few were referred to me anyway, and when I saw the speed with which some of them recovered, I became much more interested in the problems of childhood disorders. By this time my colleagues, especially Allan Cott, had also started to treat children, and their reports were very encouraging. Dr Bernard Rimland joined our orthomolecular group in 1962 and became a powerful supporter after he had studied large numbers of autistic children treated by different methods. Dr Rimland founded the Autism Society after writing his classic book *Infantile Autism*.

We soon discovered that children tolerated these large doses of vitamins very well and could be started on adult doses. I had received a research grant from the Canadian Mental Health Association, Saskatchewan Division, which allowed me to do a controlled study, using a placebo crossover design, to see how many of the varieties of childhood disorders could be treated successfully. To my surprise about 80 percent of the children responded well, provided they followed the program long enough. The failures were children who would not or could not remain on the program.

In the summer of 1973 John Hoffer, my son, had completed his second year of medicine at McGill University in Montreal. In order to encourage medical students, the Government of Saskatchewan offered medical students a two month stipend, provided to the physician who retained this payment. I employed John to follow up every child I had seen in the district around Saskatoon and in the city between July 1967 and August 1973. His report confirmed my belief that nutritional medicine was effective in treating a wide variety of children's disorders and diseases. Many of these cases are presented later in the book along with more recent accounts of orthomolecular therapy.

During this time I also made the acquaintance of Dr Linus Pauling, winner of the Nobel Prize for Biochemistry and for Peace. With Dr Osmond I had published a small book *How To Live with Schizophrenia* which Dr Pauling discovered while visiting a friend. The book had been given to her by the father of a patient who had recovered from schizophrenia on vitamin therapy after five years of failure on standard treatment. Dr Pauling was surprised that we were using such large doses of vitamin B-3 and vitamin C, and after some investigation into our research, he joined the cause, soon becoming the most eloquent spokesman for nutritional medicine. For Dr Pauling, our approach was a logical extension of his previous interest in molecular medicine. In a speech given at the California Institute of Technology in 1938, he observed: "Organic chemistry was developed into a great science during the nineteenth century, and it seems probable that all or nearly all its fundamental principles have now been formulated. There is, however, a related field of knowledge of transcendent significance to mankind which has barely begun its development. This field deals with the correlation between chemical structure and physiological activity of those substances, manufactured in the body or ingested in foodstuffs, which are essential for orderly growth and the maintenance of life, as well as of the many substances which are useful in the treatment of disease."

In 1968, Dr Pauling wrote a landmark review of our medical research in *Science* magazine entitled "Orthomolecular Psychiatry" which delighted those of us who were practising megavitamin therapy but offended many others. The American Psychiatric Association subsequently tried to suppress the publication of any information about the value of high dose vitamins in the treatment of schizophrenia. They eventually called Dr Osmond and me before their committee on ethics in 1971 because a California psychiatrist had complained about my paper describing the patient who recovered and whose father had indirectly introduced Dr Pauling to our concepts.

Dr Pauling became very supportive of the work being done by our colleagues. Within a few years we agreed that we were in fact practising "orthomolecular" psychiatry and that we should officially adopt this term as representative of what we were doing. In 1973, Dr Pauling co-edited with Dr David Hawkins a book called *Orthomolecular Psychiatry* which collected in one volume many of our reports. By now Dr Pauling was fully identified with the new paradigm and with orthomolecular psychiatry and medicine. In 1971 he established the Linus Pauling Institute of Science and Medicine in Palo Alto, where he and his colleagues began to study the relation between vitamin C and cancer, which has resulted in several books, including Ewan Cameron's *Cancer and Vitamin C* and *Healing Cancer: Complementary Vitamin and Drug Treatments*, which I co-authored with Dr Pauling just before his death.

Dr Pauling proposed the word "orthomolecular" to describe the use of optimum (often large) doses of molecules naturally present in the body to treat poor health and to promote good health. The practice of orthomolecular medicine recognizes that most chronic diseases are due to metabolic fault which is correctable in most patients by good use of nutrition, including the use of vitamin and mineral supplements. In sharp contrast, drugs are synthetics which are not naturally present in the body and for which the body does not have ready made mechanisms for their destruction and elimination. They are called xenobiotics – that is, foreign molecules.

As Dr Pauling explained in his study of orthomolecular nutrition in his celebrated books *Vitamin C and the Common Cold* and *How To Live Longer and Feel Better*, the human body has lost its ability during evolution to make certain nutrients. This precept is the basis of my two previous books on nutrition, *Orthomolecular Nutrition* and *Hoffer's Laws of Natural Nutrition*, which I have integrated into this book on children's natural nutrition. About 20 million years ago, man, other primates, the guinea pig, and an Indian fruit-eating bat lost the ability to make vitamin C, Dr Pauling argues. In my opinion, man is going through a process right now when we are losing the ability to make vitamin B-3 from tryptophan. People suffering from the various schizophrenias, for example, are a group who have gone far in this direction. As diets have become less natural, more high-tech, the amount of vitamin B-3 has been lowered, and those people who no longer have the machinery for converting enough trypto-phan to the vitamin are becoming sick. I have been convinced for a long time that if we were to add 100 mg of vitamin B-3 in niacinimide form to our diet for every person, there would be a major decrease in the incidence of schizophrenia and many other diseases such as hyperactivity and learn-ing and behavioral disorders in children.

Dr Bernard Rimland, author of *Infantile Autism*, further explains the meaning of orthomolecular and contrasts the practice of 'orthomolecular' medicine with 'toximolecular' medicine: " 'Ortho' means straight or cor-rect and 'molecular' refers to the chemistry of the body. 'Orthomolecular' thus means correcting the chemistry of the body. To contrast the philoso-phies of establishment medicine and orthomolecular medicine, I have coined the word 'toximolecular' to refer to the common practice of trying to treat disease (or at least the symptoms of disease) through the use of toxic chemicals. It doesn't make much sense to me; it is dangerous, expen-sive, and not very effective. But it is profitable. Most vitamins are quite safe, in contrast to the drugs in widespread use which can be and all too often are lethal in large amounts. Traditional medicine consists largely of giving lethal drugs in sub-lethal amounts, it seems to me. Orthomolecular psychiatry is not only much safer, it is much more sensible. Its emphasis on the use of substances normally present in the human really makes sense."

The practice of orthomolecular medicine and nutrition, unlike conventional medicine and nutrition, recognizes the principle of individuality in recommending the optimum diet of nutrients for each of us. No two patients are the same; no two treatments are the same. Everyone knows that every person is unique. Infants know this as soon as they can differentiate their mother from all other mothers. When a child first recognizes a stranger, he or she has already mastered the concept that we are all different. In appearance we are not the same. The best test for this is the interest generated when identical twins walk down the street together. When quintuplets are identical, public curiosity is enormous, for these phenomena violate the principle of individuality. I think the need for individuality was essential for survival. The outer appearance and behavior of any individual is an expression of that person's physiology and biochemistry. It therefore follows that their biochemistry and nutritional needs must also be individual. Without individuality there would be no humanity. The individuality of people was necessary for the evolution of our human societies.

We know all about the individuality of finger prints, how even identical twins do not have identical finger prints. Blood types also are unique to individuals as are dental patterns and DNA. Surgeons are not surprised when they try to find the appendix and it is not where it is supposed to be. Sometimes the heart is on the right side. Most organs of the body are not exactly where they are supposed to be, nor are they the same size and shape. Physicians and pharmacologists have known that the optimum doses for drugs can vary enormously between patients, that while there are useful guides for how much to give, many people will need much less and many will need much more. But when it came to the need for optimum nutrition, that knowledge of individuality disappeared, primarily in the medical and nutritional profession. People knew that one "man's meat was another man's poison." They knew that they could eat what others cannot, but the concept was not clearly expressed and was not acted on in developing optimum nutrition.

The manufacture and advertising of high-tech food is based upon the principle that we are all alike, however. Producers of any product will extol the virtues of their product and will not refer to the fact that many people may be allergic to or otherwise be made sick by, their product and should avoid it. It is unrealistic to expect the manufacturers of high-tech food to refer to the possibility that some may be allergic to their product, but it would be refreshing if they did place the health of their customers somewhere above their idea that this would injure their bottom line. The dairy industry touts its products very highly with support from nutritionists and physicians. But they never discuss in their advertisements that many people are made sick by milk.

We are unique as individuals and our needs for nutrients vary as do other biochemical and physical attributes. There will be a narrow range of variation for some nutrients and a wide range of variation for others. Each nutrient will have its own range. This means that most people will have an optimum range which varies about a mean for the whole group, but there will be a much smaller number of people who will need much less and another group who will need very much more.

The optimum amount of nutrients also varies, but we do not have the data for each nutrient on large normal populations. The recommended daily allowances (RDAs) generally cover a very narrow range of need. The developers of these recommended doses assumed that vitamins were needed only in very small doses and added what they considered was an ample safety factor by recommending more than they really thought were needed. However, these doses apply only to healthy people. They, in their definition, excluded people under stress, people who are sick, pregnant women, and nursing women. There are so many exclusions that these RDAs have no value for individuals. They have never been of any value for determining what individuals should be taking. Recently scientists have begun to recognize this, and some have recommended using specific doses for individual diseases. This I have done for many years.

If we constructed a large bell-shaped curve showing the range of dosage for any one nutrient along the bottom or the X axis, and plotted the area on the curve where each disease properly fell, we would find that healthy people would be in the area from the lowest doses to somewhat above the mean for the whole group. Patients would be in the high dose area, and the sicker they were, the closer they would lie to the extreme right of the diagram. Thus the average person will get along fairly well with about 3 grams per day of ascorbic acid (vitamin C). A person with any infection such as the common cold will need perhaps two to three times as much. A person seriously ill with a killing disease such as cancer will require doses ranging from 12 to 40 grams orally and may need an additional 50 to 100 grams given intravenously. Vitamin C represents the very wide variation of optimum doses. Other nutrients have much narrower ranges. Thus for riboflavin (vitamin B-2) there is little evidence to suggest that we have to give more than 100 or 200 mg per day. The water soluble vitamins are very safe because they do not build up in the body. They are easily excreted. Vitamins which are fat soluble can build up and one has to be more cautious about using high doses. But even here the dangers of these vitamins, such as vitamin D-3 and vitamin A, have been grossly exaggerated.

The concept of an optimum dose and the popularization of the word megavitamin has been confusing to many. The prefix "mega" was first applied to vitamins by my friend Irwin Stone who first summarized the world literature on vitamin C in his ground-breaking book *The Healing Factor: Vitamin C against Disease*. I met Irwin in 1966 at the same meeting I first met Dr Pauling. He told me his life had been saved by taking large doses of vitamin C. He had collected almost all the vitamin C literature, and I urged him to have this material published. A couple of years later I urged him once more to do so. In *The Healing Factor*, Stone points out that we are all suffering from scurvy which is partially controlled by the small amounts of vitamin C present in food, but these small amounts are not adequate to give us optimum health, or at least health which is much better than what most people enjoy today. He recommended large doses of vitamin C and first used the term "mega ascorbic acid therapy." He followed his own advice. One day I saw him spread liberal amounts of vitamin C on his steak until it was almost white.

Patients have come to me to ask for "megavitamins" rather than megavitamin therapy. There is no such thing, of course, as a megavitamin; megavitamin therapy refers to the use of megadoses of vitamins. Megadose refers to the use of doses which are substantially larger than those recommended by the usual government guide lines, the recommended daily doses or RDAs. The term mega is not applied in this manner to mineral or amino acid supplements.

Because the word megadose represents the new paradigm of using vitamins in therapy for diseases or syndromes not considered to be caused by vitamin deficiencies, it has been rejected by members of the old paradigm. The old paradigm insists on using vitamins only for deficiency diseases in very small RDA doses. The RDAs have been used to indicate what every person ought to obtain, though they were never designed for this prescriptive purpose, and do not apply to majority but rather to the mean of the population. They have almost been used interchangeably with nutrient need, but the nutrient need of the individual is ignored. And they have been used on a massive scale to attack any physicians who recommend more than these minimal requirements. They are, if followed, guaranteed to produce minimal good health when what we should strive for is optimum good health.

Orthomolecular medicine requires the application of both these principles, then, individuality and optimum nutrition, including the use of large doses (if needed) of vitamins as well as mineral, amino acid, and essential fatty acid supplements.

Bringing Up Joey

Perhaps the best way to conclude an introduction to this book is through the presentation of another case study, this time told in the words of a parent, where the conventional medical and educational system failed to diagnose and treat her son suffering from learning disabilities, behavioral disorders, and chronic diseases properly, leaving in the wake a sick child and a battered parent.

From his birth in 1960 "Joey" was a difficult baby. He did not eat well. He began to walk by 20 months and to speak at age 3½ years but shortly after he was fitted for glasses he stopped and did not speak again until he was 7. When I saw him he was confused, read very poorly, words appeared jumbled and numbers were reversed. He had been diagnosed as perceptually handicapped with mental retardation. He was in a special class for speech and occupational therapy.

His mother wrote an account of his illness and recovery which she entitled "Bringing Up Joey":

"I was real proud of myself with Joey born April 18, 1960, my sixth child, but the first one of two deliveries on my own. At last I knew what other mothers meant by natural childbirth. My other deliveries had all been difficult. My joy was short lived, however, as I soon realized he was different. The others were all hungry and ready to eat as soon as the nurses brought them for their feeding. Joey seemed hungry but only sucked for a few minutes and then fell asleep. No matter how hard I tried to wake him, he never ate again till the next feeding schedule, although the nurses said they had to feed him between feedings. He was only 7 lb 4 oz when he was born (my smallest baby) and had lost about 6 oz before I went home. His feeding habits didn't improve at home, and after struggling for a month trying to breast feed him, I put him on a SMA powder, hoping I could get more into him at one time. Since this didn't help, I put him on solid foods, but even then he ate very little at one time. Two teaspoons full was a good-sized meal for him.

As time passed, although I fed him often, he was not a cuddly baby and looked like an advertisement for the Hungry Children's Fund. I started visiting doctors and child specialists who checked him thoroughly but could never find anything wrong. He was a small child and thin but his blood was surprisingly good. Then he began to develop sores on his body and in his hair. These he would scratch, mostly at night, till his nighties and bed clothes were all bloody. The sores on his head would get infected, but it seemed if I washed his hair at least once a day, I could control them. So we shaved his hair off. Joey was indeed a sorry sight then, small, skinny, with his head shaved and sores on his arms and cheeks.

Of course, I did the doctor routine again with little success. We were prescribed a variety of ointments which discolored his clothes but did not heal the sores. Although each remedy did some good, he had a fresh outbreak as soon as the old one was healed.

There is a history of far-sightedness in the family. We had two children in glasses by this time, one with a very strong correction, and it wasn't very long before we realized Joey had eye problems. Whenever he was in a bright room, his eyes would cry, especially his left one. Since it seemed common sense to have his eyes attended to immediately, I made an appointment with one of our foremost eye specialists to see Joey, who was 15 months at this time. The doctor looked at Joey, took a quarter out of his pocket, and threw it at Joey's feet. Joey immediately bent down and picked it up. "See," said the doctor, "he saw it quite easily. His sight cannot be very bad, although I think he is a bit far-sighted. Bring him back in two years." I paid my $10, took my child, and went home very heart broken.

Joey was forever bumping into things. He didn't walk till he was two years old as every time he tried he was forever bumping his head into things and grew very discouraged. I began to blame his poor eating habits on his eye sight also. It seemed he noticed the food on the dish across the table from him more than his own dish. He was a very neat child, however, never messed around in his dish or dug in it with his fist to eat. At an age when most children had to be watched so they would not put things into their mouths, Joey never put anything into his mouth outside of food, and even then very little of that. He has always been a very neat tidy person, happiest only when everything was in its proper place, neatly in order.

Our children all toilet trained early and easily and Joey was no exception. When Joey was 30 months I began a very difficult pregnancy, so I do not remember his baby talk as he seemed to be babbling all the time. He got his glasses when he was three. The glasses seemed to make a great deal of difference as once Joey had them on he wouldn't take them off only to go to sleep. They are of course the first thing he reaches for in the morning. However, once his sight seemed to improve, he stopped talking. I had a new baby to look after.

Joey seemed adjusted to his new brother. However, while I had been in the hospital, he had been terrified by thunder, so for the rest of the summer we had to watch him very closely whenever a storm cloud appeared, even sitting up at night till they blew over.

As Joey approached his 4th birthday we realized his speech was not developing and that he was actually using a sign language all his own to get what he wanted, using words of his own which we understood but no one else could. He could not even say water. It was then I decided something had to be done, so I asked questions and read articles till I came to the conclusion the MacNeill Clinic was perhaps where I should take him. Since I had to have a doctor's prescription to go there, I went to our family doctor and got one, though he didn't seem too enthusiastic about the clinic.

On our first visit, I went upstairs with Mrs C., who took down Joey's history while Joey was taken to another room. The personnel at the Clinic seemed very concerned and willing to help. They mentioned that Joey was not using his eyes properly and he had very poor hand-eye coordination. The reason for this they felt was that he should have been fitted with glasses right after birth and couldn't understand why the eye specialist would leave his eyes unattended for 3 years, which had in fact caused Joey a certain amount of retardation.

We now began driving Joey once a week to speech therapy at the Clinic from February 1968 to July 1968. Mrs S. seemed a very capable person, but I found myself listening to her Scots accent instead of her words and wondered if Joey could understand her. Joey seemed very happy at the Clinic and looked forward to his visits there, but as Joey drew near the end of the school year Mrs C. spoke to me and said unless Joey attended kindergarten he would make little or no progress at school – why, I did not know.

I asked that Joey be tested again. Mrs S. called me into her office and told me that although Joey was a lovable little fellow, he was retarded. I, of course, cried as this came as a great shock to me. Mrs S. thought he had a physical problem and suggested I put him under Dr G.'s care to see if it could be diagnosed. She suggested it had something to do with his inability to digest protein and I should get his urine analyzed.

Joey's speech had not improved very much, but we were now trying to help him at home. Sometimes we used a mirror, sometimes his "Cat in the Hat" alphabet book. His tongue did not seem to function properly and his muscles in his mouth were very weak. Chocolate had never been a favorite food of his. We now noticed when he did eat a piece his tongue could not clear it out and the chocolate stuck to his teeth. He could not curl his tongue or blow, so now we concentrated on developing his mouth muscles; no opportunity was passed by to tell him the name of articles, things on TV, etc. Our speech was slowed down and we began to enunciate words. Whenever Joey had to say anything, we never rushed him, giving him time to collect his thoughts and present them.

Then we noticed his hands were not functioning properly. When his fifth birthday came, he could not rip off the paper from his gifts, he had no idea how to do it. One day as the family were sitting in the front room watching TV, I asked Joey to take off his socks. He couldn't, so I made him take off everybody's socks, and by the time he had removed 18 socks he had mastered the skill. Now we began a program of teaching him to use his fingers and hands for his feet were as nimble as one could wish for.

Joey had another malady – all his life he would vomit without a real cause or reason. Often it was when we were entertaining people with small children and all had been playing hard, running around. Joey would become flushed, his hair would become wringing wet, and he seemed to get very hot – though I never took his temperature he seemed to be burning hot. Then he would bring up all his food with enormous burps. He usually cooled off and after an hour of sleep and seemed completely normal again. This vomiting habit seemed to follow no set pattern: sometimes he was just playing by himself, sometimes when he went out to the barnyard and complained about the smell. He often became nauseated, refusing to eat for as many as three days in a row, sometimes being so nauseated he couldn't take a drink of water.

Joey became a peanut butter and jam sandwich child, eating this for breakfast, dinner, and supper and often before going to bed. He never tired of it, and as my doctor said, peanut butter was a good nourishing food, so I let Joey have all he wanted. Sometimes he drank milk but preferred water. I, however, insisted he get at least two glasses of milk a day, often over his protest. I have little patience with children who refuse medicine, so at our house when our children had medicine to take, there never was any argument, you either took it immediately or your nose was held till you had to open your mouth to breath and down went the medicine. They learned early it was much easier to take the medicine when first offered.

I couldn't get Joey to take food, however. Potatoes he wouldn't taste till he was about five, meat he didn't like, soup he wouldn't eat, pancakes he could, also greens. If I forced him to eat anything against his will, it usually came back up faster than it went down.

After Joey's classes at the MacNeill Clinic, I was very depressed. Both my husband and I phoned back to verify that Joey was not retarded and we were told he could never speak more than one word at a time, never a sentence. He was unable, they said, during the test to go across the room and pick up a pencil when asked. We made up our mind that the MacNeill Clinic didn't know what they were talking about. Joey was normal at home, functioning a little behind the older children, but this didn't disturb us as they were all performing above average at school, so that if Joey was a bit slower we figured he'd be about average. Our rural school had no kindergarten facilities at all, but I realized Joey would need some instructions soon if he would perform at all when he started school.

I contacted the principal of our school to see what he thought of Joey attending school a day or two a week just to get used to school. Mrs S.

agreed with me; however, the Grade 1 teacher put her foot down. She had more than she could handle. I spent one evening at her home and she tried to show me her method of getting children started. I realized that I was not professional enough and had no natural inclination in this direction, so after a great many phone calls I had Joey enrolled in kindergarten classes in Sutherland after Christmas thanks to the ladies of Sutherland School Home and School Association. Mrs W. was a capable kindergarten teacher but her class of 25 was quite advanced at this stage. Joey was eager to take part in all activities, but soon realized they had learned things he still was very ignorant about. Mrs W. said his coordination was poor. Although he was a willing learner and easy to please, there were days he just sat or lied down, making no effort to take part in anything. By the time the classes finished Mrs W. said Joey was just coming around and beginning to perform. She recommended another year of kindergarten, which we felt was quite impossible as we had to drive him in and it was just too costly and time consuming.

Joey developed a great dislike for coloring, he couldn't recognize colors and couldn't follow lines. He began hiding under the table when asked to color and complained about headaches.

I tried to teach Joey to do up his buttons and was astonished when he seemed to find it just as hard to find the button hole as he had putting the button through it. Did you ever see a child trying to put a button through a button hole that wasn't there? No matter how peeved I became with him he always smiled and tried harder. The same applied to lacing his shoes; he found it just as difficult to find the large holes in finding the right ones. We began to wonder again if he could see properly as we now noticed he squinted at the TV and complained about headaches whenever he tried coloring or other kindergarten type of work.

In June 65 I had taken him back to Dr K. for the fourth time. Joey's first glasses were +300 in April 1963, +400 on July 1964 ,and now were increased to a +475. Even after this fitting I wasn't happy, so in December 65 I took him to another eye specialist who said he agreed with me that Joey didn't see properly but he would have to learn to use his eyes himself. He didn't find anything wrong with his eye prescription. I felt I had wasted another $10 and gotten absolutely nothing for it.

It was now June 1966 and Joey would be going to school in the fall. I phoned our school superintendent to inform him of Joey's forthcoming school entrance, asking his advice on what would be the best procedure to follow. He visited our home. On seeing Joey he said he appeared quite normal in behavior, etc. and perhaps we should enroll him in fall classes. Prior to his visit I had asked our psychologist from our Regional Health Office to come and see Joey. She came but was not prepared to offer any advice, test him, or even give us constructive criticism. She seemed quite anxious to leave, saying that a child that was loved as much as Joey would manage to make out no matter what.

When our preschool clinic was held at our school, Joey had not been admitted. When I asked our superintendent why, he told me the nurses had informed him that I was contacted and had refused to have Joey tested. This was indeed a surprise to me as the only thing that they had contacted me for was to vaccinate Joey again, but since his body sores were so bad at this point, his doctor advised me against it. I was now down in their books as an uncooperative mother, so I phoned them and I gave them a piece of my mind. Nevertheless, Joey started school with an unfavorable record and a mother no teacher would dare contact.

Our second son developed a wart on his vocal cords in the summer of 1966, so I had to take him for physiotherapy to the University Hospital. On the way to Miss H.'s office I saw a sign "Eye Dept" and immediately made up my mind I would phone them once I got home. Yes, said the voice as the other end of the line, we help children with visual problems but need a prescription from the family doctor before we can see them. I knew that this was no problem as Dr H. was very interested in helping Joey. After our visit to Dr S. in the eye department, Joey's prescription was increased to +725. Now at last I felt that Joey could see, no more headaches. He could distinguish colors and was much more interested in books and close work.

The same summer our third son had an attack of asthma, and since our doctor was on holiday, we went to Dr G., taking Joey with us as his sores were extremely bad at this time. Dr G., upon examining Joey, thought he had scabies so I was sent home to boil clothes and wash and scrub Joey down with medicines – to no avail as the sores did not heal. Dr G. sent me to Dr K., a skin specialist, who said Joey had a skin allergy. This I couldn't believe as whenever I had suggested this to other doctors before they all said allergies did not break out in this form. Dr K. put Joey on a diet, gave him some medicine, and instructed me how to care for him. It was indeed an allergy as the sores began to clear up.

Joey was talking quite nicely now. His speech was slow and his vocabulary small but he spoke nice long sentences and we were very happy at the progress he was making. This improved even more now that he could see more clearly. We had in fact reached a milestone: Joey's speech was improving every day, his sight was greatly improved, and I at long last could control his body sores. Joey's vomiting bouts continued, however.

Joey had been attending school for about a month when we decided to visit his teacher as he didn't bring anything home. We went with fear in our hearts and left with tears in our eyes. His teacher, Mrs N., did not have one good word for Joey, had no patience with him and made it quite plain she didn't intend to waste any time on him. He had been put in a desk about three sizes too large at the back of the room facing a row of windows on the south of the room. The light over his desk was burnt out; the janitor had been notified but hadn't got around to fixing it. The woman screamed at the children, something we had never done to Joey. As time went on whenever we visited, Mrs N. had only one thing to say to us, "Get that child out of here," but our school superintendent insisted he be left there. I phoned Mr S., our principal, and asked that Joey be transferred into the other Grade 1 room, but this other room teacher flatly refused to teach him (she was the same one that had refused to have him attend before); in fact, this teacher advised me to give up on Joey. His speech was so poor no one could understood him at school and he would never learn to read or write.

This year was disastrous for Joey. By June his speech had even slipped backwards. Joey would come home at night and the first thing he would say was, "Do you love me mummy?" One night he cried because all the children had learned to print their name but the teacher wouldn't show him how, so I took him to our blackboard (nailed on the hall wall) and started to teach him to print. Now I was really shocked. Joey thought he could print with his hand while he watched whatever activity he wished, so I worked out a routine, calling his right hand "Joey" and his eyes "Mom," telling him Mom had to watch Joey closely so that Joey would do good work. He had great difficulty learning how to form the different letters – even an O came out wrong. So ended Joey's first year at school; he hadn't ever finished the first unit. Very discouraged, he couldn't understand why the teacher didn't teach him to read and to print as he very much wanted to be like the other kids.

Since we didn't have any other choice, we sent Joey back to school in the fall. All summer I had got some reading readiness books from our school unit Reading Consultant and in my spare time taught Joey words that rhymed and words that started with the same letter.

This takes Joey up to age of 7. Over the next two years, he was diagnosed with purpura and chorea and we learned he was allergic to just about everything, including the hospital and city water. By the time Joey was 11, he was attending the Children's Rehabilitation Center at the airport. After being tested at the Institute of Child Guidance and Development at the University of Saskatchewan, he had been placed at the C.R. Center. The doctor at the university hospital knew there was something wrong with him but didn't know what. He had been tested for allergies: out of 80 tests he had strong reactions to 55. His physiologist told me I should be glad he had survived at all and to forget about his schooling. The doctors also told me he had had a septic throat all his life.

By spring of 1971 Joey had been at the center since September and we had noticed no improvement in his condition. I asked my doctor to make an appointment with Dr Hoffer. After Dr Hoffer put Joey on megavitamin therapy we soon noticed a change. Joey started to come alive. Before he was always tired and very passive, now he became much more active. He started eating foods he was allergic to, drinking milk, and eventually after eating egg salad I tried him on fried eggs. Previously he hid in his room wherever eggs were served as the smell made him sick. Now he started having two fried eggs for breakfast. Ham, he couldn't tolerate at all. It came up as fast as it went down. You can imagine our surprise when he had a healthy serving of ham casserole and no after effects. Joey started to venture into the barnyard. For the first time in his life he explored the chicken coop and barn.

In the spring of 1971, Dr K. of C.R.C. told us Joey would never be discharged as his health was not improving. After school started in the fall, Dr K. asked us what we had done to Joey as he had suddenly come alive. In fact, he was now too rambunctious for the center, although when we said Joey was on vitamin therapy, Dr K. said it couldn't possibly be responsible for Joey's recovery. Nevertheless, he told us to keep him on them.

Most of Joey's body sores were gone but it wasn't until he was put on vitamin E that they disappeared. Joey always held on to me wherever we were shopping or in a crowd of people. I was told I was babying him and to stop holding his hand. However, if he couldn't hold my hand he would cling to my skirt or whatever he could grab. Suddenly this stopped that behavior, too.

Something was happening to *my* eyes. Every time I went to the store or was in a crowd, my sight would start to fade away, just as if I was a flashlight and my battery was getting weaker. My sight would get so dim I couldn't see the bills in my wallet to pay for the goods I was buying. I went to our doctor but was only told he couldn't help me as it was sign of old age and I would have to learn to live with it. My vision got worse and soon it took me about five minutes to focus in on the TV picture, etc. Since Joey was going back to see Dr Hoffer, I explained this to him. He suggested I try nicotinic acid, which I did. Much to my surprise, my vision improved. Now I knew why Joey had clung to me in crowds and why at times he couldn't read at all.

Joey has a long way to catch up on his school work, though at home he now behaves the same as his four brothers. His speech isn't perfect but normal unless he is nervous (when he was four we were told he never would speak more than one at a time). He has come a long way in the last three years, much further than in his previous eleven years of medical treatment and education, and he is still improving. He no longer walks the floor at night or needs his night light on. The night noises don't bother him as much and he doesn't insist on all the cupboard drawers and closet doors being closed tight before he goes to bed. He will stay at home by himself at night and even goes shopping by himself. Joey is no longer a passive child but will stand up for himself. As one of his playmates said, "You can't hit Joey and get away with it as he hits back."

I had started Joey on niacinamide (vitamin B-3) 1 G tid, ascorbic acid (vitamin C) 1 G bid, pyridoxine (vitamin B-6) 250 mg od, and a natural diet free of sugar and processed foods. One month later words stopped moving, reading was better, language was better, and he enjoyed reading. In December 1971 when I saw him during a follow-up appointment, Joey was better. He rarely saw figures reversed. Previous allergies were clearing.

He was in a opportunity class in a regular school. His mother then considered him normal. By 1973 he was evaluated as much improved. He was symptom free and got along well at home and at school. He was friendly and happy, despite his treatment at the hands of conventional medical and educational professionals for almost 14 years.

The success of orthomolecular treatment for children like Ben and "Mike" and Joey has encouraged me to write this book, to share my experiences with parents and physicians who see no or little hope for children suffering from the so-called learning disabilities and behavioral disorders as well as other chronic diseases. Following the pattern of this foreword, I shall present my ideas about the current state of the art of diagnosing children and how it can be replaced by one which is simpler, more practical, and effective. Treatment programs will be suggested and illustrated by case histories and clinical studies. Finally, I will provide a guide to the nutrient value of common foods.

Idiots, Morons, Imbeciles, ADD, and Other Misnomers

In an interesting report entitled "Suffering Fools," J.W. Trent Jr. describes the changing diagnostic criteria for the so-called "mentally retarded" over the past 100 years. People who were considered mentally subnormal or dull were called "idiots" until around 1840 when humane pedagogic methods were developed which produced amazing results in turning some of them into productive citizens. After 1850 schools for idiots had trouble finding places for their graduates, and the state began to keep them in institutions. About 1870 the term "feeble-minded" began to replace idiot. The feeble-minded were now seen as needing protection from society; however, the development of the eugenics movement produced yet another change as the feeble-minded were now seen as a menace to society. Adolf Hitler found ample justification for his views from the eugenics movement. With the advent of intelligence quotient or I.Q. tests, they became the determiner of the diagnosis. The normal intelligence range is considered to be between 70 and 130. Individuals scoring below 25 were "idiots," between 25 and 50 "imbeciles," between 50 and 75 "morons," and between 75 and 100 "low normal." On the basis of an I.Q. test, people who could have been kept in the community were locked up, for the protection of society.

If the nineteenth century ended with the movement to keep these patients in institutions, the twentieth century will end with the release of these people from institutions. The deinstitutionalization movement, which began about 1955 and reached its zenith over the past ten years, has brought another change. Justification was needed to *not* keep these patients in institutions. In 1992 the American Association of Mental Retardation introduced a revolutionary way of defining mental retardation. These people were not mentally retarded; rather, they had different intensities of "functional needs." Communities could restructure themselves to meet these needs and thus could cure mental retardation. As Trent observes, "a person ceases to be mentally retarded the moment people quit defining him as such."

Over the past 40 years psychiatrists have played the same nomenclature game with children. The diagnostic labels developed 40 years ago for children were derived from the older psychiatric textbooks, and children were classified primarily on the basis of their intelligence as measured by the intelligence tests. However, these terms were soon cast as epithets and parents would not accept such labels. In response, child psychiatrists started to use a more neutral term, one that could be used in polite company. No longer would doctors have to tell the parents, "Your child is a moron;" instead, they used the term "minimally brain damaged." The old terms idiot, moron, and imbecile fell out of fashion, except for the variation of the *idiot savant* popularized by Dustin Hoffman's role in the movie *The Rain Man*. The term brain damaged may have been more socially acceptable to the diagnosticians but no more reassuring to parents. At least the old terms suggested that with proper teaching methods something could be done, but what could one do with brain damage even if the diagnosis was softened by the term minimal. Damaged brains cannot be repaired. After a few years this term came into disrepute and was replaced by the less disturbing but highly clinical term "minimal brain dysfunction."

Eventually the word brain was removed from the diagnosis and replaced by "hyperactive," which described one symptom of the problem. And unlike the brain-damaged, hyperactive children could be treated with drugs like ritalin which address the symptom, though not the cause of the illness. Ritalin is the accepted treatment for the American Psychiatric Association diagnosis of "hyperactivity," as described in the *Diagnostic and*

Statistical Manual of Mental Disorders (DSM), Fourth Edition, published by the American Psychiatric Association in 1994. Although ritalin acts like an amphetamine (speed) in adults, for many pre-pubescent "hyperactive" children this drug has the paradoxical effect of calming them down as if it were a sedative and improving concentration span. Ritalin has many undesirable "side-effects," however, such as interfering with growth due to loss of appetite and causing possible drug addiction. In his book *A Dose of Sanity*, Dr Sydney Walker adds that although ritalin has been given to over one million children in the United States, it has no long term beneficial effects.

Dr Walker blames the current devout adherence to ritalin drug therapy for hyperactive children on the American Psychiatric Association DSM system of classifying mental disease. Citing the nine criteria used by the APA system to diagnose hyperactivity, he concludes, "I would worry about a child who didn't exhibit five or six of these symptoms." As a result of this broad classification system, too many children are treated with ritalin. The problem with the term "hyperactivity" is that it is too broad. There are many children who are more active than their peers but are not pathologically hyperactive and certainly do not need any ritalin. Ritalin has become a method for controlling activity within the normal range by physicians who do not know what else to offer these children, by schools who cannot tolerate even minor degrees of increased activity, especially when more than one boy in the class is this active, and by parents who do not have the energy or skills to deal with their active children.

The term hyperactivity still remains in use but has become a component of a multi-word diagnosis such as attention deficit hyperactivity disorder(ADHD). The latest classification of the American Psychiatric Association Diagnostic Manual has developed many dozens of descriptive labels with a corresponding diagnostic code number. Many are considered variants of developmental disorders in cognition, language, motor, and social skills. For example, in the area of cognition the new diagnostic scheme includes retardation, ranging from mild to profound, and pervasive developmental disorders (PDD). There are specific development disorders (SDD), developmental arithmetic disorder (DAD), development expressive writing disorder (DEWD), developmental reading disorder (DRD), developmental expressive language disorder (DELD), developmental receptive language disorder (DRLD). In the area of motor development they have coordination disorders, disruptive behavioral disorder, and an attention deficit hyperactivity disorder (ADHD). In the area of deviant behavior they have oppositional defiant disorder (ODD).

In her book *They Say You're Crazy*, Paula J. Caplan questions the scientific foundation for the many categories of mental illness described in the DSM, arguing that the system is politically motivated, if not incorrect. The APA authors are mostly white male professionals very jealous of their power to determine who is or is not mentally sick. For example, they coined a new term called "self-defeating personality disorder" for women who enjoy suffering and "pre-menstrual dysphoric disorder" (PMDD) for PMS (pre-menstrual syndrome). Caplan advised them to include a term "delusional dominating personality disorder" for men as the corresponding personality disorder related to their hormones. The APA rejected this classification, but after considerable adverse publicity, the new premenstrual term was dropped from the DSM. Caplan also claimed that the standards of scientific proof the APA authors used varied according to the desires of a small group of powerful authors, the scientific foundation for many categories was shockingly weak, tiny subject samples were used with clear self selection, and reliability was ludicrously low. She did not add one of my main criticisms – the diagnosis has no value in determining what type of treatment should be given and the outcome of the illness with or without treatment.

The DSM system has little or no relevance to diagnosis. It has no relevance to treatment either, because no matter which terms are used to classify these children, they are all recommended for treatment with ritalin drug therapy in combination sometimes with play therapy and behavioral therapy. Even as this system multiplies its use of diagnostic terms with each revision, it has no value in determining cause – in fact, is opposed in principle toward determining cause and ignores the frequent cases where causes are easily correctable physical diseases. These cumbersome terms may be excellent ways for describing the behavior of sick children, but they fail in the most important function of diagnosis – that is, they do not lead to any specific treatment. This supposed diagnostic system does not tell us anything about the diet these children should follow, nothing about supplementation with nutrients, nothing about the best kind of social situation or learning situation they should be in. If the entire diagnostic scheme were scrapped today, it would make almost no difference to the way these children are treated or to the outcome of treatment. Nor would their parents feel any better or worse.

Dr Bernard Rimland in his classic study of *Infantile Autism* concluded that modern diagnoses of children with behavioral disorders were meaningless, after examining the first and second diagnosis made on 373 children by other psychiatrists. The first diagnosis found 183 of the 373 children autistic, for example, but only 32 of the original 183 diagnosed autistic remained so on the second diagnosis by another psychiatrist. The balance were now diagnosed schizophrenic (49), emotionally disturbed (14), brain-damaged (21), and retarded (45). Only 1 of 29 schizophrenics remained schizophrenic on second diagnosis, and only 4 out of 20 retarded were still diagnosed retarded. Rimland concluded that the assignment of diagnostic labels to these children was almost random. It is impossible to argue against his conclusion.

I avoid these futile exercises in diagnosis by simply classifying them as children with learning disabilities and/or behavioral disorders. To varying degrees, they are overactive, easily distracted, impulsive, excitable, friendless, and therefore cannot learn as quickly as their normal peers. They become under achievers with all the psychosocial consequences of not being able to keep up. They are children with varying degrees of symptoms – in perception, in memory, in developing concepts, in impulse control. They have high levels of motor activity, short attention span, low frustration tolerance, aggressive behavior, and hyper excitability. No definition or brief description is adequate to describe these sick children. And no such definition or description is effective in treating their problems and recovering their good health.

Perception, Thinking, Mood, and Behavior Dysfunctions

We can describe these children suffering from learning disabilities, behavioral disorders, and brain dysfunctions in detail by calling upon Dr Karl Menninger's description of the "mental state." The mental state can be described under four categories: perception, thinking, mood, and behavior. Perception is the process by which information from the external and internal environment is received and processed by the brain. It involves the usual sense organs and internal receptors. Thinking is the process by which the brain processes the information and comes to conclusions how to deal with or respond to the information. Mood describes the feelings of the individual ranging from apathy to excitement, depression to euphoria. Behavior is the outcome of the first three processes and has to be expressed either in thought or in motor activity such as speech or physical actions.

Of course, the brain cannot be divided into four fragments, one dealing with perception and so on. This is simply a convenient way of describing what is happening and in determining whether there is a malfunction somewhere in the entire system. This is what a mental disease is, a dysfunction somewhere in the system. It is convenient to consider perception both normal and abnormal as the function of the senses alone, and there is no harm in doing so as long as we remember that in most cases of abnormal perception it is due mainly to a fault in the processing organ, the brain, and seldom in the senses, except for such disorders as blindness, deafness, errors of refraction, and pain disorders.

About thirty years ago, when computers had not yet invaded the average home, I realized after reading a book by pioneer orthomolecular psychiatrist H.L. Newbold called *The Psychiatric Programming of People* that the computer was modeled on human behavior and thus could be used to describe behavioral problems. Animal behavior had millions of years to evolve and adapt to the environment; it makes good sense to take advantage of this long experiment of nature in developing something like the computer which increases our capabilities. As I noted in my review of this book, a model is a device for examining and clarifying phenomena. Thus a model of an airplane in a wind tunnel helps the engineer design a real plane which flies better. No one should confuse the model for the real object. Models can also be used to educate people about complex phenomena by highlighting and simplifying basic aspects of the phenomena. Again no one should believe that having mastered the model he has mastered the real process but he will be much closer to this objective.

A computer consists of hardware and software. The hardware has a mechanism by which information is entered into the central processor.

The simplest pocket calculator has keys which one uses to enter information. For example, to add 2 plus 2, one first punches the number 2 which enters the memory. This input is analogous to the senses. Input is to the computer what perception is to the animal. The computer has a central processor which receives the information, stores it, and reacts to it. The brain is the animal's central processor. The computer also has a mechanism for letting its operator know what has been the outcome of what it has done. This is the output. The output is the printing on a screen or numbers on a pocket calculator or printed pages of material. Humans also record output by writing, painting, building, etc. The animal also reacts to what its brain has done by motor activity, sounds or speech, fight or flight, or other forms of reaction. But the computer must be told what to do with the information it has received. It is programmed. The program may be built into the computer or it may be altered according to the uses to which it will be put. In the same way we are programmed, first by our genes and secondly by everything that has happened to us as we developed. We are aware of the environment through our senses and how we experience them. We respond or react to these experiences according to the way we have been shaped by life. We have been shaped by our relationship to our parents and family, by the way we are fed and what we are fed, by our economic and social position, by our education and the immense variety of life experiences.

To return to our calculator. We have put in the number 2. Now we instruct the calculator to add by pressing the add button. Then we enter more information by pressing the number 2 again. Finally, we instruct the computer to proceed with its mission by pressing the go ahead button. The computer responds by showing the number 4. The computing task has been completed.

Here is a computer model of how the individual lives:

PERSON	COMPUTER
Perception	Input
Life	Program
Brain	Processor
Action	Output

If there is a failure in the hardware, the processor (brain) will be unable to respond appropriately to the software (perception). This will lead to one sort of mental illness, schizophrenia, for example. The program or the life experiences may be faulty. The wrong rewards and punishment may have led to a program breakdown. The diet may be toxic or deficient. Again the performance of the computer will be wrong and another kind of mental illness is produced, perhaps hysteria or some personality deformation. It is possible there is a defect in software, hardware, and program, which leads to a very complicated form of mental illness. In most cases there is a major breakdown in either hardware, software, or program with a minor reactive dysfunction in the other two. The result of such a disorder is seen in behavior.

Treatment therefore depends upon the site of the breakdown. If the hardware is malfunctioning, no amount of software tinkering will repair the computer. Even if tinkering is partially successful, one is still left with a faulty program or damaged hardware. In schizophrenia, no amount of software tinkering will repair the computer because the hardware is poisoned and cannot function properly. The schizophrenic patient simply cannot respond except to the simplest sort of reprogramming. The appropriate treatment is to restore the integrity of the brain, which means to correct its biochemistry. Similarly, if the software is faulty, no amount of tinkering with the hardware will be of any help. To attempt to correct the biochemistry of the brain when it is already functioning normally is foolish and futile. What is needed is a thorough reprogramming, a thorough revision of the program – that is, by the application of behavioral or other forms of therapy.

Every general disease of the brain will change one or more of these main functions. There will be changes in perception, in thinking, in mood, or a combination of changes, often resulting in disturbed behavior. These systemic changes may be caused by drugs and by major changes in the nutrition of the brain. The most common mind-changing drugs are xanthine stimulants such as tea, coffee, cocoa (chocolate), and sugar in large quantities. Unique brain changes are produced by the hallucinogens LSD, mescaline, tetrahydrocannabinol (marijuana), and the derivatives of adrenalin, adrenochrome and adrenolutin. These drugs produce disturbances in perception, thinking, mood, and behavior. Nutrient deficiencies include vitamin B-3, vitamin B-6, and zinc which can cause pellagra and schizophrenia, while excessive levels of such minerals as lead and cadmium can cause severe brain dysfunction and disturbance of the mental state in children.

Perception Dysfunctions

Perceptual disorders are very important factors in influencing and determining learning and behavior. If children are to be diagnosed properly, it must be established that these disorders are present, and if we are to understand why they behave as they do, we must understand how these perceptual changes do influence thinking and behavior.

The five main senses of the body are seeing, hearing, tasting, touching, and smelling. There are also proprioceptive senses or somatic senses by which the person is aware of his body, its size, its configuration, and the relationship of the body to space and to gravity. The senses sample the environment and convey information to the brain, where it is interpreted and stabilized. This reduces the impact of a shifting environment and produces a stable world in which it is possible to live. The act of perception requires a coordinated interaction between the senses and the brain of which they are an intimate part. Misperceptions or dysperceptions may arise from a defect of the senses, the nerves connecting them to the brain, or the brain itself. These are caused by anatomical or functional changes in any portion of the these systems.

The dysperceptions are of two kinds: illusions and hallucinations. Illusions are perceptual distortions of objects which are real and can be sensed by others but will not appear in the same way. Any one who has experienced the hallucinogenic reaction, as with LSD, will understand what illusions are. Most hallucinogens produce illusions rather than hallucinations. Hallucinations are more pathological, usually present in advanced stages of the illness.

Vision

There may be changes in form, shape, and color. Objects may be slightly distorted, angles may be slightly off, colors may be too bright, or more commonly, become too dull. Sometimes color disappears entirely. Unusual movements may occur. For example, objects may pulsate, floors may heave and roll, faces may appear older, younger, frightening, or malicious. Children usually have trouble describing these changes and may require special direct questions such as are provided for in some visual perceptual tests. Most often they see changes in the semi dark when shadows take on the appearance of things, animals, people. If they see letters or numbers reverse or stand upside down, they will have difficulty reading. This is called dyslexia. They will describe words moving about on the page, lines sliding off the page or running into each other. When words become alive, they lose their abstract properties.

Visual illusions will create serious reading, spelling, and comprehension difficulties. It is hard to concentrate on the symbolic meaning of words when the letter or words themselves are alive. Letters may be upside down, backward, or reversed as in mirror writing. Words may be distorted the same way. They may become larger or smaller, or appear to come toward the reader or to recede from them. They may collide with each other. Lines may no longer be parallel and may roll off the page. Parts of words may disappear. Some-times these changes occur only when the child is tired, either toward evening or after trying to read for awhile. It is common for parents to have the child's eyes examined frequently by optometrists or ophthalmologists, but glasses will not solve the problem. They will be diagnosed as dyslexic or being reading disordered. There is no connection to intelligence except that intelligent children will find it easier to cope in other ways. Many discover they can learn more readily by listening because they do not have a hearing dyslexia. Less intelligent children will not be able to compensate as well. They appear to be slow learners (which they are because of their perceptual handicap) and may be labeled retarded.

Reading disorders have a major impact on the child in many functional areas. The disability increases the time required to master a given amount of material. The amount of material that would be learned by a normal child in ten minutes will require many times as much time for the learning disordered child. This creates boredom, decreases confidence, and uses up time that would be available for other activities, including playing with other children. A few children are highly motivated and will spend the additional time. For example, "P.M." saw me in November 1970 complaining that he still suffered from a reading disability, that it was hard to reason and to understand words, but at age 17 he had reached grade 10 and was doing reasonably well in school. He had walked at 1½ years, began to speak at 3 years, but did not use sentences until age 5. He was given speech therapy which helped. At age 7 he began psychiatric treatment and continued for the next 7 years. He had to repeat grade 1. His psychiatrist diagnosed him mentally retarded with irreversible brain damage and advised the family that he would never be able to go through the normal school system. The brain damage was apparently confirmed by EEG changes, but I was not able to confirm that since the psychiatrist would not reply to me when I asked for his records. Nor would he reply to the patient's mother or to his former patient. The family were both surprised and disillusioned by his attitude. I suspect he considered that they had committed heresy by getting him referred to me.

With great determination P.M. worked extraordinarily hard and was able to learn enough to obtain a B average in high school. I started him on niacin 1 G tid, ascorbic acid 1 G bid, and pyridoxine 250 mg od plus eliminating sugars. Three months later he was much better. He reported that for the first time in his life he had been able to read three books through, but he still found it hard to comprehend some words. He continued to improve, completed high school, worked for a year to save money, and when I saw him last, was a first year university student, getting on very well. He worked so hard at his studies he had no time for anything else. With the use of the megavitamins learning became much easier, he had more freedom, and had a chance to learn social and other skills necessary for normal development. Most children with such perceptual disorders do not have this kind of motivation, however, and avoid reading as much as possible.

Visual illusions can be very disturbing and may be responsible for unexplained behavior. If the child has fearful nightmares which are still there for some time after he awakens (ghosts, monsters), they will cover up and cower under their bed clothes, or run from their bedroom to seek help, or will awake screaming. Clothes hanging in the closet or on a chair will look like animals or monsters. Many children insist on having their closet doors closed before they will go to sleep. I have heard young patients describe all sorts of monsters and even ghosts to the immense surprise of their parents who had not thought about asking them why they were afraid. The best way to ask about these illusions is to find out if they fall asleep without a night light. If they can, it is unlikely they have any visual illusions. If they must have a light on, or an open door, then ask them why and in most cases they will frankly tell you what it is they are afraid of.

A question about monsters seems to strike a responsive chord in many. If monster dreams are present, one should find out what is the impact on the child. Some are rarely disturbing, others so vivid the child will awaken screaming. They are said by parents to have night terrors. Sometimes the dream does not go away after the child awakens. One boy would find himself in his dreams surrounded by huge black vultures flying about the room. He was convinced that they not only would be after him but that they also wanted to eat his parents. Fortunately, the vultures never left his room. One girl saw a ghost walking through her room every night. She finally lost her fear of this apparition when she came to believe that the ghost was only her mother with a white sheet over her. When she told me this, her mother in surprise blurted out, "Dear, I do not walk through your room at night." Immediately the girl became very agitated and distressed. "You do too," she exclaimed. "You do too." Her mother had unwittingly removed her daughter's comforting solution to the presence of this vision.

Children hallucinate as often as adults, but one would not suspect this from the psychiatric literature. Few psychiatrists ask their patients who are children about these changes. Patients react to these hallucinations with behavior appropriate to what they experience, but it will be inappropriate to any observer.

Hearing

Hearing samples a narrower segment of the environment than does vision; in contrast to vision, which can be more readily controlled by shutting one's eyes, for example, hearing is more sensitive and under less voluntary control. For this reason, auditory changes are more difficult for patients to deal with. Auditory illusions are distortions in sounds. These include changes in acuity. One may become much more sensitive to sounds which become unbearably loud or the auditory senses may decrease to the extent that patients are almost deaf. There may be a defect in localizing the source of sound. For this reason some children appear deaf. It is not unusual for mothers to take their children suffering from auditory illusions to a hearing specialist who usually finds they are not deaf.

An infant must learn to locate the source of sounds or they will not become meaningful. Sounds coming from mother speaking are localized and develop meaning. If the infant cannot tell where the sounds are coming from, they will not attach any particular meaning to them. They will find it very hard to develop speech. Perhaps this is one of the problems of the autistic child. They will also have difficulty distinguishing fore-ground and background sounds and will be easily distracted. I have seen children who responded to almost every random noise as if they had fore-ground meaning. These children find it very difficult to concentrate. They are at the mercy of their environment.

Many children hear voices but usually they are innocuous, not hallu-cinations. They will hear their name and will often turn toward where they think the sound is coming from and will see no one. They will often ask their mother if she has called. Sometimes they hear footsteps walking behind them and often are afraid of walking outside in the dark for this reason. Creaks in the house may become the basis for hallucinations. They will hear voices talking to or about them. Sometimes they think out loud. This is considered one of the hallmarks of adult schizophrenia, but in my opinion is rarely used in making diagnosis. Hearing one's own thoughts is merely one step toward hearing voices. After hearing one's thoughts inside one's head, the next step in the progression of disease is to hear thoughts from outside of the head, followed by hearing voices. During recovery the reverse sequence is followed. Sometimes voices and visions retreat to the world of dreams. This is a good indication that the patient is improving.

Many years ago Dr L. Bender, a highly respected New York psychia-trist, followed a series of childhood schizophrenics for ten years. She had used classical adult criteria for diagnosing them – that is, visions and voices were present in every one. But ten years later when she examined them again, half were chronic adult schizo-phrenics living in the state hos-pital system, still suffering from voices and visions. This is not surprising. What was surprising was that the other half were typical psychopaths, members of street gangs and so on. None of this group could remember ever having had these perceptual changes, and when questioned about them, denied them. In other words, some childhood schizophrenics when they grow up are mislabeled as personality disorders because they cannot remember having hallucinated. Dr Karl Menninger aptly described schizophrenia as a prolonged delirium. When one has recovered from a delirium, it gradually fades from memory and may be completely forgotten after awhile. Children have carefully described these perceptual changes to me, but after they had recovered several years later, they did not remember them. Even if they do not recover, they still may not remember having had them. This will create diagnostic difficulties later on. If they become schizophrenic during their adolescence and do not remember these perceptual changes, they will not be diagnosed correctly and therefore will not receive the correct treatment. Many are diagnosed as personality disorders, psychopathic personalities, and, more recently, as borderline personalities. How many multiple murderers and criminal sexual psychopaths are examples of childhood schizophrenia who have outgrown their hallucinations but have not been able to develop any empathy or feeling for anyone else? They are supremely selfish individuals who have no regard for any one else and will do what they can to satisfy their own urges. Their major perceptual difficulty is that they do not see other people as human, but rather as animals or inanimate objects to be used and disposed of as soon as possible.

Touch

Illusions and hallucinations of touch are very rare. I have had a few schizophrenic patients who felt fingers touching them and concluded they were being touched by angels.

Taste and Smell

Illusions and hallucinations of taste and smell are not common in adults and even rarer in children. They are closely related. Often the change in smell is misinterpreted as a change in taste. With a cold, smell may be affected and foods may taste different for that reason. Wine and food tasters prefer to use the sense of smell first. For survival smell is more important since it will provide the first warning that certain items which appear to be food are not or are dangerous or are spoiled. The most common finding in children is a change in the sensation of taste, probably due to a zinc deficiency. They will not report this but will lose their appetite or develop very finicky appetites eating certain foods only. The deficiency of zinc is a factor in teenage eating disorders. It is not uncommon in elderly patients with zinc deficiency. Here food tastes flat or bitter, and they simply stop eating. This can be life threatening. The taste illusion that foods are bitter has been one of the main factors in the paranoid symptom which used to be more common in the past when medicine tasted bitter. These patients got the idea that someone was tampering with their food and putting poison into it. With the use of modern drugs, which are almost always sweetened, this paranoid delusion has almost disappeared. I have not run across one in the last ten years.

Pain

A few schizophrenics are not as sensitive to pain as they are when they are well. I suspect this is also true for a few children.

Clinical Pathology

Potentially there are thousands of illusions and hallucinations possible and innumerable combinations. It is not necessary to get a complete inventory of all the changes patients will have, but one must have enough information to help establish the diagnosis and to understand why the child is behaving the way they are. Children do not readily describe their perceptual world, however, and will need help. Direct and clear questions are necessary. There is no need to fear these questions will persuade the child to admit to changes that are not there. I have questioned over 1,500 children under the age of 14 and have found them to be very resistive to admitting symptoms that are not there. I am not referring to fantasies about events that can be induced in children when pressed long enough by people who already know the answers, using leading questions. If they have not experienced a perceptual change, they will not admit to having experienced one. They may readily admit having seen monsters of one sort if they have seen them, but will resist any suggestion they have seen any different types of monster.

A few key questions will initiate the exploration of perceptual disorders:

1. Do you think people are looking at you? This elicits
   information about the patient's sensitivity to people. It is a
   symptom only if the child believes he is being singled out for

special attention, both good or bad, and behaves as if it were true by avoiding going to school, for example, or by hiding.

2. Is it hard to read? This will open up possible reading disabilities, dyslexias, etc. One should also ask about hearing dyslexia. Children who learn more readily by hearing than by reading may have a visual dyslexia, and children who learn more readily by reading than by hearing may have a hearing dyslexia.

3. Do you find things about you appear strange? This will open up the area of visual illusions.

4. Do you see visions? With children it is best to first ask about bad dreams and nightmares, then shadow illusions and hallucinations. These may be present only in the dark or in the day time as sometimes nightmares still stay withthe child for many minutes after they are fully awake

5. Do you hear yourself think, do you hear voices, do you feel unreal?

After a perceptual area has been opened up it may be explored further. If the patient denies any of these changes, the chances are pretty good they are not having perceptual changes unless they are very paranoid and suspicious of the questioner. Most children and adults know that talking about these phenomena is generally a bad idea because of the reactions it generates in people about them. Many children have already seen visions or hallucinations at night which they think are dreams and have tried to describe to their parents. They have been rebuffed or discouraged by parents who do not understand what they have experienced. Even adults are reluctant to inform their relatives and friends that they have seen visions or heard voices. Or the child may have been told that they have been imagining things. This is the most common explanation given children by their parents, or by the doctors to the parents who have been worried. Children quickly realize their parents are uncomfortable with this type of conversation. Most children consider these phenomena to be normal and experienced by other children so they do not even discuss it with them.

I have seen a few adults who hallucinated all their lives considering that this was normal. One of my patients over age 30 came in to complain about hearing voices. She had recently discovered that it was not normal to hear voices. She was also depressed and wanted to be rid of the mood disorder. She did not want her voices to go. They were friendly company.

Dreams, or more appropriately, nightmares, are not the royal road to the unconscious, as Freud believed, but they certainly provide one royal road to a useful discussion of illusions and hallucinations. After talking about dreams it is easy to ascertain whether visual illusions are present. After exploring the illusions and hallucinations, it is appropriate to determine whether these are seen in the day time. If they are, it is much more serious and indicates a further extension into full hallucinations. By this time the child in most cases will have confidence in the psychiatrist, perhaps for the first time, and will be able to talk about other perceptual changes. This is often the first time they have been able to talk about these matters.

Unfortunately, people tend to be unaware that they may not perceive the world alike. Many people find it incomprehensible that others can see visions, until it happens to them. They would rather believe the hallucinated individual is imagining or faking his or her visions. Psychiatrists who have not hallucinated, either by having had schizophrenia or an hallucinogenic experience, may find it equally difficult. I have seen many patients who had vivid visual hallucinations but had not been believed when they reported them. Their psychiatrists had diagnosed them as being hysterical or psychopathic. These people generally have a tough time getting others to take them seriously. It is clear that no behavior, normal or abnormal, can be comprehended without some awareness of the perceptual or experiential world of the individual. The hallucinogenic drugs such as LSD produce a schizophrenic syndrome in normal subjects, and I have observed that nurses and psychiatrists who have experienced the effect of these drugs are better therapists, more understanding and sympathetic with their patients. Parents become too impatient with their children as do teachers. I think that children with learning disorders should be taught by teachers who have themselves had learning disorders in their childhood. They would be more patient and more sensitive to their students needs.

When a person becomes aware of an unusual perception, his response is tempered by his judgment of how real the new percept is. If the new perception is judged to be unreal, not true, something coming from one's self, the reaction will be different than if the perception has been judged to be real, true, resulting from a change in the environment. The ability to make this judgment depends upon whether or not thought disorder is present. The thinking person must be able to compare previous experience with the present one and to decide the probability that the perceptual change is real or whether it is an illusion, a distortion of what is experienced, or an hallucination. It is the faulty combination of experiencing and judging which is the hallmark of psychosis.

This was first clearly recognized and described by John Conolly who in 1830 defined madness (insanity) as a disease of perception combined with an inability to judge that these changes were unreal. A person might have visual illusions or hallucinations but as long as he knew these were unreal, according to Conolly, he was not insane. Such a person might be one who has experienced hallucinations in the past and has discovered they were not real, a psychologist or psychiatrist who has studied these phenomena, or a person who had experienced the reactions of some hallucinogens. I have seen patients who had taken hallucinogens and when later they experienced similar perceptual changes they were much less terrified. They would not have been concerned with transient changes or flashbacks but they did become anxious if the experiences became prolonged or repeated themselves too often. The previous experience with these drugs prevented them from becoming psychotic, although it may have accelerated their drift into schizophrenia.

The ability to judge that perceptual changes are illusions or hallucinations and therefore are not objectively real depends upon the intelligence, age, and personality of the individual. A person from a culture which accepts these phenomena as common or even valuable will be less apt to decide they were not real, whereas in a culture such as ours it would be more simple to consider these changes unreal. It depends also upon one's past experiences with abnormal sensations and upon one's ability to reason.

Perhaps more important than all of these is the type of information given to the individual by her senses and the number of senses involved. It may be relatively simple to decide that a short-lived vision was an hallucination, while a vision present continuously might be more difficult to rule out. It can be done, however. One of my patients was followed about by an hallucinated dog for several days which she believed was not real but reacted to as if it were by joking about it. If, however, a second sense provides information about the same object – that is, if the vision is a person who is heard to speak – then both the sense of vision and of hearing are providing information. It would be much more difficult to disbelieve this hallucination of two senses, but it is possible. If, however, a third sense also agreed – say, the person being hallucinated came over and touched the patient – then he would be unable to resist his senses and must conclude the person seen, heard, and felt must be real. John Conolly claimed that no person could disbelieve the evidence of three senses.

The concept that perceptual changes were the hallmark of psychosis was current in English psychiatry for several hundred years. Dr Conolly provided the best illustration of this concept. He described a woman who was very depressed in hospital because she had concluded that her husband was dead. No amount of reasoning could persuade her that he was alive. Her belief was based on seeing his ghost outside her window on a tree where she saw a shadow. When he heard about her delusion, he wanted to go to see her to convince her he was alive. The psychiatrist would not permit him to do so, pointing out this could be very dangerous if she were confronted with the fact he was not dead. However, her husband could not tolerate this and went into her room on his own. She promptly fainted, came to, and calmly said she would like to go home with him. Her depression was gone. Not all delusions are so easily dispelled, though.

A person who has suffered hallucinations may in time discover they were false if he recovers. The transitional phase is very interesting to the student of these changes. "Percival," described in Gregory Bateson's book *Percival's Narrative: A Patient's Account of Psychosis*, began to test his hallucinations by correlating the prophecies given him by his voices with what actually happened. When he discovered they were mostly incorrect, he concluded they were voices, hallucinations. He later observed bitterly that had his relatives told him in no uncertain terms he heard voices, then he might have come to the normal conclusion more easily. Many delusions are reactions to misperceptions. Thus the inability to judge that people are or are not looking directly at you may lead to the delusion that people are watching you all the time and may lead to withdrawal, reclusiveness, and paranoid delusions. If food tastes bitter because of a taste misperception – for example, because of a deficiency in zinc – it may lead to the delusion that some one has tampered with the food or put poison into it. If due to a misperception of smell, one smells an odor normally not present, it is easier to conclude that someone is surrounding you with poison gas. If you feel unseen fingers touching you, it is not too difficult to conclude that spirits are touching you. It is possible to produce nearly any delusion by altering the appropriate sense, including catatonia by hypnotic suggestion. Such delusions are incomprehensible to people who have never experienced them or the perceptual changes which have helped create them.

Patients may not tell their doctor about these perceptual changes and too often the doctor will not ask them. For a long time it was taught that certain lines of questioning must not be followed lest they produce signs that were not there before. For example, it was not correct to ask patients if they heard voices because they might then begin to hear them. I have seen many patients, even recently, who have not told their psychiatrists about these perceptual changes because they were not asked about them. I have heard psychiatrists call their patients hallucinations "pseudo" hallucinations because they thought their patients were hysterical.

Thinking Disorders

The presence of sensory or perceptual illusions or hallucinations is in itself not sufficient to determine the level of illness of a person or whether or not they are psychotic. To be psychotic they must also have a thought or cognitive disorder, that is, conclude these perceptual changes are real. Patients may know they are not real, that they are present because they are sick. Normal subjects under the influence of hallucinogenic drugs will most often accept their perceptual changes as drug induced. If the perceptual changes are judged to be real, the patient will react to them as if they are real. This will distinguish them from imagination or fantasy.

Two people who perceive an event more or less alike will respond to it in different ways depending upon these other factors which we might term personality, a combination of experience and heredity. If a fire breaks out, one person will run from the fire but another might run toward it. The visual experience is the same, but the response is determined by personality. This is, of course, self evident to most people. But what is less self evident is that the same event may be perceived in two entirely different ways and this would call forth entirely different responses even if the personality of the two observers were identical. Or even if the same event objectively were experienced differently by the same person but at different times. One person would perceive a setting sun, for example, as a beautiful image to be admired or photographed. Another might see it as a violent explosion, perhaps the atomic bomb, and react with fear and horror. Or a person who had always seen the setting sun with interest might one day misperceive it as the explosion of a bomb.

There are two main aspects to thinking: the process of constructing ideas which when made evident by a flow of words are intelligible to the listener; and the content of that process. There is seldom a clear distinction between these two aspects of thinking. If the first process is disturbed, it is called thought disorder but should be called a thought "process" disorder. If the second aspect is disturbed, it is a thought "content" disorder. The process disorder indicates a more serious disease process and usually occurs later in the history of the illness. Thought process changes are a direct expression of the disturbance in the brain caused by the presence of chemical toxins. Thought content is determined by personality. These are the thought disorders sensitive to perceptual disturbances. In children it is very difficult to measure thought content disorder, and if the child is not speaking, this is impossible. Intel-ligence tests are of little help.

Any type of brain disorder will cause changes. Content disorder is usually the earliest manifestation of cerebral disorder. It includes delusions and other paranoid ideas. Thus, the earliest changes in thinking as a person becomes drunk are delusions. Many alcoholics express these only when they have been drinking. But in the late stages of the inebriation thought process disorder is present and they may not be able to speak intelligibly, nor will listeners be able to make any sense out of what they are trying to say. LSD at lower doses causes delusionary thinking. Only with very high doses will it cause a process disorder. Whether an idea is a delusion or not has to be determined by studying the background of the patient and the family. If everyone in a community has a certain belief, the presence of this belief in a patient's thinking cannot be a delusion. Families must be questioned about the reality of the delusions as well.

Content disorders come on much earlier in the course of these diseases than process disorders. Content disorder takes the same form it does in adults but children are less experienced and sophisticated and will have simpler forms of thought disorder. Paranoid ideas are common but childish. Everyone hates them, their school mates are their enemies, the teachers pick on them more than they do on the other children. Their possible hyperactivity and lack of social skills will indeed expose them to the type of attention that feeds these paranoid ideas, but they do not accept any responsibility for eliciting these responses from the people about them. Rarely do they have more bizarre ideas typical of adult schizophrenics, though some children are full of hateful, even murderous ideas, about their parents, brothers, sisters, or friends. One child set fire to his neighbor's fence because he wanted to set the whole world afire. This is not much different from the action of a Charles Manson who wished to provoke a nation-wide cataclysm by murdering a few people. Later this child, grown into a schizophrenic youth, was found not guilty of capital murder by reason of insanity after shooting and killing the son of his employer and severely wounding the father. He had been treated with tranquilizers only with no response. There are no simple tests for eliciting thought content disorders, but it can be estimated by careful examination of the child and comparing that with information gained from the parents. The older the child the simpler the task.

Thinking process disorders are also distorted. In the process of thinking ideas are logically connected in a sequence so that they are comprehensible to others. Anything which interrupts this flow of words is a process disorder. There may be changes in the rate and rhythm. The stream of thought may be interrupted by frequent pauses (blocking) or by other ideas intruding. Thinking may be too slow, too fast, halting, characterized by long pauses and difficulty in finding the right word, confused. The child may experience difficulty in concentration. Ideas may come too slowly, too quickly, or may be interrupted by long pauses. Random or near random ideas may flood into consciousness. Any of these changes will interfere with expression of ideas and with their communication. These and other changes will make it difficult to communicate. They will also create problems in learning. This can be measured by intelligence tests, but they are crude, often unreliable, and measure merely the process of thinking or of learning and not the content. A thought content disorder has less effect in determining the intelligence test results, while a change in process will have a major impact. Generally intelligence tests of the standard type should not be used to measure intelligence in sick people.

I have become convinced that many students who test in the low intelligence range of the I.Q. tests are not retarded at all. They appear to be retarded because they have been unable to learn due to a thought disorder. Many of these children, diagnosed retarded, both by intelligence tests and school performance, become normal when they are treated. One boy, age 9, was slow and perplexed and simply could not keep up with his class. He was at the bottom of a class of 20 in the fall. By next spring he was the first in the same class. His apparent retardation vanished after he was given niacinamide 1 G tid and pyridoxine 250 mg od. Another patient, a young woman, complained that her mind was always confused. As a child she had been very slow and had been diagnosed retarded. She slowly worked her way through special classes for the retarded. Her confusion was a symptom of her undiagnosed schizophrenia which had not been investigated. A year after she started treatment, she was able to learn normally. She went back to high school and took an accelerated course. She had never been retarded.

The usual diagnostic terms, including mental retardation and the more modern and more pleasant euphemisms for it, are of little value. These diagnoses do not lead to effective treatment; they are very pessimistic since they are accepted as permanent and nihilistic, they are dead-end diagnoses. Once this diagnosis has been made all active treatment ceases. The unfortunate patients are promptly banished from the "sick" role and installed into the "impaired" role. Attention swings from what could be appropriate biomedical and nutritional treatment to a number of psychosocial treatments, ranging from neglect to the most intense form of special education and behavioral modification.

Nevertheless, severe brain damage of any kind can lead to neurological and to behavioral changes. According to A. Towbin, fetal and neonatal anoxia (lack of oxygen) may reduce and distort brain function causing retardation, palsy, epilepsy, and behavioral disorders. He believed a large proportion of the children called hyperactive or minimally brain damaged do suffer from the residual effects of lack of oxygen. Birth is one of the most traumatic experiences. The fetus is compressed and forced through the birth canal and must make rapid adjustments from one way of life to another. Hypoxia and mechanical injury of the central nervous system, the most vulnerable part of the body, is almost inescapable. The degree of disturbance caused by hypoxic damage depends upon the severity of the hypoxia and the area of the brain injured. Deep damage occurs in prematures and newborns and leads to spastic cerebral palsy. At term and in the newborn, the surface of the brain mainly is affected. If the frontal cortex is injured, intelligence is reduced. If the occipital (back) region is injured, the infant will be blind. On healing a scar may be left which may cause epilepsy. Early during gestation the deeper areas of the brain are growing very quickly and therefore this area is very susceptible to lack of oxygen. Later on the cerebral cortex is growing rapidly so it is more sensitive.

In an earlier report, Towbin referred to the 300,000 premature children born annually in the United States. Infants born very prematurely have a very high incidence of mental retardation, the degree of impairment generally being proportional to the degree of prematurity. When birth weight was under 2,500 grams 10 percent of the group had an I.Q. less than 70, almost twice as common as in normal term babies. Anoxia is not necessarily due to mechanical damage during birth. Towbin believes that in a large proportion of cases the cerebral lesions are imprinted early, in the last trimester of pregnancy. This accounts for the number of children with uncomplicated birth histories who are retarded.

It is possible that anoxia might so alter the respiratory enzyme system of the brain that a vitamin B-3 dependency is formed. Nicotin-amide adenine dinucleotide, the active anti pellagra enzyme made from vitamin B-3 in the body, is one of the most important respiratory enzymes. This could explain why so many need extra amounts of this vitamin.

There are children who have various degrees of brain damage which is anatomical – that is, due to defects in the structure of the brain whether caused by congenital defects or anoxia. There are also children who have no damage of this sort whatever and still show various forms of behavioral disorder. This group must have biochemical lesions primarily. Therefore, there must be a large number who lay somewhere in between. It may be very difficult clinically to decide exactly where on the continuum a patient falls. Since a large proportion of children respond to megavitamin therapy, this suggests that some of them, even if brain damaged by anoxia, are able to respond. It suggests that some of the anoxia still present is due to a need for extra vitamins, that genes for vitamin dependency made these children more vulnerable to anoxic damage and that megadoses of the correct vitamins correct some of these pathological biochemical lesions.

A.D. Rossi has suggested that demylinization caused by excessive methylation could be a factor in causing cerebral dysfunction. Mylin is an essential component of nerve sheathes. Evidence supporting this possibility is that methionine made 70 percent of the children worse, while niacinamide improved 50 percent. Niacina-mide could divert methyl groups and decrease excessive loss of mylin, while methionine would increase the amount of methylation. Other conditions which can lead to hyperactive behavior are encephalitis, especially if associated with delirium, severe head injury, intracerebral calcification, epilepsy, and brain allergy.

The primary examination and diagnosis of every child with a learning or behavioral disorder must therefore include a thorough physical and neurological examination. Every organic thought defect must be given the best possible treatment, for even these brain damaged children can improve significantly.

Mood

Mood disorder symptoms can be classed on a continuum ranging from depression to euphoria and may be judged appropriate or not appropriate. In normal people, mood is a response to situations or ideas or events but the mood itself may determine how people react to real events. A person in good mood will face situations with humor and skill, whereas on another day, faced with a very similar situation but in a bad mood, may respond with irritability, anger, or despair. By way of experiment, Dr Fogel and I hypnotized normal subjects and suggested that when they came out of their trance they would be depressed. One of the subjects was then asked why she was so depressed. She described the reasons. She was working hard as a housewife and was way behind in her work, her husband made little money, the world situation was precarious (in 1960 she was worried about the atomic bomb). How could anyone not be depressed? She was then re-hypnotized and told that this time she would be very happy in the post trance state. When she was out of her trance, she was classically hypomanic and cheerful. When asked why, she said that she had a good husband, felt great, the sun was shining. Why would anyone not be happy? Here the same woman in a matter of minutes was made depressed or euphoric by post hypnotic suggestion and in each case reacted appropriately in describing why she was depressed or euphoric. The mood was the motor which drove her explanation for her mood. Very few people realize how important mood is in determining how they respond to situations or people about them.

Children's moods may be very labile, alternating quickly from depression to excessive good feeling but the latter is rare. Children may be very depressed, even suicidal, and will show the usual characteristics of a depression – sadness, crying spells, irritability, tension, and retardation of movement. Mothers will report that their child has not smiled in months or years, nor laughed. Depression is a very common symptom of vitamin B-3 and B-6 dependency; it is also the earliest symptom of pellagra. The first indication of recovery is when the child can smile again. Euphoria is very rare, though often assigned, incorrectly, to the hyperactive child. Hyper-active children are typically oblivious of their mood, even though they are aroused, more excitable, and apparently euphoric. This mood is common among manic patients who will often say that they were not happy in their manic state even they appeared to be so. It is important not to confuse activity with mood. Normally one tends to equate hyperactivity with euphoria and hypoactivity with depression. They may coincide but they are unrelated. A depressed child may be either hyper or hypo active. The modern TV ads for junk foods, especially the sugary beverages, equate hyperactivity with good cheer. They are what I call hyperactivity ads and truly represent the effect of these drinks upon behavior. They have recognized that there is a connection and have turned what should be inappropriate behavior into something which should be considered desirable and which can be induced by drinking these beverages.

Behavior

Behavior is the culmination of the interplay of perception, thinking, and mood with personality. Behavior can be judged on the basis of two continua: the degree of activity from too passive (hypoactivity) to too active (hyperactivity); and from inappropriate to appropriate. There are, therefore, four extreme states. Most children fall somewhere in between. Behavior is measured by observing the child and by interviewing those who know the child well, such as parents and teachers. Behavior can also be evaluated by special using behavioral tests such as the "Hyperactivity Scale."

How behavior is modified by changes in perception, thought, and mood depends, of course, on the other psychosocial experiences to which the person has been exposed. But assuming that individuals are more or less in the same environment, then one can begin to understand why the behavior of children may be different. A child seeing monsters in the shadows will respond depending upon all these other factors. The usual reaction of a child seeing monsters in the shadows is to try and get rid of them by covering up, by having a night light on, or by running away from them if they are judged to be real or even suspected of being real. If the child realizes they are illusions, there will be little change. Children hearing voices of their parents will seek them out until they realize that they are hallucinations. Children seeing and hearing other children no one else can see will play with them and call them imaginary if that is what their parents have told them. There is an endless variety of perceptual disturbances and the impact on behavior is also very variable. But in each case it is important to try and understand why the abnormal behavior is present.

The behavior, not the perceptual disturbance, will bring the child to the doctor. Abnormal perception may be excessive, not merely distorted. One of my adolescent schizophrenic girls began to see faint lines around her eyes that no one else could see. She was a beautiful girl but began to think of herself as ugly because of the lines. As a result she refused to go to school and eventually secluded herself in her bedroom. Many children have an inordinate craving for sweets, usually caused by a diet too heavy in sugar which does not provide enough of the important nutrients and which may induce an allergy to the sugars. This craving may also be due to a deficiency of zinc in the diet. The craving for sugar can be overpowering. One mother told me about her son whom she saw one night carefully and slowly going into the kitchen, on his hands and knees, to the sugar bowl and eating handfuls of the stuff. This craving and the need to satisfy it can have enormous behavioral consequences; I believe that the seeds of major antisocial behavior may be traced to an extraordinary craving for sweets. I wonder how many people who break and enter started out as children with this apparently innocuous habit of stealing for sweets. Older children with these addictions may swing over to alcohol and steal that for several years. I have seen alcoholics who began to drink by stealing from bottles in the home and became alcoholic by the time they were age 8. Drug addicts depend upon stealing in order to satisfy their craving and habit.

Paranoid thinking also leads to abnormal behavior. A child who thinks all the students are picking on him and hating him will not want to go to school, and when forced to, will fight with and resent the parent or teacher. It is difficult to imagine that child doing well academically. A child who cannot keep up with his peers and is forced to try and do so may respond by playing hooky, not going to that school. A child who has to spend all the time on studies will have no time for playing and will resent having to work so hard. Failure to develop empathy by the child will result in behavior which ignores the feelings of other children and create many difficulties. These are just a few examples of how thought disorder will influence behavior.

Abnormal mood also influences behavior. A child depressed will behave in the way depressed people behave and a child too manic will behave in a too exuberant way. Some children's mood is so abnormal a few minutes in their presence is sufficient to begin diagnosis. But other children may be very subdued, quiet and well behaved in the doctor's office. These children are anxious about meeting a new doctor and I think are sedated by their own adrenalin. After several interviews when they are no longer made so anxious, their abnormal behavior will become obvious. If there is a discrepancy between what is observed and what has been reported, it is advisable to see the child several times. If this is not recognized, the doctor on the first visit may conclude that there is nothing wrong with the child and that the parent is unduly worried. This was common many years ago when parents were much more apt to be blamed for their children illnesses. Many mothers have told me that after the first visit the psychiatrist found nothing wrong with the child, told the parents so, and then accused them of being the problem. They never had another chance to see that child.

Hyperactivity (Subclinical Pellagra)

Perceptual, thought, and mood disorders make it very difficult for the child to grow and develop properly. The difficulty of keeping up with their peers and with their parents' expectations for them creates so much stress on these children that they develop psychosocial techniques for dealing with the problem, for example, not going to school or running away. They may also lack energy, except for those that are driven to excess activity by their illness.

Slight over activity when appropriate is not pathological but it may be difficult to live with these restless children. When the hyperactivity is great, it is almost always inappropriate since they are so out of tune with their environment. My working rule is that if the parents are exhausted from trying to keep up with or to control their child's behavior, then that child is pathologically hyperactive. Passive behavior is not as disturbing and may be recognized later as a problem. A common picture is a very anxious, disturbed parent who appears tired, trying to control an hyperactive child who cannot be controlled. Simply watching them for a awhile will exhaust many.

The first recorded description of children with hyperactivity or attention deficit disorder was the description of "subclinical pellagra" presented by T.D. Spies and his colleagues in 1938. They wrote, "mental changes as a part of the pellagra syndrome have been recognized by many physicians, and in areas where the disease is endemic, these symptoms are so common and so striking that they have become associated with pellagra even by the lay observer. Various abnormal psychic states have been described in medical literature on pellagra and some writers have thought that one or another psychosis was typical of this disease. . . . Subclinical pellagrins are noted for the multiplicity of their complaints, among which are many that are usually classified as neurasthenic. The most common of these symptoms are fatigue, insomnia, vertigo, burning sensation in various parts of the body, numbness, palpitation, nervousness, a feeling of unrest and anxiety, headaches, forgetfulness, apprehension, and distractibility. The conduct of the pellagrins may be normal, but he feels incapable of mental or physical effort even though he may be ambulatory. . . . It is noteworthy that many physicians who wrote on pellagra before the publication of Goldberger's work contended that pellagra should be classified in the group of neuroses. Every pellagrin has one or more symptoms which might be considered those of a neuroses." For the medical diagnosis and treatment of hyperactivity, one footnote in this article is particularly important. "Preliminary studies on 75 children with characteristic pellagra have shown that the majority of them have dizziness, irritability, stomach upsets, flight of ideas and inability to get along well in school or with other members of their family. These symptoms usually disappeared promptly following the ingestion of tablets of nicotinic acid."

There is also an experiment with animals conducted over 50 years ago that relates hyperactivity to a deficiency of the B vitamins, including nicotinic acid. G. Wald and B. Jackson reported that a deficiency of B vitamins increased the daily running distance of rats. Wald later received the Nobel Prize for his work with vitamin A. They recorded the average distance run by rats in running cages when their diet was normal and when deprived of calories. On the starvation diet they increased the distance run from 1.5 to 7 miles per day. This is not surprising. Animals are motivated by hunger to search for food. A running animal is much more apt to run into or after food and a fish that swims faster is more apt to find a meal. Animals tend to rest and relax or sleep after a meal. But the second part of their experiment was much more important. Rats deprived of their B vitamins but given normal amounts of calories – that is, starved of B vitamins but not of calories – ran 7 miles daily. They ran as if they were hungry, even though they ought not to have been. In natural settings animals may often be hungry but seldom do they suffer a deficiency of B vitamins in the presence of adequate calories unless they are humans or human pets like cats and dogs. Nature has not made any provision against this kind of deficiency. When it exists, the animal therefore responds as if it were calorie deprived. It runs more, as if it were looking for food.

This is a excellent model for human hyperactivity. The deficiency of B vitamins (chiefly vitamin B-3 and vitamin B-6) activates this basic animal reflex for increased activity when hungry. Hyperactive children are literally running looking for more food. The hyperactivity is a replacement for the food hunting activity of the hungry animal. In adults the same primitive reflex may lead to the increased food intake. More food does in fact provide more of the B vitamins but the price probably will be obesity and the variety of techniques humans use to avoid this such as laxatives and vomiting. But these are futile gestures until the B vitamins or other nutrients are replaced to balance the calories which are eaten. Whenever I see an hyperactive child, I visualize a child trying desperately to obtain more B vitamins using the only means nature has built into our genes to provide for hunger, a hunger for the vitamins and not just for calories.

Human experiments have been carried out unwittingly. Pellagra, a deficiency of vitamin B-3, makes these children hyperactive. Giving them this vitamin cures their hyperactivity. And in this book I have given ample evidence that at least two B vitamins, B-3 and B-6, markedly removed hyperactivity in children. Adults are not spared this kind of response. Hyperactivity in children, running about and ceaseless activity, is gradually replaced by more adult type of hyperactivity seen during adolescence and adulthood. I have seen many adults who cannot tolerate any inactivity. They are constantly on the move, restless, tense, unless under the influence of alcohol or other drugs.

This thesis has been amplified by Dr Glen Green in his studies of subclinical pellagra (SP), which in my opinion is the best term to describe behavioral disorders such as hyperactivity and attention deficiency disorder, much better than any of the more than 50 diagnostic DSM labels now available. In a seven-month period, Dr Green, a general practitioner in Prince Albert, Saskatchewan, diagnosed over 100 cases. These children were overly active. Some suffered from dyslexia. Words blurred or moved and many wore glasses in an attempt to correct what could not be corrected. They were tired, moody, irritable, and many had perceptual illusions and occasionally hallucinations. About one-third wet the bed. Yet these children all responded to vitamin B-3 within a few days or weeks. They did not have any of the classical symptoms of pellagra, no gastrointestinal problems, no skin changes. They were really cases of pellagra *sine* pellagra, a term used many years ago for patients who responded to this vitamin but had not shown any of the classical symptoms.

Holistic Diagnosis

Consider a typical child with subclinical pellagra (SP). The diagnosis would certainly be missed unless all four areas of the mental state were examined. This is what might happen to such a child with different therapists. Perceptual clinicians or counselors would find and try to treat these perceptually handicapped children calling them dyslexic. If reading was difficult because the words were moving about on the page, they would be given remedial reading. If they could not concentrate on the written page or on the black board, they might be called attention deficit and treated for this. Treatment would be directed at improving perceptual performance but these would be difficult and not usually successful. Those interested in learning deficits would find one or another form of retardation and would "treat" them in special schools or classes. More polite terms for these children would be slow learners, underachievers, intellectually impaired, etc., terms more considerate of their parents feelings. The clinician primarily interested in mood would treat the mood disorder with drugs for anxiety or for depression. Finally, the behaviorist would diagnose hyperactivity, one of the many forms, and use ritalin to slow them down or one of the many kinds of behavioral or conditioning therapies. The treatment that child received would depend almost entirely upon the orientation of the treating doctor. The diagnosis would be random and so would the treatment given them. None would diagnose them subclinical pellagra or needing large doses of vitamin B-3, unless they were familiar with pellagra and its variants and had taken time to examine all four areas of the mental state.

The possible range of possible diagnoses combining the four categories of perception, thought, mood, and behavior with the nomenclature of the American Psychiatric Association DSM would look like this:

CHANGES IN	DIAGNOSIS
Perception	perceptually handicapped
	dyslexia
	reading disorder
	minimally brain damaged
	hallucinosis
	pseudo-hallucinosis
Thinking	retardation
	intellectually handicapped
	slow learner
	underachiever
	attention deficit disorder (ADD)
	developmental arithmetic disorder (DAD)

CHANGES IN	DIAGNOSIS
...Thinking	developmental expressive writing disorder (DEWD)
	developmental reading disorder (DRD)
	developmental articulation disorder (DAD)
	developmental receptive learning disorder (DRLD)
Mood	depression
	bipolar
	emotionally disturbed
Behavior	autism
	hyperactivity
	conduct disorder
	oppositional defiant disorder

The reason for this wide range of diagnostic terms is now clear. Take chronic pellagra or schizophrenia, for example. Medical experts in only one aspect of brain dysfunction will miss much of the symptomatology. It is like the six blind men who examined the elephant and came up with six different diagnoses of the phenomenon they were examining. Suppose we ask each of four psychiatrists to examine only one of the four different aspects of the mental state of a chronic pellagra or schizophrenic patient. The first one would restrict his examination to the perceptual area, the second to the area of thought processes, the third would be interested only in mood disorders, and the fourth would be a behavioral therapist. The perceptual psychiatrist would elicit illusions and/or hallucinations and might diagnose hallucinosis. The thought psychiatrist would be interested in intelligence and in abnormal thinking processes and content. He would be interested in the delusions, paranoia, etc. The third, the mood disorder expert, might diagnose any one of the mood disorders, bipolar disorder, for example, formerly manic depressive. The behavioral expert would find one of the common behavioral diseases such as immature personality (currently better known as borderline personality disorder or BPD), psychopathy, criminal behavior, and, in children, hyperactivity or the older term, hyperkinetic syndrome. Not one would diagnose pellagra or schizophrenia. Currently many schizophrenic patients are misdiagnosed bipolar because their psychiatrist has not studied their perceptual changes or thinking processes; they are treated with lithium, the treatment of choice for bipolar conditions. Each diagnostician is using criteria derived from only one aspect of the brain dysfunction. Much more is derived from the orientation and bias of the diagnostician. The disease is single, pellagra, but the number of ways of describing it has no limit.

The only way to simplify and make more accurate diagnosis is to examine the complete mental state, all the four aspects of brain functions – perception, thinking, mood, behavior – and to explore the biomedical and nutritional causes of brain disorders and dysfunctions.

Food and Ecologic Allergies, Additives, and Toxins

When I take a history I never forget to take an allergy history in the hunt for clues. With children or young adults it is vital to examine for the presence of the common allergic diseases as a factor in causing their psychiatric problems, for any food allergy can reproduce almost every known psychiatric syndrome from infantile autism and schizophrenia to mood and behavioral disorders. Allergic reactions tend to develop against staple foods such as milk, wheat, and rice. Thus in wheat consuming countries, wheat allergy is much more common than it is in rice consuming countries where rice is a greater problem. In tea drinking countries, tea will more often cause allergic reactions than coffee, while the converse is true in coffee consuming countries. I have seldom seen allergic reactions to tea but coffee allergies are more common in Canada and the United States, where dairy food allergies are much more common than in South American countries where dairy foods are seldom consumed.

Any patient who has a history of allergy, who has the signs of allergy, and whose food patterns are such that allergy is possible, should be examined by a dietary test. Limiting exposure to allergens during infancy will protect children from developing major allergies later in life. As Dr Hide, Director of Asthma and Allergy Research Center, St. Mary's Hospital, Newport, England, has noted, "The newborn is particularly vulnerable to sensitization." He studied 120 high risk children over a four-year period. Of this group, 58 were breastfed or given hydrolyzed formula and the mothers avoided dairy products, eggs, fish, and nuts and they took vitamins and mineral supplements. In addition exposure to house dust was minimized by using anti-house mite dust four times each year. The control babies were breastfed but no other measures were taken to minimize exposure. After four years the control group had 2.7 times as many allergies and 5.6 times as many allergy symptoms. They had 3.4 times the amount of eczema and 3.7 times as many positive skin reactions to pricks. He concluded, "Families at high risk for allergic disease should use dietary and environmental control measures to reduce the risk in infants."

Cerebral Allergies and Ecologic Mental Illness

Even though we have known for over 75 years that cerebral allergy can cause mental state dysfunctions such as learning disabilities and behavioral disorders in children, there is little reference to this knowledge in the psychiatric literature – even less in psychiatric treatment of these children. Undesirable reactions to food have been more or less ignored in most medical curricula, and the majority of physicians ignore the possibility of cerebral allergy when diagnosing and treating children with these problems. A review of research into these allergies induced by food ingested or by the environment suggests the importance of this knowledge for diagnosing perception, thinking, mood, and behavior disorders in children properly.

In 1916, B.R. Hoobler first described the allergic tension-fatigue syndrome in children which left them restless, fretful, and sleepless, then in 1922, W.R. Shannon described seven patients with disorders of the nervous system which were out of proportion to the primary allergy. These children were described as unusually irritable, peevish, and out of sorts. I.S. Kahn in 1927 found that allergy to pollen was often associated with languidness and restlessness, alternating with spells of intense temper and fury. A.H. Rowe reported in 1930 that allergies produced drowsiness, irritability, fatigue, weakness, and slowness of thought; in children he observed irritability and incorrigibility. In 1932, W.D. Alvarez considered a variety of gastrointestinal symptoms produced by food allergies, but also added, "in severe cases of food sensitiveness there may be sick headaches, mental dullness and depression." Out of a series of 500 food allergic patients, over 25 percent were allergic to onions (raw), milk, and apples. Wheat did not appear in his table.

Dr Alvarez was a famous gastroenterologist at the Mayo clinic who wrote a very popular column on health syndicated in daily newspapers reaching up to 40 million readers. He became a supporter of our work in nutritional medicine because he was extremely critical of psychoanalysis. During lunch with him in Chicago he told me about his first experience with food allergy and how it nearly cost him his job at the Mayo Clinic. In the early 1920s, he was puzzled by the fact that every Monday he could not think clearly, his mind felt foggy. He described himself as being dumb. Eventually he realized that because his family was so poor, they could afford to eat chicken only on Sundays. He deduced that the chicken on Sunday made him dumb on Monday, and when he stopped eating chicken, he no longer suffered from "dumb" Mon-days. He published this report in the medical literature, which created a wave of hostility among his staff associates because they all "knew" that no one could be allergic to any food. The pressure was mounting to have him fired when the senior Dr Mayo, one of the founders, met Dr Alvarez in the corridor of the hospital and congratulated him on writing one of the best "goddam" reports he had ever read. After reading that paper, Dr Mayo discovered he, too, had a food allergy.

Dr T.G. Randolph probably has had more experience with cerebral allergies to food than any other physician. His interest became greater between 1939 and 1944 when he tried to diagnose sensitivity to common foods by feeding single food items. When patients were fasted one day and given single foods, a few mild emotional changes were seen. However, after Dr H.J.Rinkel developed the "Rinkel Method" of fasting 4-10 days followed by introducing individual food items, many more severe psychiatric reactions were seen. As Dr Alvarez described this elimination diet, "the simplest method would be to eat nothing for a few days. If then the distress continued, it would be clear that food could not have much, if anything, to do with it. If, however, the distress promptly ceased, then the patient could try out one new food each day, keeping the good ones and rejecting the bad ones." With this technique, the relation between foods and mental illness became clear, but only to a small number of clinicians and hardly any psychiatrists, unfortunately for children.

Around the same time we were exploring the effects of vitamin B-3 on behavior, Dr H.M. Davison reported that children with allergenic foods in their diet are like Mr Hyde, but when those foods are removed from their diet they are like Dr Jekyll. Children suffering from food allergies were sleepy, sluggish in their thinking, had difficulty in concentration, could not be pleased, and were generally unhappy. On the basis of his experience with 500 cases of food allergies, he concluded:

1. Any food can produce a cerebral reaction;
2. Multiple food susceptibility is the rule;
3. Usually foods consumed every three days are involved;
4. Other chemicals in the environment such as insecticides, hydrocarbons, sprays, perfumes, and so on can produce similar allergic reactions;
5. Such cerebral reactions are often labeled neurotic or emotional.

Dr Randolph called these cerebral allergies "ecologic mental illness" in a report for the Third World Congress of Psychiatry. During the fast, the avoidance of the allergenic food accentuates the symptoms, Randolph discovered. The subject may feel much worse, especially during the second day. Then the symptoms gradually disappear. The specific adapted stages of the reaction revert to a non-adapted stage. Reexposure induces acute test reactions. He also provided a diagnostic scheme showing the relationship between the allergenic food and the intensity of the reaction:

Relation Between Effect of Allergenic Food and Depth of Hangover

PICK UP INTENSITIES	DEPTH OF HANGOVER
1. Active, buoyant, alert, stimulated	A. Sniffly, itchy, queasy, absent-minded, tired
2. Hyperactive, keyed up, energetic, irritable	B. Wheezy, rash, cramps, brain fogged, aches, puffy
3. Jittery, argumentative, aggressive, drunk-like	C. Confused, indecisive, morose, lethargic
4. Uncontrollably excited, agitated, maniacal	D. Depressed, stuporous, disoriented, amnesic

Slightly susceptible children and adults reacting to frequently consumed foods may remain at levels one, two, and three. Levels two and three describe the hyperactive syndrome. Later on, lower levels of hangover become more common. When symptoms of hangover persist in adults, this is said to represent the onset of the illness. However, my experience is that levels two and three will cause parents to take their child to a doctor. Levels C and D are rarely recognized as allergic reactions.

Patients can alternate between the pick up intensity or hangover, much as an alcoholic will swing from a state of intoxication to a hangover state. There are also vertical alternations, and starting anywhere in this table there are counter-clockwise changes. Thus a patient may start from A, move to 1, then to 2, to B and back to A. However, as the process becomes chronic, patients tend to settle into C, 4, and D. Randolph concluded that "any mental or behavioral aberration in which causation has not been demonstrated deserves to be investigated from the ecologic standpoint."

Dr W.G. Crook in 1970 further clarified the allergic tension-fatigue syndrome as part of a primary allergic disorder of the nervous system. It can occur alone or in conjunction with other allergic syndromes. He described the reactions as follows:

1. *Tension*
   (a) Motor: overactivity, clumsy, unable to relax
   (b) Sensory: over-sensitive, irritable, photophobia
2. *Fatigue*
   (a) Motor: tired, achy
   (b) Sensory: sluggish, torpor
3. *Less Common Mental Nervous Symptoms*
   unreality, depression, bizarre and irrational behavior, inability to concentrate, nervous tics
4. *Associated Systemic Manifestations*
   (a) Always present: infraorbital circles, stuffy nose
   (b) Common: infraorbital edema, increased salivation, increased sweating, abdominal pain, headache, enuresis

Crook concluded that "the net result of this hyper group of symptoms is to make the unfortunate youngsters who manifest them definitely unpleasant little people to have around. They are apt to be reprimanded and punished by parents and teachers, and rejected or ignored by their siblings and contemporaries."

He found that the most common allergic foods were consumed every day: milk, chocolate, cola drinks, eggs, cereal grains, especially corn. He recommended a 5-14 day period of food elimination. After that re-introduction of the offending food would cause a reaction. He recommended three trials to establish the relationship clearly. In one case, an 8-year-old child showed schizophrenic behavior while on a diet containing large amounts of chocolate. She suffered from fatigue, pallor, infraorbital circles, abdominal pain. Mentally she showed obsessive-compulsive behavior, had periodic hysterical screaming spells, or was moody, withdrawn, seemingly in a trance. After seven days on a chocolate-free diet she was normal.

After visiting an institute in Moscow where a prolonged fast is used for treating chronic schizophrenia, Dr Alan Cott introduced this approach into North America. Basically, patients were fasted under carefully controlled conditions in hospital for up to between 20 and 30 days. This treatment had been developed over a 23-year period by Dr U. Nickolayev and his staff at the Moscow Psychiatric Institute. The treatment had been effective in 64 percent of cases of chronic schizophrenia; 47 percent remained well over a six-month period. Following the fast the patient is kept on a vegetarian diet with dairy products for at least six months. Since then Dr Cott has treated a substantial number of chronic schizophrenics and has corroborated the findings of the Russian physicians. I have treated a small number of patients with this form of fasting and have seen dramatic changes, often appearing on the 4th or 5th day. A few illustrative cases will be presented further on.

In 1973, H.L. Newbold, W.H. Philpott, and M. Mandell reviewed the history of ecologic mental illnesses. Apparently Richard Burton in 1621 was aware of allergic depressions when he wrote in his *Anatomy of Melancholy*, "Milk and all that comes from milk increases melancholy." Newbold and colleagues have been prominent in introducing the allergic mental syndromes to psychiatrists and using the "deliberate food ingestion test" (a four-day fast followed by introduction of a single food). They found that two-thirds of 53 schizophrenics were allergic to wheat, one-half to corn and milk. Other common offenders were tobacco, coffee, eggs, chocolate, potatoes, and peanuts. Neurotics had a similar high frequency of allergies, as did manics and depressives. These authors suggested that the antihistaminic properties of tranquilizers might account for some of their antipsychotic effect, and the histamine-depleting properties of nicotinic acid might similarly be involved.

Over the past five years Dr E.L. Rees has emphasized the important role of allergy in the production of hyperactive behavior in children. In this report Rees provides methods for determining which are the offending food allergens and how to deal with them. They must be removed from the diet. Rees describes five different types of children suffering from cerebral allergy or ecologic mental illness: the severely malnourished normal child; the allergic child exhibiting the tension/anxiety syndrome who is often a bottle-fed child with a runny nose, colic, frequent respiratory illness, and occasionally eczema, with dark circles under the eyes and a generalized pallor and with a family history of allergy, especially to corn and milk; the schizophrenic and autistic child; the minimally brain damaged child; and the truly retarded child. Children with Down's Syndrome should also be included in this group suffering from cerebral allergies.

Dr Philpott, in a series of papers, has suggested that in some cases hypoglycemia is a consequence of the allergic reaction and provides an excellent explanation of the addictive power of certain allergens. "A most valuable perspective is that of Randolph's observations about addiction being based on a physiological compensation to an allergy," he writes. "Food allergies are often missed since the frequent use of an allergic food produces an addiction. An allergic food may be used frequently to relieve withdrawal phase symptoms. Therefore, the patient's favorite foods are often proved to be the allergic culprits behind chronic physical and mental illness. Testing the glucose level of a series of patients at the time of addictive withdrawal phase symptoms has convinced me that a mild, and sometimes severe, degree of hypoglycemia quite routinely occurs as a physiological expression of the state of stress. Quite frequently the same set of symptoms can also be evoked as an allergic reaction without hypoglycemia being evoked. It is important to understand that a four-day fast changed a food addiction state with symptoms occurring some hours after ingestion to an allergic response with the symptoms occurring within a few minutes after ingestion of the food. Spot sampling of glucose levels during deliberate food testing of single foods has revealed both hyperglycemia and hypoglycemic responses to be sometimes occurring at the time the observable hypersensitive symptoms are occurring, which is usually between 30 minutes to one hour after the feeding period. These observations reinforce the concept that disturbances in carbohydrate metabolism, whether hypoglycemic or hyperglycemic, should be given the benefit of a systematic allergy-ecology study. Any organ of the body can be the allergic shock organ. Certainly the adrenals, pancreas, liver, pituitary, and hypothalamus are no exception. In the list of possible causes of disturbed carbohydrate metabolism it is imperative that allergic and similar hypersensitive reactions be considered in the differential diagnosis.

"A further surprise comes when we discover that a protein rather than a carbohydrate can sometimes be demonstrated to be the culprit disturbing carbohydrate metabolism. In some hard-to-manage hypoglycemics I have found them allergic to some of the high protein foods they were frequently using in an attempt to manage their hypoglycemia. They were literally addicted to the high protein foods, and frequent use of these foods provided a partial relief of withdrawal phase symptoms. They were remaining chronically ill while frequently eating high protein foods to which they were addicted. This is why it can sometimes be a mistake to treat hypoglycemia as viewed only in terms of carbohydrate metabolism. Any food addiction, no matter what type of food, can be the culprit. Thus to the program of high protein, low carbohydrate, sugar-free, caffeine-free, frequent feeding, there must be added that of any other food to which the person is demonstrated to be hypersensitive. This can only be discovered by a broad spectrum testing of reactions to foods. The frequent between-meal feedings become unnecessary when a proper allergy survey has been made and implemented."

Bed-wetting is a common problem for children and for their parents, of course. A large proportion of the children I have seen have suffered from enuresis, but fortunately as they have recovered this has subsided. Rarely is it the primary symptom leading to a referral to a psychiatrist, but I have seen several whose enuresis was so troublesome it was responsible for a number of psychological problems. There have been a large number of etiological explanations for bed-wetting, ranging from far-out psychoanalytical theories to behavioral conditioning ideas which resulted in the use of electric bells and flashing lights to arouse children when the first drop of urine fell upon a sensitive blanket. This device was more successful than psychoanalysis. Dr G.W. Bray in 1931 was the first person to suggest allergies were responsible for many cases of enuresis. More recently, several allergists and urologists have established that a large proportion of children with enuresis are allergic to foods or to other chemicals. According to Gerrard, the main problem in enuresis is a small capacity bladder caused by a spasm in the detrusor muscle in reaction to an allergy. Many of the children were cured by removing offending foods from their diet. Imipramine, an antidepressant, and antihistamines are helpful in the short run; for example, when a child is away from home. They relax the detrussor muscle and allow the bladder to enlarge its capacity. When children recover, there is an increase in bladder capacity. In girls, enuresis predisposes to recurrent bladder infections. One of the more common offenders is milk and dairy products. W.W. Anderson found that many of the hyperactive children he examined had early histories of colic (usually milk allergy) and irritability during infancy. Indeed, dairy products are a primary cause of cerebral allergy.

Dairy Food Allergy

The most informative single study that describes dairy products and human nutrition is Frank Oski's book entitled *Don't Drink Your Milk*. Milk and its many derivatives are the most widely promoted and advertised food product in North America and major parts of Europe. According to Dr Oski, at the time his book was written, 14 percent of all food dollars went for milk and its products. This made up the second major food expense following the combined costs of meat, fish, poultry, and eggs. These products are promoted by the vast majority of physicians, by almost every dietitian and nutritionist, by most professors of nutrition and bio-chemistry when they teach nutrition in medical schools, by Departments of Public Health, and of course by the most powerful group of all, the various national, provincial, and state dairy organizations. It has become an article of faith that unless children are given copious quantities of milk, best of all three glasses each day, they will not grow, they will not develop, their babies in turn will not get enough calcium, and the women will all get osteoporosis after menopause.

I invariably get a startled reaction from mothers when I advise them their children or even they must stop drinking milk. The first question is where will I get enough calcium, how about osteoporosis. The public is confused about the various mammalian milks. I believe we should have different names for human milk and for cow milk so that they will not be equated as equivalent good products. Cow milk is good for calves but has never been shown by any independent experiment to be good for human babies or for adult women to protect them against osteoporosis. Against the position taken by the dairy industry are a few dedicated individual physicians such as Dr Oski and a growing band of supporters who main-tain that milk is not a perfect food, that it is not even a good food, and that milk must be used with extreme caution. I would support the idea that all dairy products be labeled with the warning sign applied to ciga-rette packages, something like "Warning, This Product May Be Hazardous to Your Health."

The vast majority of people in North America and in Europe can con-sume dairy products with few problems, especially those who have been consuming it for many centuries, because they have been adapted to this as a major food supply. Others can use it in small amounts with no harm, but for those who suffer any of the above conditions milk is as poisonous as any other food causing similar reactions would be. Dr J. Gerrard, Professor of Pediatrics at the Medical School, University of Saskatchewan, after a series of careful studies, concluded that 59 infants out of 787 were milk allergic, or 7.5 percent. He reported that the frequency depended upon how soon the infants were started on milk. One quarter of the babies started on milk before they were three months became milk allergic. The active defence of dairy products by the dairy industry dismisses airily the findings of legitimate research scientists and nutritionists, including the eminent pediatrician Dr Benjamin Spock. The Dairy Bureau of Canada labels him a "radical animal-rights activist," thus dismissing his attempts to improve our health. This arrogant dismissal of the harm caused by dairy products to many people will simply delay recognition by many patients that they are sick because they cannot tolerate dairy products.

Most mammals feed on their mothers' milk until they have tripled their birth weight. In human infants, this takes about one year. Of all the mammals, the human species alone never gets weaned from milk. Since formula is rich in sugar and milk is rich in lactose (another sugar), it is more accurate to say that only humans never get weaned from milk and sugar. As will become clear later these are two of the most common and most injurious food allergens. Americans and many Europeans have developed a taste for milk which is not natural, while most people in East Asia, Africa, and South America regard milk as not fit for human consumption. They are in better tune with the rest of our mammalian cousins. We have broken the adaptation between our need and the food by depending so much on cow milk. Nature never intended that children should forever be dependent on their mother's milk, and the loss of the enzyme lactase is a reflection of this adaptation.

Gastrointestinal disorders may be due to lactose intolerance. After infancy, many people no longer make enough lactase, the enzyme that splits lactose into galactose and glucose. The lactose cannot be absorbed and stays in the intestine where it is fermented by bacteria creating a lot of gas and intense bowel discomfort. The frequency of lactase deficiency varies enormously between various peoples. Over 80 percent of Filipinos, Japanese, Taiwanese, and Thais lack this enzyme. Over 60 percent of

Blacks, Arabs, Jews, and Greek Cypriots also lack this enzyme, while under 10 percent of Danes, Swiss, and American Whites have the same problem. Peoples who had to depend upon milk to survive have, by a process of natural selection, retained the ability to create lactase long after it was natural for the same people who did not have to consume so much. Thus, in Nigeria, tribes that did not raise cattle had a 99 percent deficiency of lactase, while other tribes where milk was a traditional food had only a 20 percent lactase deficiency. This is good news for the dairy industry, for if milk consumption can be maintained long enough, no matter what the cost, most groups will have developed the ability to retain lactase production. However, it is now possible to swallow lactase tablets before the milk is drunk and to drink lactase treated milk and thus avoid most of the symptoms of lactase deficiency.

This will not solve the problem for the milk allergic individual. For allergic reactions to dairy products are very common and can cause an amazing variety of allergic reactions anywhere in the gastrointestinal tract and very often in the upper respiratory system. I am an expert in dairy allergy, one among many, because I have a fixed allergy to these foods. Many years ago I got a common cold, at least that is what I thought it was. I did what I should have done to bring it under control, including taking large quantities of vitamin C and vitamin A, but there was no relief. For two years I had a constant nasal drip which was so bad that when I gave a lecture I would have to hold a kleenex in one hand and my notes in the other. I always carried pockets full of kleenex. After two years I had given up hope. At that time, for other reasons, I did a four-day water fast. To my amazement, I was well by the fourth day. On a retest with a little milk my drippy nose promptly returned in about 15 minutes. For the next few years, whenever I was exposed to dairy products, whether I was aware of it or not, I would get another four-day cold. Since then, for about 35 years, I have not had any colds and have been inadvertently exposed to dairy foods only on a few occasions. My dairy allergy expressed itself as a runny nose, congested sinuses, sore throat, with difficulty in clearing my ears with changes in air pressure.

The most common gastrointestinal reaction, though, is chronic diarrhea, ranging from frequent soft stools to numerous, watery, explosive stools, occasionally showing traces of red blood. The diarrhea impairs the absorption of nutrients. If there is chronic slow bleeding, a protein deficiency will develop leading to swelling of the abdomen, hands, and feet. It will also lead to iron deficiency. Half the iron deficiency in infants is a result of feeding infants cow milk. Iron deficiency will make many babies irritable with impaired attention span. This has caused a common problem called the "blue bottle syndrome." The child walks about with a plastic bottle of milk from which he drinks now and then. When only glass bottles were available they would drop these so often and break them that mothers would stop giving them bottles. With plastic bottles there is no relief for the child. Blue bottle babies are usually iron deficient. Colic is a common manifestation of milk allergy. In adults peptic ulcer is another reaction. As well as causing iron deficiency due to chronic bleeding in the gut, excessive intake of milk also is associated with other nutrient deficiencies. Excessive intake of dairy products crowds other foods out of the diet, foods which are richer in vitamins and minerals. Another factor is chronic inflammation of the intestine which decreases absorption of nutrients. I have already referred to protein deficiency caused by the milk. Another common deficiency is zinc and pyridoxine. I have been surprised at the large number of children I have seen who had white areas in their finger nails. This is due to a deficiency of pyridoxine and zinc. Most often these children are heavy consumers of dairy products. In some cases 50 percent of their calories came from this source. Milk tends to be low in zinc and in pyridoxine.

The related psychiatric and behavioral changes caused by milk are also numerous. Any food allergy can cause almost every known psychiatric syndrome and milk is no exception. One dramatic case I have seen was a chronic paranoid schizophrenic who had been resident in a mental hospital for years. He suddenly could not urinate. He was brought to City Hospital in Saskatoon from the mental hospital and came under my care when it was found he was physically normal. After a fast he was normal. The next day after a test dose of milk, he became violently ill with nausea, vomiting, severe diarrhea, headache, and more. He had been mentally normal after the fast but after milk he was once more the same psychotic person I had known for many years. The case ended sadly, though. He refused to keep away from dairy products because, he told me, if he remained well he would have to get a job and try to make his way outside the hospital. He was too old for this and preferred to remain in a mental hospital where he would be looked after. He died there two years later from leukemia.

I had one young boy as a patient who in the fall was at the bottom of his class of 20. On a milk-free diet he was at the top by the following spring. Another youngster diagnosed with infantile autism by a clinic specializing in these disorders became normal on a diet free of dairy and sugar products in one month. His mother had placed him on this diet against the advice of his therapists, who laughed at her when she first discussed it with them.

I have seen other dramatic improvements in many children who were placed upon a dairy-free diet. Over a period of about three years I fasted over 100 patients who had not responded or had responded only partially to the orthomolecular treatment I was using. More than 75 percent were much better after the four-day fast. Of these many were milk allergic. The syndromes produced by these allergies included learning and behavioral disorders, depressions, and schizophrenias. One female had been depressed for over 20 years. She had not been helped by medication or even one series of electroconvulsive treatment. She went onto a dairy-free diet on a Friday and by the following Monday her depression was gone. Another good example of this type of response occurred with Rhonda (born 1959). I was asked to see her in October 1973 while she was in hospital. She stated she had been ill for the previous year, irritable, upset, not like herself. She disliked school and claimed that she was involved with a group of girls who had a code of ethics requiring she take LSD. The school could find no evidence for this. She was seen by a psychiatrist and admitted because of severe depression and suicide intention. She also had suffered a series of convulsions for which no organic reason was found. An examination of her mental state showed perceptual changes, including illusions and very clear visual hallucinations. She saw people killing each other, ghosts, tigers, etc. She heard voices, mostly nasty, telling her that someone would kill her. She had withheld this information from her psychiatrist because she found it difficult to talk about this, even though she liked him. She was paranoid and believed that a gang of girls was plotting against her. Her memory and concentration were poor. I diagnosed her as schizophrenic and started her on orthomolecular therapy. But she could not take the vitamin tablets because of nausea and vomiting. She had been discharged but was readmitted in December for five weeks for a series of seven bilateral ECT. There was no improvement then or during follow up.

On March 2nd she started a four day fast and eliminated medication. She was alert and active, hungry at supper. On the second day, she awakened at 3:30 a.m. suffering from terrible dreams. She was depressed, cried, and felt weak. On the third day, she was very tense, nauseated, but in the afternoon the voices suddenly left her and she felt good. On the fourth day, she was normal. On the fifth morning she had a small glass of milk. One hour later she was tense and heard voices for a few minutes, but later these cleared. On April 22nd she remained well. She had required no medication since the beginning of her fast. Between March 2nd and April 10th that year, I placed 30 adult patients on the four day fast. Twenty-one were all well at the end of the four day fast. In most cases milk was the offender, but others were allergic to peanuts, beef, smoking, aspirin, and food additives.

Food Additives

Renowned pioneer allergist Dr S.F. Feingold has described a salicylate-free diet for aspirin-sensitive patients. However, food flavors which contain a salicylate radical also cause similar problems. Later he found that chemicals used as dyes, such as tartrazine (a yellow dye), induce similar reactions. In order to eliminate this color additive from the diet, he eliminated all artificially-colored foods. His final salicylate-regime excluded:

1. Food: almonds, apples, apricots, blackberries, cherries, currants, gooseberries, grapes and raisins, nectarines, oranges, peaches, plums and prunes, raspberries, strawberries, cucumbers, tomatoes.
2. Flavorings: all artificially flavored foods and drinks.
3. Drinks: all drinks containing alcohol, sugar, additives and caffeine.
4. Drugs: all drugs containing aspirin as well as all perfumes and toothpastes.

Feingold also found that many children were cured of their hyperactivity syndrome when placed upon such a diet and thus opened the exploration of the effect of food additives on children's health.

Over 75 percent of our current diet consists of processed food. This diet is deficient in fiber, too rich in processed fats, too rich in simple sugars, and deficient in vitamins, minerals, and essential fatty acids, the omega-3 type. It is also too rich in additives. The average person consumes about 140 pounds of additives per year. Of this, 102 pounds is sucrose, 13 pounds is dextrose, 15 pounds salt, 8 pounds pepper, mustard, baking soda, citric acid, and 26 other common kitchen substances, and 2.1 pounds comes from 2400 synthetic cosmetic additives. Trace additives coming from processed products used to make food mixtures are not included.

Food additives decrease the nutritional quality of foods. The refined sugars, for example, dilute the food with a pure energy source totally free of all the other essential nutrients. Even the highest quality foods do not contain a surplus of these nutrients. If a substance is added which dilutes these to half the original amount, there will not be enough of these nutrients to provide for the caloric needs of the body. Any additive simply dilutes food and increases the burden on the rest of the diet to make up the deficiency. The food industry defends their practice by claiming that in a balanced diet these nutrients are provided. However, using the optimum definition of balanced diet, it is impossible to provide balance when additives are used. Thus the criticism that breakfast cereals do not provide enough nutrients is countered by the claim that they are not meant to be eaten alone and are usually mixed with milk. The presence of additives in food is equivalent to the presence of a parasite at the dinner table, a person who consumes but never makes any contribution to the food supply. If 90 percent of the diet is whole food, it can to a degree compensate for 10 percent junk food. If 80 percent of the diet is junk, the remaining 20 percent cannot cover for the complete deficiency of nutrients generated by that diet.

Today in high technology societies about 80 percent of the diet is processed. A recent survey in England showed that 63 percent of the children obtained over 35 percent of their calories from fat and 88 percent consumed 11 percent from sucrose. When the average sugar intake is 125 pounds per person per year, half the population must ingest more than that, and since the estimate includes the entire population and children do not eat as much as adults, then there are many, including children, who are using over 250 pounds per person per year. The favorite foods are chips and crisps, white bread, confections, processed and preserved meat, biscuit, cakes, buns, and soft drinks in decreasing order of preference. The term balanced diet is meaningless today although it might have been useful before junk foods corrupted the national diet.

There are two ways to correct this intolerable situation. The best way is to eliminate all junk foods. The second way is to add to the child's diet a mixture containing all the essential amino acids, essential fatty acids, and vitamins and minerals with enough fiber. Adding these substances to a good food will diminish their nutritional value. It is even worse when they are added to processed foods which have already lost a good deal of their nutritional value. Other additives such as processed fats and oils distort the diet in the same way as do the sugars. Pure protein, protein hydrolysates, and mixtures of amino acids will have the same destructive effect but they are too expensive so far and are generally not used as additives to the same degree.

A good example of what is wrong with our diet is the doughnut. This is made from white flour, fat, and sugar. It is a combination of everything which is undesirable in our diet. The fat and sugar contain no other nutrients and the white flour consumed by itself could not sustain life very long. The doughnut would be the perfect food for killing someone if you wanted to do so by giving them excess amounts of this type of food they love to eat. They would eventually die obese and sick but grateful to you for having been so kind to them.

Refined Sugars

Many years ago a mother brought two of her sons to see me. One was adopted. Both were seven years old, both suffered from severe hyperactivity, and both were having learning difficulties. I suspected that the amount of sugar and junk food they were eating was a factor and advised the two children and their mother that they should go onto a sugar-free diet. The two children were horrified. One month later one child was well and the other remained as hyperactive as he had been before. The boy who was well had been following the diet, while the other refused to do so. He told me in no uncertain terms that he would never ever stop eating sugar and stamped his foot to emphasize his decision. I then advised them to go on to plan B. They both asked me what was plan B, expecting something even worse. I asked them, would they follow the no sugar diet on week days if they could have all the junk they wanted on Saturday? They both agreed. When they came back after another month both boys were well. Their mother then told me what had happened.

In preparation for junk-food Saturday they had gone to a store. The boy who had been cooperative before was very upset because his brother was going to get all those sweets. His mother agreed he could also go onto the same program. But then the five other children in the family complained that they were being left out. Mother finally said the whole family could do so. The following Saturday one of the children became violently ill with nausea and vomiting after consuming sweets. Pretty soon every child in that family was sick with either headaches, nausea, or vomiting. After that the little boy who had been so determined he would never give up sweets told me, adamantly, that he would never ever eat sweets again.

Two common sugars circulate in the blood: glucose, which is very essential and safe when the concentration is not too high, and fructose, which is not safe. All carbohydrates are broken down or hydrolyzed during digestion into the simple sugars. The simple monosaccharides are then absorbed through the intestinal wall and enter the bloodstream. This sugar provides energy for all the cells of the body. If the concentration of glucose in the blood drops too far, cells become starved for food energy, and the brain may suffer enough deficiency that the person will faint and go into a coma. This is what happens when a diabetic takes too much insulin. This drives the blood sugar too far down by increasing the amount of glucose which the cells take up. Glucose released by digestion and absorbed into the blood will not cause any harm if the food being digested is whole food, such as whole wheat, carrots, brown rice, and so on. The rate of entry into the blood is slow, controlled, and accompanied by the nutrients in the whole grain. Each molecule of sugar released in this way comes with a package of other nutrients, vitamins, and minerals, and these are available to the body for the processing of the sugar molecules into energy and into other products.

In sharp contrast are the so-called free sugars which have already been refined, liberated from every nutritional component of the foods in which they were made. They can be eaten very quickly so that in addition to the quantities consumed, which are excessive, they are absorbed too rapidly. This throws an enormous burden on the body which has to deal with all the sugar.

Whole foods contain very little free sugar. Even ripe fruit will contain less than 20 percent, and fruits which have not been altered by plant breeders contain even less. Natural fruit tends to be less sweet, but plant breeders have selected for sweetness since this appeals to the taste of the public. The major source of sugar before the advent of the chemical age was the honey that our ancestors gathered. With the development of cane and beets as good sources of sugar, it became possible to consume huge amounts of free sugars. This has had a major impact on the health of the populations which follow the high-tech diet.

The combination of high sugar and low fiber in the processed food diet creates the condition called the Saccharine Disease. The symptoms are peptic ulcer due to a deficiency of protein when gastric juice is secreted while eating. Drinking a sugared, carbonated drink stimulates secretion of acid which finds no protein to which it can be attached. The excess of calories, sugar, other simple carbohydrates, fat, and lack of exercise are factors in causing obesity and diabetes mellitus, especially the late maturity or adult onset type. It is probably more accurate to consider this type of diabetes a variant of hypoglycemia. Relative hypoglycemia afflicts nearly two-thirds of all psychiatric populations and 100 percent of all addict populations. Out of several hundred tests, I have yet to find one alcoholic with a normal five-hour glucose tolerance curve.

Excess sugar also provides a medium for yeast which inhabits our gastro-intestinal tract. The combination of too much sugar, antibiotics which destroy normal bacterial flora and allow yeast overgrowth, and birth control medication which encourages vaginal overgrowth of yeast is largely responsible for yeast infection that troubles so many people. In addition, chemotherapy or steroid therapy decreases the immune defense system. A combination of yeast overgrowth and decreased immune defense may be responsible for a number of auto immune diseases, such as multiple sclerosis, perhaps lupus, muscular dystrophies, rheumatoid arthritis, and many gastrointestinal diseases.

The proof that sugar additives affect children's health adversely is overwhelmingly clear in the medical and scientific literature and persuasive to everyone except the sugar industries who provide these sugars. Unfortunately, the sugar industry is supported by nutritionists and dietitians of the old school who still believe, as did Dr Fred Stare, formerly of

Harvard University, that the more sugar the better. He once recommended we should all double our sugar intake. Investigators seem reluctant to accept that sugars and other food additives cause attention deficit hyperactivity disorder (ADHD). A recent National Institute of Health study attempts to dispel the "myth" that these contaminants cause ADHD. Part of the evidence for this argument was derived from a 1980 study that was financed by the National Advisory Committee on Hyperkinesis and Food Additives for the Nutritional Foundation, a lobby for the major food, chemical, and pharmaceutical companies. I expect similar articles every year from food-industry supported research.

Pure sugars used as individual nutrients are probably not as pathological as processed foods which contain sugar plus a large variety of other additives. I thus advise parents and children to avoid foods containing added sugar, not simply to get rid of the sugar but also to lessen the ingestion of other additives. It is rare to find processed foods which contain added sugar alone. I have seen many children who were not disturbed by adding sugar back into their diet and perhaps many more who were improved when it was avoided.

Excellent controlled studies have shown a direct relationship between an excess of refined sugar consumption and anti-social behavior. Noting that children's health is a primary concern among politicians, Dr Tuormaa notes that "crime is also presently on top of the political agenda. In fact the present rising trend of the criminal statistics and violence resembles today more of an epidemic disease, with symptoms including mental disarrangement combined with a complete lack of any behavioral or emotional control. While crime statistics relentlessly rise, the government and the media are trying to put the blame on varied sociopolitical influences such as TV and film violence, poverty, lack of parental guidance, alleged child abuse, frustration, lack of motivation, lack of appropriate prisons or institutions, the police, etc. In fact the blame has been pointed at most things, but never on faulty nutrition. Yet, as this paper has shown, an inappropriate nutrition can modify brain function resulting in susceptible individuals, to a severe mental dysfunction, including manifestations of criminal and violent behavior.

"The following fundamental dietary factors must be taken into consideration when confronting anyone displaying an inappropriate behavior pattern: is the person concerned living on a high sucrose, high food additive diet which lacks an appropriate amount of good protein? Is the diet completely lacking in foods high in vitamin and mineral content such as fresh fruits and/or salads? Could the person have an allergic intolerance to any foods he or she is consuming regularly? Could the person suffer from a toxicological burden of heavy metal contamination, such as lead, cadmium and/or aluminum, which can be easily diagnosed by current hair mineral analysis testing methods."

The Medical Post recently reported on a paper delivered by Dr Leonard McEwen who studied the hyperactivity level of nine juvenile delinquents by changing their diet. The "devil" in our children appears to be food allergies, he said. The police had regarded these children as the worst young criminals in Shipley, England, near Leeds. Most had 10 or more offenses and the cost of their vandalism in the previous years was $200,000. They were all hyperactive. As long as they stayed on their nutrient enriched diets they were crime free. Three abandoned their diets and went back to a life of crime with their gangs.

Replacing sugared drinks and junk food with fruit juice and fresh fruit and nuts in these studies decreased the incidence of aggressive acts up to 50 percent. These sugar rich foods worsened behavior of young offenders and increased the restless and destructive behavior of hyperactive children. Mothers of these children are not surprised since in most cases they have already seen what these foods have done. Schools close the day after Hallowe'en because the children are too restless and disorganized. Teachers have told me they hate teaching on the day after this children's binge day on sugary foods.

Food Coloring and Preservatives

Dr T.E. Tuormaa has recently reviewed the literature on the relation between hyperactivity in children and the presence of additives in food. The xenobiotic or chemicals foreign to the body implicated include tartrazine, curcumin, sunset yellow, and many others. But tartrazine toxicity provides a good model for what these chemicals can do. Tartrazine is used in soft drinks and is one of the additives most often implicated in food intolerance studies. This occurs mostly in subjects also sensitive to aspirin. Between 10 percent and 40 percent of aspirin-sensitive patients react also to this dye with asthma, urticaria, rhinitis, and hyperactivity. In one study of 76 children diagnosed as hyperactive, the food color tartrazine combined with the food preservative benzoate caused abnormal reactions in 79 percent of the group. Tartrazine increased loss of zinc by increasing excretion in urine and decreased the amount in the blood and saliva with a corresponding deterioration in behavior.

Other dyes cause similar toxic reactions, including curcumin (mainly in confectionery and margarine), sunset yellow (used in biscuits), carmoisine (in jams and preserves), amaranth, poncea 4R (found in dessert mixes), erythrosine (in candied cherries and sweets), and caramels (found in cola drinks, beer, in crisps, bread, and sauces). Caramels contain the impurity 4-methylimidazole which is toxic. Preservatives and antioxidants include benzoates, sulphites, nitrates and nitrites, butylated hydroxyanisole (BHA), monosodium glutamate (MSG), saccharin, and aspartate. Aspartate contains phenyl alanine. In rats it doubles the level of phenyl alanine, increases tyrosine in the brain and reduces tryptophan. Reducing tryptophan will decrease the amount of NAD in the cells, decreases the amount of serotonin, and makes it more difficult for the pineal gland to make enough melatonin.

The adverse reactions to these substances may be allergic or toxic. For every individual more than one substance will create these reactions with a synergistic effect. Dr Egger found that of 76 children 79 percent reacted to artificial colors and preservatives. But for these children, 48 different foods were found to cause symptoms. Thus 64 percent reacted to cow's milk; 49 percent to wheat; 32 percent to peanuts; and 16 percent to sugar. On elimination diets, the children's behavior improved with the removal or reduction of many symptoms. In subsequent studies he obtained similar results.

Glutamate

Glutamate is a neurotoxin that can destroy central neurons but it is still one of the most widely used food additives. Other compounds with glutamate type toxic activity are aspartame, l-cysteine, and other related sulfur-containing amino acids. Protein hydrolysate contain large amounts of glutamate, aspartate, and sulfur amino acids. These are called excitotoxins. Young animals are particularly sensitive: a single feeding of glutamate to a young animal will destroy neurons. Glutamate is present in commercial soups which may contain up to 1,300 mg of free glutamate per 6 oz cup. A twenty pound baby eating one cup would get 130 mg per kg of body weight. The toxic dose for immature mice is 250-500 mg per kg. This is too small a margin of safety. But humans are 5 times more sensitive than mice and 20 times more sensitive than monkeys to brain damage from glutamate. Aspartame is equally toxic in destroying brain neurones. These excitoxins are being examined for their possible role in causing degenerative brain diseases like Alzheimer's and Huntington disease.

Toxic Metals

Another large group of food additives are the toxic metals lead, aluminum, arsenic, copper, nickel, tin, mercury, cadmium, and aluminum, among others. Every disturbed child will need to be examined for the presence of heavy metal toxicity. These metals may also enter the body by inhalation. Lead is the most widely distributed and researched toxic element. Lead was poured into the atmosphere by the ton by motor cars burning gasoline enriched with lead additives. Lead levels in the atmosphere are now 200 times greater than they were 3,000 years ago The amount of lead in the oceans has increased more than ten times. And the average person in North America has 100 times as much lead in his body. In spite of overwhelming evidence of its toxic properties, the industry most firmly wedded to its use resisted to the end any recognition that it was poisonous and only government legislation forced it out of the gasoline. Lead was also used as a binding ingredient in paint until its toxic properties were discovered. Lead intoxication produces children with learning and behavioral disorders.

In a her book *Turning Lead into Gold*, Nancy Hallaway of Vancouver describes how her twin boys began to recover from one of the most serious of children's diseases, infantile autism, when it was recognized by Dr Z. Strauts that they suffered a heavy lead burden and treatment was started to remove the lead. During my career of seeing over 1,500 children since

1960, I cannot recall children who were as sick as these boys were. They were given ritalin and anafranil, which helped a little. The boys were examined and re-examined and the diagnosis given back was what the parents already knew, they were sick and uncontrollable. With prodigious effort and the aid of some workers, the boys made a little progress in developing some human characteristics. But it was only after Dr Strauts tested them for lead burden and began to remove that burden by the use of chelation therapy (penicillamine) and by the addition of essential minerals that the boys began to recover. They are not yet well but they are improving and heading toward recovery. Zinc may be a useful way of reducing the toxic properties of lead. Zinc blocks the absorption of toxic minerals including lead and inhibits the effect of lead on some enzymes in the body.

I am not surprised this occurred in Vancouver. Some years ago I pointed out that in some places in Vancouver the amount of lead in the surface soil is so great that people growing their own vegetables would be poisoned by it if they did not wash off the soil particles very carefully and thoroughly. There is more lead in the surface soil of some places in Vancouver than there is downstream from the lead smelters in Trail, British Columbia.

There is less lead about since it has been removed from the gasoline but plenty is left. It is found in some tinned goods from the lead solder, in houses with old lead based paint and lead galvanized plumbing, in some dishes, and some old toys. Since lead particles are heavy, they tended to occur within three feet of the surface of the soil so that children playing in this atmosphere would be getting a heavy load of lead while adults walking in the same atmosphere would have their heads above it.

The diagnosis is relatively simple. Thinking about it as a possibility is most difficult for most psychiatrists who are not educated in the importance of biochemical factors in causing psychiatric disorder. Hair analysis for lead is important, blood analysis less important, but a special test may be needed to demonstrate the burden of the heavy metal using a chelating compound such as penicillamine to increase the excretion. In a recent letter to the *Canadian Medical Association Journal*, W.O. Robertson refers to the possibility that both zinc and iron can protect against the toxic effects of lead. Zinc may decrease the absorption of lead and iron limit the damage to the brain. He suggests that iron deficiency may be a main factor in toddlers damaged by lead.

There is no safe dose – that is, there is no level below which lead and other toxic metals are safe and above which they are toxic. The safest levels are zero; any level above that increases the toxic effects on the body. The higher the levels the more toxic they are. As Dr M. Marlowe notes, "a metal that produces subtle cognitive alterations in many children may produce a learning disability or mental retardation in those who are especially susceptible because of genetic, perinatal, or other factors e.g. malnutrition. Under-nutrition can influence susceptibility to metal toxicity. Deficiencies in calcium, iron, zinc, and phosphorus are all known to increase susceptibility, and the large majority of studies reviewed here have not examined nutritional correlates. It may be that the ratios of nutrient minerals to metals may be more important than the absolute values of the metals."

In a recent report Dr Marlowe and Dr Palmer compared the concentration of minerals in the hair of a series of disadvantaged children against a smaller control group. The first group were higher in trace toxic metals in their hair and lower in the nutritive minerals. Manganese was found, among others, to be elevated in the nutritionally poorer group. Trace elements were examined in 104 violent male criminals and compared to 83 normal controls. The violent group had more manganese in their hair. The author concluded that increased manganese levels combined with alcohol, poor diet, and psychosocial factors all combined to predispose these men to violent behavior.

Manganese may be a major cause of decreased intelligence and increased behavioral disorders. In small quantities, manganese is essential, but in large amounts will be toxic. The Violence Research Foundation in Tustin, California, funded by E.L. Red Hodges, stimulated further investigation of this relationship. Based on three independent studies carried on over three years, this research group reports that manganese levels were elevated in violent subjects. L.A. Gottschalk and colleagues reported that prisoners compared to controls had higher levels of manganese in their hair. Using a value of 0.7 ppm, 62 percent of the prisoners had above these levels while only 10.3 percent of controls were in this range. Sixty percent of the aberrant/violent criminals had four times the levels of manganese. In only 11 percent were similar hair levels found in non-violent subjects. Gottschalk's two hundred subjects had not been associated with mining and processing of manganese ores. California has one of the lowest ambient manganese levels in the Unites States, which is surprising since there is a positive association between criminal behavior and ambient manganese levels by states. In 200 counties the rate of violent crime was 200 per 100,000 with no manganese toxicity in the air, while in 13 counties with high levels of manganese discharge violent crime was six times as high.

Professor F.M. Crinella suggested in a letter to the National Nutritional Foods Association that elevated levels of manganese can develop not only from high ambient levels but also when the diet is inadequate, thus depriving the subjects of trace elements which neutralize the effect of excessive manganese. These diets are deficient in calcium, zinc, and essential nutrients. Areas with the highest ambient manganese levels combined with deficiencies of calcium had the highest rates of violent crime. Nutritional sources of manganese will contribute to the manganese burden. Human milk is comparatively low in manganese, containing about 10 micrograms per quart. But cow milk contains three times as much and soy based formulae contains up to 100 times as much. As Hodges concludes on the basis of these studies, "The Violence Research Foundation believes that manganese is not only a marker for violence as reported by Gottschalk, but is directly implicated in the destruction of serotonin, the master impulse controller in the brain. Manganese serves as a building block for monamine oxidase-A which is the key enzyme in the synthesis of serotonin, considered to be the brain's main inhibitory neurotransmitter. There have been dozens of studies which have shown that serotonin functioning is abnormal in persons with propensities for violence. Further, the scientific literature reports that newborn infants immediately exposed to cows' milk or soy based baby formula have a significant chance of neuronal damage. In addition, adults exposed to high levels of ambient manganese, especially with a low nutritional status, have a propensity for aberrant/violent behavior."

Since February 1996 the oil refiners and the company that makes a manganese-containing additive called methylcyclo-pentadienyl manganese tricarbonyl (MMT) have been trying to gain government permission to add this manganese-based element to gasoline because it is a a low cost octane booster. If MMT is allowed to be added to gasoline, we will once more face the problem of slowly gathering much more data to prove to the satisfaction of the industrial skeptics that the manganese in the atmosphere damages the health of children. As Dr H.L. Needleman and

Dr P. Landrigan conclude, "a child's brain differs in many ways from an adult's, and their daily lives differ also. As a result children are more vulnerable to most neurotoxins. Children live and play close to the area where automobile exhaust settles. The nerve cells in young brains are continually changing during the developmental process, laying down some connections and pruning back others, while cells continue to migrate to their final destinations. During these critical dynamic events, any noxious influence is likely to produce long-term effects. These effects may announce themselves years later as difficulties in learning, language expression, or in behavioral and attentional disturbances. Once again lead had provided a trustworthy model for this phenomenon; early lead exposure produces permanent deficits that appear to worsen over time. Childhood lead poisoning was first described in the 19th century. After tetraethyl lead was inserted into gasoline, raising blood levels all over the world, it required over half a century to get it out. Surely we can learn something from this costly experience. Surely, this time, before we permit the introduction of a new neurotoxin into our children's lives, we have the right to demand proof that it is unquestionably without harm to them. Our engines can certain tolerate the lack of manganese, but our children's brains may not tolerate the presence of it."

I have not discussed fluoride as a possible toxic factor in impairing learning and normal behavior. Most of the controversy about fluoride in our drinking water has centered about its toxic effects on the body, but a recent report raises the question about the effect of fluoride on the development of the brain. Different amounts of fluoride were fed to pregnant rats, weaning rats, and 3-month-old adult rats. Fluoride exposure caused sex and dose specific behavioral deficits with a common pattern. Prenatal exposure produced hyperactivity, while after birth exposure caused cognitive defects. The severity of the effect was directly related to plasma levels and to accumulation in the brain. Plasma levels which caused these changes are seen in humans ingesting 5-10 ppm fluoride in drinking water and during fluoride therapy for osteoporosis. Higher levels are found in plasma of children one hour after receiving topical applications of acidulated phosphate fluoride 1.23 percent gel. The authors of this study concluded that "because humans occasionally are exposed to high amounts of fluoride and plasma levels as high as those found in this rat study, neuro-toxic risks deserve further evaluation. This is the first laboratory study to demonstrate that CNS functional output is vulnerable to fluoride, that the effects of behavior depend on the age at exposure, and that fluoride accumulates in brain tissues."

Public Health Officers can no longer avoid carrying out their major responsibility of protecting us all against the heavy metal contamination which is present within our environment. It is probably more deadly than many infectious diseases because they are invisible whereas infections are easily spotted. I urge all parents and all personnel involved in child care to read this book and to absorb its message. It is criminal to allow our children to be poisoned by these heavy metals when the solution is so simple: suspect, test, diagnose and treat this problem – and ensure we do not keep adding to the burden of young people who will not become normal because they are being poisoned by these heavy metals.

Non-Toxic Additives and Supplements

Of course some additives are very beneficial, even essential. Nutrients, when added to food in appropriate amounts, are additives but they are non-toxic. On the contrary, they improve the health of the individual eating this enriched food. Nutrient additives have been used for many years, ranging from iodine in table salt to prevent goiter, through vitamin B-3 (niacin), vitamin B-2 (riboflavin), and vitamin B-1 (thiamine) in flour to prevent pellagra, and vitamin C in juices to prevent scurvy. Everyone recognizes these are good things to do. Nutrients used in tablet or other form but not added to food are not to be considered as undesirable additives. They are the essence of orthomolecular therapy which I have been describing in this book. Ever since I began to use these supplements in 1951, it has been clear to me that the use of these supplements improves every aspect of human functioning, ranging from improving perceptual stability and intellectual performance to improving mood and therefore making behavior better.

Behavioral, Perception, Biomedical, and Intelligence Tests

All the areas of the child's mental state – perception, thinking, mood, and behavior – need to be assessed or tested not so much because a diagnostic conclusion is needed for the purposes of treatment as because the diagnosis report becomes the base line by which one can judge improvement after treatment has started. Diagnostic tests are always helpful because they increase the accuracy and speed in making the diagnosis, but they are always secondary to the clinical diagnosis made by a skillful and experienced clinician. I use several diagnostic aids: a behavioral or hyperactivity rating scale; perceptual tests, the "HOD" test for older children and the "PD" test for younger children; and biomedical tests of the child's urine for kryptopyrole and a text for NAD deficiency. Labora-tory tests are becoming available for almost all the allergies and nutrients. They may be needed for some of the children. For diagnosing mineral deficiency and toxicity, in addition to blood and urine levels, one can use hair analyses. The latter is especially valuable in ruling out toxic minerals.

Hyperactivity Scale

In 1970 when hyperactivity had emerged as common childhood illness, Dr Mark A. Stewart developed a diagnostic test by comparing a series of 37 hyperactive children (32 were boys) with normal boys. From a large list of behavioral adjectives and phrases used to describe these children, Stewart found that 27 such symptoms appeared much more frequently in hyperactivity. These are shown in the following table, which I have adapted to prepare a rating scale. I have used this scale for the past 25 years and have given it to over 1,500 children. The test is done by marking the appropriate score after questioning parents, teachers, or any close adult who knows the child. The maximum score is 135 and the minimum is 27.

Behavioral Rating Scale for Children
Normal vs Hyperactive Children

Adjective (Symptom)	Occurrence		Score		
	Normal	Hyper	Marked	Moderate	Absent
1. Overactive	33%	100%	5	3	1
2. Doesn't finish projects	0	84	5	3	1
3. Fidgets	30	84	5	3	1
4. Can't sit still at meals	8	81	5	3	1
5. Doesn't stay with games	3	78	5	3	1
6. Wears out toys, furniture	8	68	5	3	1
7. Talks too much	20	68	5	3	1
8. Doesn't follow directions	3	62	5	3	1
9. Clumsy	8	62	5	3	1
10. Fights with other children	3	59	5	3	1
11. Unpredictable	3	59	5	3	1
12. Teases	22	59	5	3	1
13. Doesn't respond to discipline	0	57	5	3	1
14. Gets into things	11	54	5	3	1
15. Speech problem	25	54	5	3	1
16. Temper tantrums	0	55	5	3	1
17. Doesn't listen to whole story	0	49	5	3	1
18. Defiant	0	49	5	3	1
19. Hard to get to bed	3	59	5	3	1
20. Irritable	3	49	5	3	1
21. Reckless	3	49	5	3	1
22. Unpopular with peers	0	46	5	3	1
23. Impatient	8	46	5	3	1
24. Lies	3	43	5	3	1
25. Accident prone	11	43	5	3	1
26. Enuretic	28	43	5	3	1
27. Destructive	0	41	5	3	1

These questions may be answered by parents at home or in the office, though I usually ask these questions in the presence of the child. In most cases, the child is in agreement with the way their parents answer the questions. In 1972 Dr Max Vogel found a high correlation between scores when the test was administered by teachers and by parents independently of each other. This is not surprising since they are examining the same child but shows that school behavior closely mirrors home behavior. But there are many children whose behavior at home is much more active than it is in school. This happens very often with children on ritalin. The effect begins to wear off late in the afternoon and the parents then bear the full brunt of their hyperactivity.

Many years ago I examined the scores of 200 children whose files were then current. Each child had been referred, previously diagnosed with either learning or behavioral disorders, usually some of both. The scores by age are given below.

Male and Female Hyperactivity Scores by Age

Age	Male		Female	
	Number	Score	Number	Score
0 to 3	2	91	6	83
4 to 6	17	59	7	73
7 to 9	59	78	14	74
10 to 13	51	78	13	83
14 to 16	25	78	5	72

In this series, the mean scores were independent of age, and the parents' judgment of their children's behavior was also independent of the age of their children. Since then the range of scores has remained the same. The maximum score is 135 and the minimum is 27. Normal children score 45 or less and the average hyperactive child scores about 75. The same test may be given to the parents to complete at home and may also be completed by teachers. The teachers' and parents' scores, even if done independently, are very similar. As they get better the scores decrease until they reach the normal range. The rate of decrease in scores will indicate approximately how long it will be before the children recover. However, a few of the children on ritalin who appeared to be better still scored very high with this test.

The hyperactivity scale has proven to be very useful in determining the degree of pathology and in determining the rate of improvement. The test is thus a useful screening device, takes only a few minutes, and is readily accepted by the parents. I have given the hyperactivity scores for every child described in this book when it has been available.

Hoffer-Osmond Diagnostic (HOD) Test

Dr Humphrey Osmond and I developed the Hoffer-Osmond Diagnostic (HOD) test in 1960 for assisting in the diagnosis of schizophrenia, but the test has proven effective in diagnosing the mental health of children over the age of 10, though not all children will understand the meaning of some of the key words in the test.

Our research with schizophrenia beginning in 1952 convinced us that we had to know what our patients were experiencing in order to diagnose correctly and to understand how best to deal with them clinically. We could get this information by spending a lot of time with patients in order to question every possible perceptual change, but this would be very time-consuming and would tire them. It occurred to us that we could get at this information much more accurately and quickly by developing a set of questions to which patients could reply with a simple yes or no. General practitioners who have diagnosed schizophrenia very early on using the HOD test as an aid to diagnosis have been astonished with the rapid responses they have seen in their patients. Before these patients had been tested they were very difficult, with a lot of anxiety and depression and other vague complaints. They had not responded to the usual anti-anxiety or antidepressant medication.

The questions were placed on cards, one question per card, and each card was numbered, beginning with 1. Patients were given these cards in random order and asked to sort them into True or False categories. Only statements which they were certain were True were accepted; the rest were considered False. All the cards said to be True were recorded on special scoring sheets.

From these True responses we prepared 145 questions. They covered all perceptual areas such as visual, auditory, tactile, taste, smell, and time. There were also questions which dealt with thinking and mood. Questions were phrased so that normal people would place most in the False category, whereas schizophrenics would place many in the True category. We then gave the test to hundreds of subjects: to schizophrenics -— acute and chronic, sick, better, or well; to non-schizophrenics such as anxiety states, depressions, and personality disorders; to seniles, subjects after LSD, patients under physical stress, and to healthy people. We then compared the way each question was treated by groups; that is, if a question was said to be True by a large proportion of schizophrenics and only very few normals, we assigned that card a special score. We scored each patient by giving each card one point if placed in the True box, and 5 points if it was a special question. We were not surprised to find that schizophrenics scored very high and normal subjects very low. We also found that one-quarter of the non-schizophrenic patients also had high scores as if they had schizophrenia; that is, they had a large number of perceptual changes as do schizophrenics.

The HOD Test is comprised of 145 True/False questions that range from simple questions like "Most people hate me" through more complex questions like "A chair is like a table because they are usually together rather than because they both have legs" to questions like "Water now has many funny tastes." Here is a random list of other questions:

47. Some foods which never tasted funny before do now.
66. My mind is racing away with me.
81. People are watching me.
35. I have often felt that there was another voice in my head.
127. The world has become timeless for me.
17. Now and then when I look in the mirror my face changes and seems different.
90. An orange is like a banana because they both have skins rather than because they are fruit.
124. My bones often feel soft.
136. People interfere with my mind to harm me.

129. Other people smell strange.

26. I often see sparks or spots of light floating before me.

142. More people admire me now than ever before.

87. A dress is like a glove because they are articles of clothing rather than because they are worn by women.

145. I am not sure who I am.

The numbers of the cards placed in the true box are recorded on special answering sheets and scored very quickly using templates. It is not a psychological test and does not require any special skill in marking or scoring. The HOD Test is now available as a computer program and on the world wide web (www.softtac@islandnet.com).

Here is an example of the efficacy of the HOD test. This young patient became schizophrenic in the mid-1950s. He was treated at University Hospital, Saskatoon, with placebo, as part of our second double-blind controlled experiment. He did not respond. His treatment code was broken and he was started on niacin, 3 grams daily, plus a brief series of electroconvulsive treatments. He recovered. Later he completed his degree and, following that, enrolled in a medical college. As I was supplying him with the vitamin from our research supply, I kept in contact with him. I advised him to stay on the niacin for five years, after which he discontinued it. About five years later, while at medical college, he again came to see me, to tell me he was not feeling well. I had him do the Hoffer-Osmond Diagnostic (HOD) Test which showed very high perceptual scores, indicating that he was suffering from many perceptual illusions. I recommended he resume his niacin. He was so desperate to get well quickly, he took 6 grams per day instead of 3, and one week later he was well again. His HOD scores returned to normal. He has remained well since that time and is practicing medicine. Had I waited for him to again suffer hallucinations, it would have required much more intense treatment, probably in hospital, and he would have lost that year of medical school.

As part of the standardization of the HOD test Margaret Callbeck, Chief Research Nurse, and I carried on a five-year study of the relationship between HOD scores and achievement in the high-school system in Saskatoon. We administered the test to students ranging from Grade 8 to

Grade 12. We also tested students past Grade 12 in teachers' college and a smaller number in the slow learners' classes who were receiving a technical education. Al-together about 2,000 students were tested.

The scores for younger subjects were much higher than were adult scores and the decrease with age was linear. We thought at first that younger children, even if normal, were more apt to show perceptual problems because they had not yet reached the adult stable relationship between the senses and their interpretation by the brain. But later we found that children with higher scores did not do as well in school as their same age peers with lower scores. Students, age 14 for example, who had high scores performed less well in school and were one to two years behind compared to other students the same age with low scores. This was such a consistent finding that even students considered normal with high scores were handicapped in our educational system. As they matured their scores decreased until they reached low adult levels. Some children had already reached adult levels in their early teens, many only in their late teens. Students who scored low were one to two years a ahead of their peers in school. Some of the students who scored high were later referred to me by their physicians and were clearly schizophrenic by then. Treatment with vitamin B-3 invariably brought the scores down very quickly and helped the patients get well.

This does not mean that all high scorers were schizophrenic. The vast majority were not. It suggests that they need improvement in their diet with supplementation with vitamin B-3. I am convinced that the first indicators of vitamin B deficiency are perceptual disturbances. These perceptual tests can be used to select that part of the population most apt to need supplementation. Since coming to this conclusion I use the same normal scores for all subjects irrespective of age. Normal scores are 30 or less. Schizo-phrenic scores are around 65. The higher the score the greater the probability that they have schizophrenia.

We found a linear relationship between HOD scores and performance in school. Within any grade the students with the higher scores were one or more years older compared to the average for the grade – that is, these students were behind one or more years. When students of the same age were compared, we found that students with the higher scores were in the lower grades. The students in the special class scored highest of all for their age. Several students in the special class scored highest of all. Others from this class were referred for treatment. When they were placed on megavitamin therapy their scores went down. It was clear that students with perceptual changes of a severe nature were not able to function as well in the schools as were children with minor degrees of perceptual disturbances.

In a second phase of the study, a couple of hundred students from Grade 9 in six schools were selected at random. They were asked to volunteer to be tested with the HOD during each grade in the following four years. Very few refused to cooperate. By the fourth year we had lost 25 percent of the original group. The results were very similar to those found in the first phase. We concluded that HOD test results indicated an illness was present characterized by increased perceptual instability and decreased ability to learn and to remember.

For many years, I had considered that the age factor was simply due to the perceptual instability of younger children. The original study on 2,000 students had shown that average scores decreased from age 10 to age 18 when they reached adult levels, and remained low unless they became sick. Then they would increase again. I still consider it evidence of perceptual instability, but that this is due to a pathological problem which will handicap the child unless they are treated. All children with perceptual problems have a degree of cerebral dysfunction, and a search must be made to find out if this is due to a vitamin deficiency, a vitamin dependency, to other forms of malnutrition, to cerebral allergy or to other biochemical factors.

If every student with high HOD test scores were treated with vitamins and diet, there would be a substantial and significant improvement in their mental state and in educational achievement. Lloyd J. Njaa in 1975 studied 875 students in a large urban high school in Edmonton, Alberta. In this sample he did not find the same general age relationship but he did find a negative association between HOD scores and I.Q. scores. The HOD scores of underachievers and students seeking counseling were significantly higher than the HOD scores of other students. The HOD scores also differentiated students with a high rate of absenteeism from students with a low rate. He found that the mean HOD scores in his sample from 1970 were significantly higher than the mean scores for the Saskatoon sample in our 1962-1963 study. He suggested this might be due to the increased deterioration of our national diet over the decade. He concluded, "It can be stated the HOD is a valid instrument when used on an adolescent sample. It would appear therefore that the HOD and the accompanying orthomolecular therapy should be used on high school students at least on an experimental basis. The degree of perceptual and mood changes indicated by the students HOD scores do require close investigation and experimentation. The HOD test can be used to determine if vitamin deficiencies are present and the improvement in scores will indicate when adequate quantities of these supplements are being provided. Hopefully, in the near future, as is already being done to a certain extent, orthomolecular therapy can be used to bring 'help' to thousands of adolescents in our society – not only those diagnosed as having severe mental problems, but also those who have problems but seem to be coping in their present circumstances."

The HOD test is thus used to assist in diagnosis, to follow progress in treatment as the scores go down with improvement, to judge the possibility of relapse, and to encourage patients who can see how they are improving as they see the scores do down. Patients are not bored by this test because it only takes a few minutes.

The Perceptual Dysfunction (PD) Test

Because of the nature of the questions, the HOD test cannot be used effectively for children under age 10; however, Dr Glen Green has adapted the HOD test into a series of questions specifically aimed at eliciting perceptual changes in younger children. The child does not read anything but is asked the questions.

As Dr Green explains, "a long history is time-consuming and may be rambling. When questioning for physical and psychic complaints, we must follow a pattern or many things will be forgotten. Children who have dysfunctions and disorders caused by subclinical pellagra require extra time for two reasons: more questions have to be asked and more information must be recorded. Because of these prerequisites, it was necessary to develop a questionnaire which the patient could answer at his convenience and which could be filed with his chart.

"The perceptual dysfunction (PD) test consists of 100 questions which elicit physical and psychic complaints, and which are merely checked off by the patient. The parent may help. The questions are designed to make it easy for the patient to express himself and to admit to symptoms which he has without fear of being laughed at or scolded. Patients find it easier to tick off an answer than they do to vocalize their complaints, which bring the patient to the office in the first instance. Paranoia, depression, and thinking abilities are not covered by this test; the HOD test is admirable for that purpose.

"The test is a convenient and inexpensive method for eliciting complaints and recording them. It has been copyrighted as it appears. The questions are grouped loosely to cover the special senses and somatic complaints. Proprioceptive problems are even more loosely grouped. The reason behind the seemingly random questions is so the patient will not recognize a pattern, then try to figure out what answer he is supposed to give. There are three columns for answers: sometimes, yes, and no. 'Sometimes' and 'yes' have almost equal weight. The patient will often say 'no', unless the symptoms are present all the time.

1. When you read do the words seem to blur or go fuzzy?
2. When you read do your eyes seem to get blurred?
3. When you read do your eyes get sore or tired rather quickly?
4. When you read do you get a headache?
5. Do the words move a little bit when you read sometimes?
6. Do the words go double when you read?
7. When you read do the words seem to come closer thenfurther away?
8. When you read do the words seem to get bigger or smaller?
9. Do the letters get mixed up when you read?
10. Do the words seem backwards when you read?
11. Do the numbers move a little bit when you are looking at them?
12. Does your mind go blank when you read?
13. Do the lines move together or get mixed up when you read?
14. Do the words seem to disappear when you read?
15. Do you often forget what you have just read?
16. Do you have to re-read a sentence several times?
17. Do you get a pain in or behind your eyes when you read?

18. Do you sometimes think you can see animals when there are none there?

19. Do you sometimes think you see people when there are none there?

20. Do you watch television now?

21. Does the television picture look different now?

22. Does the television picture seem to move in a strange way?

23. Does watching television make your eyes sore?

24. Do you see things on television that your friends don't see on the same program?

25. Do you get a headache when you watch television?

26. Does there seem to be a fog between you and the television set?

27. Do you think you hear someone calling your name when there is no one there?

28. Do you think you hear voices when there is no one there?

29. Do you think you hear animals or noises when there are none there?

30. Do you think you hear voices talking or yelling when there is no one there?

31. Do you seem to have trouble with your hearing now?

32. Do you hear your own voice inside your head when you are thinking?

33. Do you hear your own voice outside your head when you are thinking?

34. Do some things seem to feel different now, than before, when you touch them?

35. When you pet a dog does he feel like a dog should feel?

36. When you write does the pencil feel other than normal?

37. Do you think you feel someone touching you when there is no one there?

38. Can you tell where your hands are when your eyes are closed?

39. Can you tell where your feet are when your eyes are closed?

40. Do you seem to feel that you get bigger when you walk?

41. Do you seem to feel that you get smaller when you walk?

42. Do you feel that your feet seem to get big when you walk?

43. Does it seem that you are walking off the ground sometimes?
44. When you are walking on level ground, do you feel as though you are going up hill or down at times?
45. When you walk does the ground seem to go up and down?
46. When you walk does the ground seem to move ahead of you?
47. When you walk does the ground seem to go sideways?
48. Do you get dizzy when you walk?
49. Do you feel that the stairs seem to get higher or lowerwhen you climb them?
50. Do trees or buildings seem as though they move or lean over?
51. Do you feel that your sense of taste has changed lately?
52. Have you noticed that your food has no taste?
53. Have you noticed that your food seems to taste rotten or too sweet?
54. Have you noticed that you can't smell your food?
55. Do some foods smell different than they used to?
56. Do some foods smell rotten?
57. Do you often get a sore throat?
58. Do you bite your fingernails?
59. Do you often get a headache?
60. Do you often have painful joints?
61. Do you often get pains in your stomach or your chest?
62. Do you often suffer from cramps?
63. Do you often get an earache?
64. Do you sometimes wet the bed?
65. Do you often feel more tired than you think you should?
66. Do you often lie down after school or work?
67. Do you often feel so tired you quit your play or work to lie down?
68. Do your bones feel soft or rubbery at times?
69. Does your school work seem to tire you more than it used to?
70. Does your school work seem harder than it used to?
71. Do you find it harder to learn now?
72. Do you have trouble breathing quite often now?
73. Do you feel like throwing up?

74. Do people seem to have a light around them at times?
75. Can you see all of your face when you look in a mirror?
76. Does it seem sometimes that your face gets bigger or smaller when you look in a mirror?
77. Does there seem to be a fog in front of the mirror so it's blurred or hard to see yourself?
78. Does your face seem to get wavy when you look in a mirror?
79. Do you get scared or feel nervous most of the time?
80. Do you feel afraid to go to school or work sometimes?
81. Do you often wake up at night for no good reason?
82. Do you find it difficult to go to sleep?
83. Do pictures seem to move a little bit, at times, when you look at them?
84. Does a chair seem to move at times or change shape?
85. Do people in pictures seem to breathe or to watch you?
86. Do you feel afraid to look at yourself in the mirror?
87. Do people frighten you when they look at you?
88. Do objects seem to change shape at times?
89. Do you feel sad most of the time?
90. Do you feel that people watch you more than they used to?
91. Do people seem strange or different when you look at them?
92. Do objects seem strange or different when you look at them?
93. Do letters seem to change shape?
94. Do numbers seem to change shape?
95. Do numbers seem to change direction?
96. Do numbers seem to change around?
97. Do pictures or objects seem to change color at times?
98. Do you have to look to see where your arms or legs are?
99. Do you have to pinch part of your body to know it is there?
100. Does your skin feel like fur or plastic, etc. at times?

"This test is useful in my hands as a rough screening for a multiplicity of symptoms. If one is interested in the clinical situation of the patient and how the medication affects a patient, this test also gives a good idea of what is happening," Dr Green adds.

Hypoglycemia Questionnaire

Dr Green has also developed a hypoglycemia questionnaire, based on the work of Dr John Bumpus. As Dr Green explains, "here again a high score indicates not only a sweet tooth but the cerebral signs of allergy – fatigue, irritability, anxiety, depression, and others. This test can also be used as an index of progress in treatment. The patient's score goes lower as he improves. The usefulness of this index varies directly with the comprehension of the questions. Many seemingly literate persons have difficulty interpreting the questions, especially as to the degree. It is not uncommon for a patient to deny liking sweets. What they really mean is they have their sweet tooth under control. A score higher than 60 should prompt the doctor to check the answers with the patient to make sure everything is understood. It is not uncommon when a mother answers for a hyperactive child to attain scores over 115. It is not uncommon to see this total drop by 50 points just by eliminating sweets, bread, cake, and other highly refined carbohydrate foods."

Instructions: To show degree of severity, use figures (1) Mild, (2) Moderate, and (3) Severe. Use (0) if the answer does not apply.

1. Do you now have a craving for sweets?
2. Did you used to have a craving for sweets?
3. Do you take candy, chocolate bars, coffee, teas or pop for quick energy?
4. Do you think you feel better if you eat candy or cookies between meals?
5. Do you drink alcoholic beverages?
6. Were you ever a heavy drinker?
7. Do you drink tea or coffee?
8. Do you eat when you are nervous or upset?
9. Are you a compulsive eater?
10. Do you eat before you go to bed?
11. Do you feel tired all the time?
12. Do you need eight hours of sleep or more to feel right?
13. Do you wake up feeling tired?

14. Do you have trouble getting to sleep?
15. Do you feel dizzy if you get up too fast?
16. Do you feel sleepy after you eat?
17. Do you feel weak, shaky, sick, or tired if you are late for a meal?
18. Do you get a headache if you don't eat?
19. Do you get ravenously hungry if you do not eat?
20. Do you get sweaty if you go too long without eating?
21. Do you sigh or yawn a lot?
22. Do you have shortness of breath or feel as if you are smothering?
23. Do you tire easily for no obvious reason?
24. Do you have any allergies – eczema, hay fever, asthma, etc.?
25. Do words blur when you read?
26. Do words seem to move a little bit sometimes when you read?
27. Do you get chest, stomach or low abdominal pains?
28. Does your heart pound, or go fast, or skip beats?
29. If you get light-headed and trembly, does sugar make you better?
30. Does your stomach make a lot of noise?
31. Do you have to force yourself to work?
32. Do you have bad dreams?
33. Do you feel frightened or tearful for little or no reason?
34. Do you feel cranky, irritable, sad, or miserable for no good reason?
35. Do you get upset or worried about little things?
36. Do you cry easily – often over silly things?
37. Are you hard to get along with?
38. Do you have 'bad nerves'?
39. Do you have to read something several times before you understand?
40. Do you get confused easily?
41. Do you have trouble making up your mind?
42. Do you lack interest and ambition to do things?
43. Are you more forgetful now?
44. Do you have trouble concentrating now?
45. Do you prefer to be alone?
46. Do you sometimes think of suicide?
47. Do you feel anxious and/or depressed?

Kryptopyrroluria (KP) Test

During our research with schizophrenia, it occurred to me that we could discover the biochemical problem in schizophrenia by using the LSD experience as a model. In 1951 when we first began to use LSD there were very few people in the world who knew anything about it. LSD is widely used today as a street hallucinogen, of course, and millions of people have experienced what it can do in distorting perception, thinking, and mood. The restrictive legislation introduced in panic by the governments of the United States and Canada in the early 1960s completely eliminated valuable research with this substance and made it much more appealing to the street.

In 1960 it occurred to me that in the same way that LSD produced a psychological model of schizophrenia it might induce a chemical model – that is, it might induce biochemical changes in the body of non-schizophrenic subjects which were similar to what was present in the schizophrenic body. If true, this would give us a lead into searching schizophrenia for abnormal substances.

Our biochemical team had been working with paper chromatographic studies of urine to try and identify any difference between schizophrenia and normal controls. I decided that we should examine the urine of subjects before and after they had taken LSD. Since we were routinely treating large numbers of alcoholics with psychedelic therapy, it was simple to arrange for this. The first patient we studied excreted a compound in his urine at the height of the LSD experience at noon which was not present in his first morning specimen taken before 9:00 am. We found that the substance was not LSD itself and therefore was a chemical the body produced in response to the LSD. The next test was whether the same compound would be found in the urine of patients who had not been given LSD.

The paper chromatograph test is relatively simple in principle. A long piece of filter paper is dipped into the solution to be tested and stands there for several hours in a carefully controlled environment. The solvent moves up the filter paper by a wick action and as it does, sweeps with it the other molecules which are present in it. The smallest least adherent molecules move the fastest while the large molecules move more slowly. Thus at the end of the run the upper level of the wetted paper will contain only the solvent and trailing behind will be the other constituents. The paper is dried and developed – that is, sprayed with a chemical which brings out the compounds on the paper. The distance traveled by the compound is recorded as a ratio of the distance it has traveled over the distance traveled by the solvent. If the solvent travels 20 centimeters and the substance in it 16 cm, it is said to have an Rf of 0.80. The new chemical induced by the LSD stained a mauve color at Rf 0.80. We called it the mauve factor.

I then collected 12 samples of urine from schizophrenic patients, non-schizophrenic, and normal controls. They were numbered from 1 to 12 and taken to the laboratory for analysis. I was the only one who knew the code. At the end of the day we examined all 12 chromatograms. The differentiation between schizophrenic and other patients was perfect. The papers were read by the chemist doing the analysis who did not know the code. Every schizophrenic had the mauve factor at Rf 0.80 and none of the controls had it. The odds this was due to chance were so low that I was certain we were on to something.

We then expanded these studies to include thousands of subjects and we found that the highest correlation between the presence of this factor and disease was in schizophrenia. Normal controls, stress free, did not have the factor. In normal controls under a lot of stress it was present in 2 percent of the subjects. In subjects under severe physical stress due to physical disease, like cancer, it was present in 10 percent. In non-schizophrenic patients, including those suffering from depression and alcoholism, it was found in 25 percent and in acute schizophrenic patients it was found in about 75 percent. Patients who recovered no longer excreted this factor. We also found that patients who excreted mauve factor clinically resembled schizophrenic patients much more than they did non schizophrenic patients. They were similar to schizophrenics in having high HOD scores, in their response to megavitamin therapy, in clinical outcome after treatment. We concluded we could use this urine test as a diagnostic test for all patients who shared these properties whether or not they were diagnosed schizophrenic or anything else.

Once we examined the properties of the mauve spot, we discovered it was not LSD itself or a breakdown fraction of LSD. The substance was identified as kryptopyrrole (KP). Many years later, after we had examined urine from thousands of patients at our four research centers, we found KP was present in different psychiatric groups as follows:

Acute schizophrenics	75%
Chronic schizophrenics	50%
All non-psychotics	25%
Physically ill patients	5%
Normal subjects	0
Recovered schizophrenics	0

The following table shows the relationship between diagnoses and presence of urine factor:

Diagnoses	Number Tested	Positive Percent
1. Schizophrenics		
a) First episode	50	90
b) Second and more	300	75
c) Chronic-at home	300	50
d) Chronic-in hosp <20 yrs	300	40
e) Chronic- in hosp>20 yrs	25	10
f) Recovered	100	0
2. Alcoholics, neurotics, mood disorders	100	30
3. Down syndrome	100	60
4. Physically ill	300	10
5. Normal subjects (four were first order relatives of schizophrenics or had KP)	100	5
6. First order relatives of schizophrenics and KP excretors	100	35

We could now discover how many patients with schizophrenia excreted KP, but we had to show whether non-schizophrenics who did not resembled schizophrenics more than they did non-schizophrenics without KP. If they did, we could then assume that patients with KP were in fact schizophrenics. To study this, we compared large numbers of patients using clinical descriptions (diagnoses) and the HOD test. We concluded that patients who excreted KP (the mauve factor) were similar and called them "malvarians."

In a 1963 study we compared 75 patients without malvaria to 104 patients with malvaria. The malvarians were 104 consecutive patients tested routinely over a two-year period. The non-malvarians were tested the same way. The only differences between the groups before testing were the sex ratio and the number of people who were single. The malvarian group contained more males than females, while the other group had the reverse ratio. Malvarians were more often single, and the non-malvarians were most often married.

The urine test divided 179 patients into 2 groups. A higher proportion of the malvarian group suffered from perceptual symptoms, thought disorder, and inappropriate behavior. These symptoms occurred in only 5 percent of the non-malvarians. Only in the proportion suffering from depression were they the same. Psychiatrists would have no difficulty identifying which group most closely represented schizophrenia.

On the HOD scores the malvarians had mean scores identical to schizophrenic scores, and non-malvarian scores were identical to non-schizophrenic scores. It was obvious to us that malvarians were, in fact, undiagnosed schizophrenics. If all the malvarian non-schizophrenics had been examined for perceptual changes, and had their psychiatrists taken these changes as indicators, they would have been diagnosed schizophrenic. However, their psychiatrists had no interest in our research and never asked me to divulge to them what their patients' HOD scores were.

After the mauve factor was identified we dropped the term and used Dr Carl Pfeiffer's more appropriate word, kryptopyrroluria, or pyrroluria, for the same group. Dr Pfeiffer discovered that KP binds both zinc and vitamin B-6 and produces a double deficiency of these two nutrients. KP combines with pyridoxine and zinc to produce a double deficiency by carrying these nutrients out of the body into the urine. Later, while working with Dr Osmond at the Brain Bio Center in New Jersey, he established pyrroluria as a schizophrenic syndrome and developed a simple calori-metric test for diagnosing this syndrome. Some children with learning and behavioral disorders excrete this factor in their urine. I have found the KP test very useful in identifying children who need supplementation with these nutrients.

Measuring KP in Urine (2.4 Dimethyl-3-Ethyl Pyrrole)
Urine is collected in a container containing 1 tablet of vitamin C, 500 mg. This preserves the KP.

A 2 ml urine sample is placed in a glass stoppered centrifuge tube and extracted with 4 mg of chloroform by shaking either by hand or on a Vortex shaker for about 2 minutes. After centrifugation the top aqueous layer is carefully removed and 100 to 200 mgm of anhydrous sodium sulfate is added to the chloroform and shaken briefly to remove traces of aqueous globules.

2 ml of the clear chloroform extract are placed in a clean test tube and 0.5 ml of a 1 percent solution of p-dimethylamino benazal-dehyde (Ehrlich's reagent) in Methanol containing 5 Vol percent sulfuric acid are added and shaken briefly. After 30 minutes a deep pink color will develop if KP is present. The intensity of the color is read in a spectrophotometer at 540 mu. The normal range is 0 to 20 u percent — patients may read as high as 200 to 300 u percent.

A standard Kryptopyrrole solution containing 1 ug to 15 ug is prepared for establishing a standard curve.

Notes:

1. The Ehrlich's reagent is prepared once weekly and it is stored in a brown bottle.

2. Kryptopyrrole is a liquid obtained in an ampule from Aldrich Chemical Company, and is very sensitive to air. Once the ampule is broken a few drops of the Kryptopyrrole should be distributed in several ampules sealed under nitrogen and stored in the freezer. For preparation of the standard an

appropriate amount is weighed and dissolved in 1 percent aqueous ascorbic acid solution. This stock solution is stable for 72 hours if kept in the cold.

3.   For preservation of the KP, ascorbic acid should be added to the freshly obtained urine (approximately several hundred mgm).

4.   Porphobilinogen, which gives the same color reaction will not interfere, as its complex with the Ehrlich's reagent is chloroform insoluble.

Obviously the presence of KP is not a diagnostic test for schizophrenia or for any known diagnostic group. But it does select a group of people who are all homogeneous with respect to the presence of the abnormal chemical in their urine. This "new" disease is caused by the excess formation in the body of products which are excreted as KP. These products, including KP, bind pyridoxine and zinc, producing a double dependency. Clinically they resemble the majority of schizophrenics no matter what criterion one uses to make the comparisons. I think we should use this diagnostic term "kryptopyrroluria" or simply pyrroluria as developed by Dr Pfeiffer, but it will take decades to break the tradition of using the old clinical diagnosis, useful many years ago, no longer useful, even detrimental to the health of the patients who are said to have it. Children will be diagnosed on the basis of their chemistry and kryptopyrroluria will be one of the easily diagnosed conditions and just as easily treated.

Vitamin B-3 Deficiency (NAD) Test

I have already discussed the problems with our modern psychiatric classification of diseases or nosology. They are descriptive only and do not indicate what treatment should be used. And there is a wide disagreement between psychiatrists with respect to how they diagnose. The same patient seeing five different psychiatrists may come out with five different diagnoses. But they will all receive the same treatment, tranquilizers or antidepressants and one of the many psychotherapies which are being used. We need objective diagnostic tests which can be used to make the diagnosis, much as we have them for diabetes mellitus, syphilis, and so on. Only then will it become possible to sort out the patients into homogeneous groups who will receive similar treatment and will respond to specific treatment. The urine test for KP is such a factor for it finds patients who excrete too much of this factor and therefore have a deficiency of vitamin B-6 and zinc. The response to vitamin B-3 therapy is another because it sorts out patients who respond to this treatment. Since it is the NAD $\longrightarrow$ NADH system which fails, it seems appropriate to diagnose these patients NAD (which will stand for both forms) deficient. NAD deficiency is synonymous with subclinical pellagra and Vitamin B-3 deficiency.

The NAD/NADH deficiency is the result of four possible contributing nutrient deficiencies:

1)   Tryptophan deficiency due to low protein diets. This is one of the factors in causing pellagra.

2)   Excess leucine and deficiency in isoleucine. Isoleucine is deficient in corn and was one of the major factors producing pellagra.

3)   Deficiency of pyridoxine. This vitamin is needed for the conversion of tryptophan into NAD.

4)   Deficiency of essential fatty acids leading to a deficiency of prostaglandins. Dr D.O. Rudin has shown that the essential pathology in pellagra is a deficiency of prostaglandins. This can arise from a deficiency of essential fatty acids from which the prostaglandins are made or from a deficiency of nutrients needed for the conversion of the essential fatty acids to the prostaglandins. These include vitamin B-3, vitamin B-6, and others.

About 30 years ago I tested the idea that it should be possible to define a population of children who were vitamin B-3 responsive. I gave a large number of children vitamin B-3 in order to see what the children who responded had in common. I examined all seriously disturbed children referred to me. They were also evaluated by Dr B. O'Regan, a psychiatric colleague in practice in Saskatoon. These children were then given niacinamide or, rarely, niacin if there was no response to the niacinamide. The dose was increased from 500 mg tid to 2 G tid. They were also given ascorbic acid 1 G tid and, rarely, small doses of medication. They were seen every three months but they were not given psychotherapy or any other form of psychological counseling.

As soon as the child recovered, whether it took three months or two years, he was taken off the B vitamin and this was replaced by equivalent placebo tablets. The child was not aware there had been a change, though his parents were. By then I had concluded that double blind experiments were not ethical. Thereafter, as long as the child remained well, he was maintained on the placebo. But as soon as the parents were convinced that the child had regressed to a substantial level, they stopped the placebo and started him back on the niacinamide. After three years I made a final evaluation of each child, taking into account his family's reaction and the presence of symptoms. They were again evaluated by Dr O'Regan.

From 38 children entered into the study, 6 had to be withdrawn before they had finished their three years. One was a Down syndrome child whose father was schizophrenic. The child had shown no response after 6 months and there was no point trying any further. A second child made excellent progress but would not keep her appointments. Her parents were quite disinterested and she was dropped from the study. A third child would not take his vitamin tablets. When he was forced to take them, he would start to get better, but eventually he won the battle and did not take any more. He was sent to a home for disturbed children. The remaining three children had a schizophrenic alcoholic father who killed himself, leaving them in the care of their mother who was also schizophrenic and who was unable to cope.

Twenty-four children completed the three-year project. Every one who got well on niacinamide relapsed when placed upon placebo within one month. Many needed more time to recover when the vitamin was resumed. Eight were still in the first year of the study and had not been placed upon placebo. They were all well or nearly well. From the 32 children who took their vitamins, there was only one failure.

Twenty-seven families were involved in this study. In 13 families both parents were normal. They had a total of 47 children but only 16 were ill and required treatment. In 9 families one parent had been sick and had recovered on vitamin B-3. Six had sick fathers and three had sick mothers.

Out of a total of 29 children, 13 or 45 percent were sick. In five families both parents were schizophrenic. From a total of 22 children, 18 or 82 percent were ill.

The children who were given the vitamin B-3 regularly recovered. If they did not follow the program for any reason at all, they did not. In this small series nearly all these children were vitamin B-3 responsive – or, more accurately, vitamin B-3 dependent. This did not depend upon the diagnosis. The only thing in common to the children were they were very sick, very disturbed, and most were hyperactive. The diagnosis did not predict the response.

I concluded that these children were vitamin B-3 dependent, examples of subclinical pellagra. This syndrome, which I have called vitamin B-3 dependent or subclinical pellagra, is characterized by the following symptoms: (1) hyperactivity; (2) deteriorating performance at school; (3) perceptual changes; and (4) inability to acquire or to maintain social relationships. It is finally diagnosed by their response to vitamin B-3 used in optimal doses which in most cases are megadoses.

From the data I have, vitamin B-3 dependency appears to be inherited. In more than 100 families I have worked with over a 10 year period, I found that if one parent was vitamin B-3 dependent, it would occur in 25 percent of their children. If both parents were dependent, it would occur in 75 percent of their children. In one family it did not skip any generation. Grandfather was a depressed person with paranoid features. Of his 10 children 3 were mentally ill with schizophrenia or retardation. Of the three, one woman was under treatment with three of her nine children, and of these three children, one had an hyperactive child.

The only certain diagnostic test for pellagra was their response to vitamin B-3. This also applies to vitamin B-3 dependency. Both diseases (in fact they are one and the same but I will consider them as two in this discussion) are characterized by changes in perception, in thought, and in mood. The major difference has been in skin pigmentation. Pellagrins usually suffer symmetrical brown pigmentary changes in their skin, much less common in subclinical patients or in schizophrenics but they still do exist in some. It is likely this is due to an artifact arising from the way the patients were treated. Schizophrenics were usually locked up and not exposed to the sun, whereas pellagrins came in from the community having been exposed to sun. The skin rash of pellagra is due to photo-damage that cannot be repaired when the NAD pool is depleted.

What is not as well known is that long before pellagrins became psychotic they suffered from tension, depression, personality disorder, fatigue, and every other symptom commonly seen in neurosis, psychopathies, mood disorders, and the addictions. Mild forms of pellagra make a good model of all the other forms of mental disorder. This suggests that psychiatrists are in fact treating patients with subclinical pellagra without being aware and are applying psychosocial and other techniques that are inappropriate.

Perhaps psychiatrists should be replaced by subclinical pellagrologists. A pellagrologist was a physician who was expert in treating pellagra before vitamin B-3 was discovered to be the treatment. And in turn subclinical pellagrologists will be replaced by general practitioners who will know how to use vitamin B-3 in optimum doses and not be afraid of it. In a recent editorial in *The Lancet*, it is suggested that psychiatry may have to branch into two main areas: a neuroscientific group which would be familiar with molecular, technological, and physical treatments; and a psychosocial school, including psychotherapy, which would deal only with psychosocial problems.

These two biomedical ways (KP and NAD tests) of diagnosing children with learning and behavioral disorders are related. Using the KP urine test, one will locate those children who need extra doses of pyridoxine and zinc. But they also respond to vitamin B-3, probably because the metabolism of these two vitamins is intimately related. A B-6 deficiency will decrease the formation of NAD, the anti pellagra coenzyme. This can be corrected by giving the missing B-6 or by giving more vitamin B-3 which will force greater production of NAD. Scientifically they should be called NAD deficiency diseases. This raises the interesting speculation that anything which increases NAD concentration in the body will be therapeutic. This would mean that one might expect tryptophan to be effective as well since some of it is converted to NAD. NAD and NADH, now coming on the market in special preparations to avoid destruction in the stomach should also be effective. Many years ago I found NAD effective for treating schizophrenic patients using doses of 1 gram daily. It was more effective than vitamin B-3.

Pyrroluria (kryptopyrroleuria) is a disease homogeneous with respect to the presence of KP in the urine, by the response to treatment, and by the commonality of the clinical picture. Vitamin B-3 dependency or subclinical pellagra is another homogeneous disease characterized by the response to vitamin B-3 and also by the clinical picture. In neither of these two conditions does the usual clinical diagnosis play an important role. This again illustrates the futility of the usual descriptive diagnosis used by psychiatrists, including the once revered I.Q. tests.

I.Q. (Intelligence Quotient) Tests

I do not think that intelligence tests should be used to measure intelligence of children who are sick. They will most often yield low intelligence scores which do not reflect the real native intelligence of these children. I became very skeptical of I.Q. tests when we took into our home a schizophrenic woman who had been in a chronic mental hospital for 13 years. On admission to that hospital, her I.Q. was around 25. When she recovered on vitamin B-3 she was normal. She worked at the Royal University Hospital in Saskatoon for 30 years on their cleaning staff and lived an independent, productive life, paying taxes on the way. I have described her rehabilitation in our book *How To Live with Schizophrenia*.

I.Q. tests were developed to measure intelligence of normal people and they probably are fairly good at that. If, therefore, they are of little value for sick people and valuable for normal people, it follows that the closer the tested subject is to being well the more accurate these I.Q. tests will be. There would therefore be an apparent increase in intelligence on repeated testing if the subjects got well, and no change if they did not get well. Improved I.Q. scores are therefore an appropriate measure for improvement on treatment.

Any person with a normal brain will have normal intelligence and any nutritional deficiency or abnormality will not permit that brain to function normally. This will be expressed as a form of mental retardation. I do not think that there are truly retarded people with normal brains. Retardation is another measure of brain dysfunction. In most individuals restoring brain function will increase intelligence.

R.F. Harrell and her colleagues have reported that nutrient supplements and thyroid hormone given to mentally retarded children increase their I.Q. levels. In one issue of *The Lancet*, seven letters signed by 16 authors were published, all critical of a single report by D. Benton and G. Roberts which had been published earlier claiming that nutrient supplements increased the intelligence of school children not considered to be nutritionally deprived. Benton and Roberts completed a double blind experiment on sixty 12-year-old children. Thirty were given a vitamin-mineral supplement containing bioflavonoids 50 mg, biotin 100 mcg, choline tartrate 70 mg, folic acid 100 mcg, inositol 30 mg, niacin 50 mg, panthothenic acid 50 mg, para-aminobenzoic acid 10 mg, pyridoxine 12 mg, thiamin 3.9 mg, riboflavin 5 mg, vitamin A 375 mcg, vitamin B-12 10 mcg, vitamin C 500 mg, vitamin D 3 mcg, vitamin E 70 iu, vitamin K 100 mcg, calcium gluconate 100 mg, chromium 200 mcg, magnesium 7.6 mg, manganese 1.5 mg, molybdenum 100 mcg, iodine 50 mcg, iron 1.4 mg, and zinc 10 mg. Thirty children were given placebos. And a final thirty were given nothing. After eight months all the three groups had the same verbal intelligence scores. Non-verbal intelligence increased significantly only in the group given supplements. Verbal intelligence is a measure of the individual's unique cultural, educational, and environmental experiences, whereas non-verbal intelligence is considered to be innate or biological in nature. The answers do not require general information and vocabulary.

Seven of the critics were afraid that physicians and the public would be misled and might even start giving their children vitamin and mineral supplements. One thought children would be harmed with these very small or moderate doses of supplements.

In a second report, Benton and Cook tested 47 children using a double-blind procedure. After 6 to 8 weeks the children on the nutrients increased their I.Q. by 7.6 points. On placebo the scores decreased 1.7 points. They also found a significant correlation between sugar consumption and improvement in intelligence. The more sugar they consumed the greater was the improvement in intelligence scores. They pointed out that these children were not seriously malnourished. In another study, Benton suggested that children consuming a poor diet were most apt to benefit from supplementation. Since such a large proportion of the population of children does consume a poor diet, it would be prudent for almost all children to take these moderately dosed supplements of vitamins and minerals.

A clinical study by M. Colgan and L. Colgan provides additional evidence of the importance of diet and supplements. Each of 16 children referred to remedial reading and behavioral modification were given an individually designed program of vitamins and minerals combined with an improvement in the diet by removing sugar, refined foods, and toxic metals. An equally matched control group were given the same improved diet without the supplements. After 22 weeks the control group improved in I.Q. scores by 0 to 21 points, while the supplemented group increased their I.Q. by 5 to 35 points. "The correlation between hair concentrations of toxic metals and I.Q. scores, learning disabilities and behavior disabilities is also strong," they concluded. "Significant associations between high hair cadmium and these disabilities has now been reported in five studies. Significant disabilities with high hair lead has been reported in nine studies. The possibility suggested by results here is that brain damage caused by these metals may remit in children if the metals are removed from the body. Whatever the mechanism, if the innocuous nutritional modification used here are followed by increases in I.Q. scores over 20 weeks or more than one standard deviation and by almost doubling of the expected increase in reading skills, and also yield happier and healthier children, they are deserving of far greater attention than heretofore."

In a series of studies, S.J. Schoenthaler and his coworkers found a definite connection between the quality of the diet and intellectual performance and antisocial behavior. In one study 15 subjects on supplements gained significantly in non-verbal I.Q. compared to 11 on placebo. In a major study on 803 New York City Public Schools, Schoenthaler reported that a four-year study of improved nutrition in these schools increased mean academic percentile ranking above the rest of the nations schools by 15.7 percent. The number of learning disabled children in these schools fell from 125,000 to 49,000. Similar findings have been made by other investigators.

I recommend that I.Q. scores be used as a measure of improvement in intelligence, not as a measure of real native intelligence. I further suggest that a wide discrepancy between normal and scores achieved on testing indicates the degree of brain dysfunction. Any treatment which will improve brain function will improve I.Q.s, and of these treatments nutritional medicine or orthomolecular treatment is the best. One could use the effect of supplements on I.Q. as a measure of how important these supplements would be. If after six months there was no improvement in scores, this would suggest, all other things being equal, that child did not need these supplements.

② | TREATMENT

Optimum Diet

Most of the families who bring their children to see me are unhappy with what has happened to their children when treated by other psychiatrists. The first thing I must do is to remove misinformation they may have received. I still see families who tell me that the psychiatrist who saw their child told them there was nothing wrong with the child, that they, the parents, were the problem. I see many who have already had their children receive plenty of child play therapy, behavioral therapy, and family discussions. I let them know that my orientation is that their children are sick, that they have a learning and/or behavioral disorder, that the diagnoses that may have been assigned to them are of little value, and that I will depend upon the use of proper nutrition and supplements, rather than drugs, for treatment, but that I will use drugs if necessary until the orthomolecular or nutritional therapy takes effect.

I began to tell parents they had not made their children sick in 1960. The first time I did this the mother burst into tears. I was surprised until she told me she was crying from relief. The previous psychiatrist had given her a very rough time blaming her for having made her schizophrenic son sick. This was a bizarre idea that permeated psychiatry for several decades.

I have often wondered how any one could make anyone else schizophrenic and I still am puzzled by this, unless of course one were to make them deficient in either vitamin B-3 or B-6. The only other way is to change the criteria and/or to label anyone who doesn't agree with you schizophrenic. This was done in Russia for some time with dissidents who were diagnosed and then clapped into their special hospitals.

I also advise the parents about the prognosis, giving them an estimate conditional on the cooperation of the family and child in following the program. I discuss the reason for the special diet, the nutrients I will use, dosages, possible problems, side effects, and do the same for drugs. This approach makes the family and therapist allies in the battle against the disease. Too often in the past the psychiatrist and patient appeared to be in league against the family.

I consider the nutritional or orthomolecular model of treatment, rather than the psychoanalytical or chemical (drug) models, the appropriate one for children suffering from perceptual, thought, mood, and behavioral disorders and dysfunctions. Ortho-molecular treatment begins with a history of the patient (including nutrition), followed by the diagnostic tests when necessary, then a prescription for diet and nutritional supplements. Medication may be required to assist the child's recovery until the nutritional regimen takes hold.

Junk and Sugar Free

I immediately advise that all refined sugars should be eliminated from the child's diet as well as all "junk" processed foods. No food which contains *added* sugars can be part of the diet. This rule excludes all foods prepared with sugar and all processed foods containing sugar. This sugar-free rule has the advantage of also removing most of the cerebral allergy causing additives which are commonly found in these foods to "enhance" or disguise color and flavor. I know that most patients do not strictly follow this rule, but if they follow it 90 percent of the time, they will gain a lot.

Sugar is the pervasive food additive, present in almost all processed food, which also contains a number of other food additives to create "desirable" properties of taste, color, odor, consistency, stability, or emulsifiability. They are not added to enhance the nutritional quality of the food. I consider sugar the basic addictive substance from which all other addictions flow. The amount of refined sugar added to some foods will surprise many. Catsup contains 30 percent sugar. Some breakfast cereals have more sugar in them than do chocolate bars, containing over 50 percent sugar. The love for sweetness is so great it makes sugar the best addicting drug we have today. Overly processed food contains lots of sugar for the following reasons: (1) sugar masks the bland taste of overly processed foods which tend to remove the natural flavors of the original raw food; (2) it is addicting. If there are two competing pea soups made by different companies, the one with the most sugar in it will sell the best. There is an advantage to the bottom line if one can sell sugar in the product at the price of beans or peas when the price of sugar is low enough. There are a number of sugars. Food additives which end with "ose" are sugars, such as sucrose (table sugar), lactose (milk sugar), fructose, glucose, maltose, and so on. If companies want to avoid the intent of labeling laws, they will use several different sugars so that these sugars can be printed further from the beginning of the label. By law if sugar is the major ingredient, it must be listed first. If, however, one uses three different sugars, each one will be listed further on. It is thus possible to have a product which is 60 percent sugar but none of the sugars will appear first since individually these are not the major components.

A few children are addicted to sugar and will defeat almost every parent in pursuing their addiction. A seven-year-old boy was seen by his mother in the middle of the night crawling into the kitchen on his hands and knees to the sugar bowl and eating the sugar by the handful. They resemble adult addicts who will do the same. To solve this problem, I often then use a "junk-food" Saturday program. I invite the child to agree to eat no junk on week days on condition that they can eat all the junk they want on Saturday. Sunday is recovery day. I tell them that my idea is for them to discover for themselves how bad junk food can be. Keeping them sugar-free five days increases their reactivity to the junk they eat on Saturday. After a few Saturdays they realize that they feel rotten on these days and that they are subject to more discipline because they are so much more hyperactive. Most will volunteer to discontinue these junk-food Saturdays.

There is a natural mammalian reflex, commonly called the "vomit" reflex, not to eat anything an animals knows will make them immediately sick. That is why rats are so hard to poison. If they do not die after first eating the poison, they will not eat that food again. Adults would never become addicted to anything if the same thing happened to them. Unfortunately, addicting drugs produce an immediate pleasure or reward and only later do the bad effects appear. Humans who become addicted are getting short term gain followed by long term pain. To get them off drugs, they have to be ready to accept short term pain for the long term gain. Children have to experience the short term pain caused by the sugar before they learn it is not good for them.

If the child has food allergies, they are advised to discontinue the foods containing the known allergens. The child may be allergic to any food but usually they are usually staples including meat, potato, bread, and milk products. The most common allergy is to sugar additives, followed by milk products. The combination of milk and sugar in ice cream, for example, is a devastating combination for many children. The formula fed to so many babies contains both milk and sugar.

Primitive vs Processed Food

We should eat only foods that are pure, not processed, primitive, not high-tech, if possible. In my book *Hoffer's Laws of Natural Nutrition: Eating Well for Pure Health*, I have described in detail the principles of nutrition following the rule that we should eat those foods to which we have adapted during evolution. The idea that we should match our food supply with what our bodies have been adapted to makes so much sense there ought not to be any controversy about it. There is, however.

Most people are convinced that modern high-tech food provides the best in nutrition – a so-called 'balanced' diet . This is the message put forward by food industry advertising, by their nutritionists, and by many doctors of the old school. Overly processed food tastes very good, looks good, satisfies the sensation of hardness or softness in the mouth, and is packaged attractively. Epidemiologists have used measures of health which indicate that our society is healthier than it has ever been, namely the infant mortality rate and the increasing number of people living to retirement age. Some conclude that the high-tech diet has been the main factor in bringing about this apparent high state of good general health.

The high incidence of chronic disease (every second Canadian has one or more chronic diseases, for example) contradicts this claim, as does the ever-increasing cost of medical care. One of the chief factors in generating chronic disease is the mismatch between the food to which we have become adapted and the food which we consume. The adaptation developed over evolution has been destroyed by the changes in our foods which have come about so quickly it has been impossible for our digestive apparatus to accommodate them. Most drivers know that they must buy gasoline to operate their cars and oil with which to lubricate it. They know that cars will not work well if diesel oil or water is placed in their gas tank. They know that the type of oil will have to be changed if one drives in very cold weather as opposed to warm weather. If they do not know this they will soon discover it. They know that the cars have been made to run on these products, that these products have been designed to work in the cars, that there is a match between the design of the engine and the type of fuel which is needed. They are not surprised that their car will not work well on the wrong fuel, that it is sick. No amount of tinkering with the car's engine will make those cars well again. This can be achieved only by the use of the right fuel. The same principle applies to our bodies. They have to be fueled with the nutrients which they require to move, keep warm, grow, and maintain good health. We should not be surprised to find that our bodies do not operate properly if given the wrong fuel, if there is a mismatch or maladaptation of diet to body.

All living organisms live within an environment to which they have to adapt. The environment may be relatively constant over enormous periods of time or it may shift very rapidly. Organisms, plants or animals, that cannot adapt to the environments cannot survive. Obviously the rate of adaptation will depend upon the rate at which the environmental changes occur. When the environment changes slowly, there is ample time for the organisms within that environment to adapt and to change. When the environment changes rapidly, there may not be sufficient time and species of living beings may be wiped out very quickly simply because there has not been enough time.

The connection between food supply and survival of species is clear. Animals must be provided with food of the type their species has been consuming and to which they have adapted. There is a wide variation in adaptation, ranging from species which appear to have only one major food supply, like the anteater, to species which can consume a wide variety of plants and animals. This has been recognized by animal nutritionists, especially those in charge of modern zoos, but this recognition has been very slow in coming to human nutritionists. Lack of recognition of the need to match our food supply with our inherited needs underlies the health crises of which we hear so much today. Maladaptation is the major factor and must be corrected if ever we are to halt the inevitable increase in chronic disease and bring it back to levels which a proper match of genetics and food supply would ensure.

In a recent issue of the *Wall Street Journal,* there was a discussion of this view of nutrition and evolution. This new way of examining our health has been called "Darwinian," which Dr Jerome Kassirer, editor of the *New England Journal of Medicine*, the bastion of conservatism still fearful of the dangers of ascorbic acid, has dismissed as "just wild speculation," to which Dr Randolph Ness, author of *Why We Get Sick* retorted, "many brilliant doctors don't understand the most fundamental ideas of evolutionary biology."

An experiment conducted at Colorado State University in Fort Collins showed that the prehistoric or primitive diet was healthier than our current diet. One of the investigators on a Stone Age diet, which consisted of game meat, lots of vegetables, and fruit but virtually no dairy products and grains, brought his cholesterol level down to 160. His level on the best modern diet was 200. In his book *Nutrition and Evolution*, Professor Michael Crawford, Head of the Department of Nutritional Biochemistry at the Nuffield Institute of Comparative Medicine at the Institute of Zoology, London, has presented the hypothesis that evolution was driven, not only by random genetic changes, but also by the food supply that was available at the time these changes occurred. I am not surprised that Dr Crawford, interested in animal nutrition, came to this conclusion before most human nutritionists. They have failed to see the connection. Modern zoo keepers are wiser when it comes to feeding animals than most human nutritionists, and modern Colleges of Veterinary Medicine are much more interested in teaching and in conducting research into nutrition than are most modern medical schools. Of course, it is possible to put a dollar value on healthy hogs and chickens.

Another way to understand the differences between a "primitive" or pure diet and a modern or high-tech diet is to compare them using this table:

PRIMITIVE	HIGH-TECH
Whole	Artifact
Alive	Dead
Fresh	Stale
Varied	Monotonous
Non-Toxic	Toxic
Scarce	Abundant
Endogenous	Exogenous
Natural Flavor	Synthetic
Simple	Complex

Artifact

Much modern high-tech food is artifact. By this I mean that foods are broken down to their constituent fractions, such as starch, sugars, fats, oils, and protein, and these are then recombined to make preparations which have the appearance of natural food but are not. For example, it is possible to buy tomato soup which contains no tomatoes but in appearance and flavor would lead one to believe that it is really tomato soup. It is possible to buy overly processed cheese which has little of the original cheese in it, overly processed turkey which is turkey protein pressed out to look like slices of real turkey meat but isn't. These artifacts are dangerous because they are made to look and to taste like food. The average person eating these foods would naturally assume that they are what they appear to be and yet they would not contain the nutrient quality that was present in the original food. Overly processed foods not only fool the senses of taste and smell, but they also make it impossible to judge the quality of the food by using the subterfuge of appearing to be real food. Artifacts are pseudo-foods, preparations which are made up from a combination of artifacts or fractions of the original foods.

Dead

Much modern high-tech food is dead. Alive food does not store well. Animal products very quickly deteriorate due to oxidation, enzymatic activity, and decomposition by bacteria and fungi. These changes can be inhibited by using freezing, by drying, or by cooking the products. Cooking will slow down the rate of decomposition. The food is also preserved by the addition of chemicals which retard the growth of bacteria and fungi and which are antioxidants, thus retarding the oxidation of the food. Milk can be heat treated at such a high temperature that it is stable even at room temperature for a long time. It does not turn sour because the lactobacilli which ought to be present to sour the milk are destroyed. Modern bread has many chemicals in it which prevent it from aging and turning hard. One of the main additives used to improve the baking quality and cosmetic properties of white bread, potassium bromate, is being disallowed in Canada. Canned foods can be stored for years as can frozen foods. The least damaging way of storing food is to freeze it, followed by canning. Removing the enzymes and the reducing compounds will decrease the rate at which these foods oxidize. Removing vitamins and minerals will discourage bacteria and fungi, which must also have these nutrients to grow. The more a food is deprived of its easily lost and destroyed nutrients the more apt is that food to be stable. This is why starch extracted from wheat or potatoes is much more stable and can be stored much longer than the original plant material. But the price for the increase in stability is an equal decrease in the nutritive quality of those products. The price, however, is paid by the consumer, not by the high-tech industry which creates these long-lived stable foods. One of the aims of processing good food like wheat or oats is to convert them to a final product which costs a lot more, is much more stable, tastes sweet — and is much more dangerous to our health. We increase the value of products by converting good food into junk. In economic terms this is value-added.

Stale

Stale is another quality of high-tech food. Most of what I have said about dead applies as well to this term. As a rule overly processed food is both dead and stale.

Monotonous

The term monotonous refers to the limited variety of foods which are available. This will be surprising to shoppers who have not thought about it, especially when they are cruising around a supermarket with 15,000 to 20,000 different items on the shelves. They must think that we have an enormous variety of foods. If the prepared breakfast section carries 50 different products, are we in fact having access to 50 different foods. We are not because they are all artifacts made from oats, wheat, rice, sugar, flavors, and other additives packaged in attractive boxes. Even if we eat a wide variety from each of the 50 items, we are still eating the same three grains and sugar.

A monotonous diet is responsible for many of the health problems present in high-tech societies. There are two reasons for this. First, there will be a shortage of vitamins, minerals, and essential fatty acids. A diet which contains a variety of cereals, vegetables, fruit, and animal products is much more apt, even if only because of chance, to provide an adequate amount of these essential nutrients. For over 99 percent of man's existence on earth, there was no need to apply intelligence towards food selection. The only important fact was whether the food was poisonous or not. Among the foods found not to be poisonous, it was good enough to eat everything else provided there was an ample variety available. Since there was no abundance of any one food, it was necessary to eat what was available from all the foods. Thus primitive tribes living as hunter-gatherers would eat everything in their path that was edible. The variety depended on what was available in their community and varied from morning to night, from week to week, from season to season. Variety, combined with the absence of high-tech food products, was adequate to maintain a reasonable state of health.

We have seen the same phenomenon closer to home. About 50 years ago the average grocery store contained few items, often in bulk, chiefly vegetables, grains, and fruit. A person ignorant of nutrition could by chance purchase what would be needed to sustain good health. Suppose one were instructed to purchase 12 different items. The number of good items would be greater than the number of poor items nutritionally. That person could be healthy using those 12 items that had been selected at random, without any intellectual knowledge of which foods should be eaten or not. This is no longer possible in the modern supermarket. Out of the 15,000 items available about 50 would be suitable to maintain health. The vast majority of items would not be nourishing since they are the product of the high-tech industry. About the only safe place in which to shop is around the walls, for that is where the vegetables and fruits, the meat and fish, the dairy products, much of the frozen goods, and the breads are found. Recently, I read a report that food processing companies were becoming concerned about the number of people who only shop around the walls, thereby avoiding most of their products. They were trying to work out a way to entice shoppers to go to the center of the store.

The second reason for the ill-effects of a monotonous diet is that the probability of developing allergic reactions to foods is directly related to the proportion of our diet occupied by that food. That is why most of the allergic reactions are to foods which are staples for that region. In England tea allergies are more common than they are in the U.S.A. In countries where rice is the main staple, there will be more allergic reactions to rice. In wheat countries, wheat products will be common allergens, and in countries where corn is used extensively and corn by-products are incorporated into prepared foods, corn allergy will be common.

Toxic

Modern high-tech foods are often toxic. By toxic I do not mean they contain poisons which will kill rapidly, but taken over long periods of time, years and decades, they produce a state of chronic ill health. Before additives can be incorporated into foods they have to pass certain toxicity tests. The test may simply be one where the additive has been used for a long time and has apparently not made anyone ill. The modern test is to add the chemicals to the diet of animals and to determine the toxic dose, the so-called LD_{50}. This is the amount which will kill half the animals given the chemical over a period of time. The chemicals are also tested to determine whether they have any effect on the growth of young animals and whether they interfere with pregnancy or the development of the fetus. These are usually short term experiments. They are seldom given to animals over a major fraction of their lives, so they do not accurately test the effect of chronic use. A second objection is that additives are tested singly. When given in combinations, the toxic properties of these chemicals can be addictive and probably are. Most high-tech foods contain more than two additives. Seldom is the exact mixture of the food used in tests to determine its long term effect. The third objection to testing is that the additives are tested on animals who are fed properly. Laboratory animals are given nutritious food of the type they have adapted to. A healthy animal is better able to resist the toxic effects of chemicals. However, the diet for most people is inadequate and they are less able to cope with the chemicals present in their food.

Abundant

Modern diets are abundant, or, more accurately, they are excessive. Before high-tech foods became available, the common problem facing mankind was starvation. We had adapted to this problem by developing mechanisms for storing extra calories which could be drawn on during these periods of inadequate food supply. It is much like the camel's ability to store water to be used when none is available. Usually what food was available was of pretty good quality. There simply was not enough. Today there is no starvation in high-tech societies, unless it is created by war and other man-made activities. There are many people who believe they are not getting enough food, but the proportion of our population which is too thin, which suffers from protein-calorie deficiency, from marasmus, is very small. On the contrary, perhaps 25 percent of the population is overweight, even among people seeking extra food from community agencies. The problem in modern times is that there are too many calories but that the foods which carry these calories are lacking in nutritional quality. They are short of vitamins, minerals, and fiber —— excessive in sugars, fat, and oils. The gastrointestinal diseases generated by the over- consumption of high-tech food – high sugar, low fiber, high fat – are almost legion.

Exogenous

Our modern diet is exogenous. This refers to foods which are gathered, grown, or raised in areas of the world which are climatically much different. An example would be the consumption of fruit native to the tropics in cold countries like Sweden or Canada, or the importation of apples grown in Canada to the tropics. The essential fatty acid composition of these exotic foods will differ significantly from the composition of the vegetables and fruits raised in the same areas. Cold climate animals and vegetables contain a higher proportion of unsaturated fatty acids relative to the saturated fatty acid. The essential fatty acids make living organisms more cold tolerant.

Artificially Flavored

High-tech processed food is artificially flavored. Chemical flavor additives have no value in nutrition except for cosmetic purposes and over the long haul will be found to be toxic. More and more additives are being removed from the market, usually after many complaints, after some testing, by government decree. Flavor additives also destroy the ability of our senses to distinguish good from bad food, and in this way add to the general burden of ill health caused by these high-tech diets. The major flavoring substance is sugar, of course, followed by salt.

Complex

The last adjective we can apply to the modern high-tech diet is complex. High-tech foods are composed of a large number of items. For example, one breakfast cereal lists the following ingredients: "whole oat flour, degermed yellow corn meal, wheat starch, sugar, salt, dextrose, vitamins, reduced iron, calcium carbonate, color, trisodium phosphate." This is one of the better cereals, containing less than a gram of sugar per serving. There is a reason for each ingredient. The major item is the oats. Degermed corn is used since germ would make this product more unstable and it could not be stored as long. The sugar, salt, and dextrose (another sugar) are flavoring agents. Color is added with phosphate to stabilize the color. The vitamins and iron enhance its nutritional quality and try to restore what has been lost in the processing.

The main problem with complex foods is that the consumer does not know what is present in the food. It may contain ingredients to which we are allergic. Many patients have a multiple allergy syndrome and are reactive to almost every chemical. The presence of so many chemicals increases the likelihood that they will have an additive effect in causing toxicity and ill health. The foods we have adapted to contain a combination of nutrients which can be dealt with by our digestive apparatus. If we were given the 50 or so pure nutrients and asked to provide the proper balance for all our needs, there would be great difficulty. The combinations of ingredients placed in these complex foods has not been worked out by nutritional tests. They have been worked out on the basis of economics, cosmetic properties (taste and smell and appearance), and the need to prepare mixtures which will not deteriorate in time.

It is claimed that the complexity of the label should not be a deterrent since a label on natural food would be even more complex if every ingredient were listed. The difference is that in whole natural food none of the ingredients are in a pure state. They are all part of a very complex series of molecules. And they have been around for so long that the body is accustomed to them and knows how to deal with them. They are "orthomolecular" products. The synthetics added to food are xenobiotic or foreign and therefore they present major problems to the body.

Just as we are able to describe the problems of the modern high-tech diet with nine adjectives – artifact, dead, stale, monotonous, toxic, abundant, exogenous, synthetic, complex-— so we can describe the natural or orthomolecular diet with opposite attributes – whole, alive, fresh, varied, non-toxic, scarce, endogenous, naturally flavored, and simple. The adequacy of these adjectives can be assessed by anyone who has any familiarity with the way animals eat in the wild and the way they are fed in zoos. Natural food is whole. Some fish eat other fish swimming less rapidly and they eat them whole. Lions after the kill eat the whole animal provided they can protect the kill against other predators. A tiger does not cut a steak from its prey and store it either cold or dried or otherwise preserved. Herbivores naturally graze on living vegetable material, although domestic horses and cows are fed grasses which have been cut, dried, and stored.

Whole

Animals that eat their prey will ingest all the available minerals, vitamins, and other food components whole. Carnivores often eat the internal organs first and later go after the muscle meats. With plant material there is a tremendous difference nutritionally between the various fractions of that food. Whole wheat is comprised of the germ, the bran, and the white endosperm. The outer coating of the wheat berry or the bran is rich in minerals and vitamins and the richest source of nutrients is the germ. In milling white flour both the bran and the germ are discarded, and by eating the white flour (bread, pastry, pasta) we are depriving ourselves of the most nourishing part of the wheat berry. Nearly 200 years ago it was shown by a French army surgeon that dogs fed on whole meal bread alone were kept alive and healthy, while similar animals fed on white bread quickly sickened and died. Eating whole grain foods provides all the nutrition available in that plant.

Alive

Natural food is alive. Even scavenger animals eat meat which has not been stored very long. The main advantage to eating food which is or has recently been alive is that all the nutrients present in that food are available for use. Fresh food, alive or recently alive, has not had time to deteriorate or to develop infection or infestations with organisms and insects that are harmful. Fresh food which has deteriorated loses substantial amounts of vitamins and enzymes. If live food is not always available, the best means of preserving food value is freezing at very low temperatures, and next best is canning. None of the stored and preserved foods can compare in nutritional quality to the original fresh food. Remember that when animals do store foods, it is food like nuts and seeds which are alive but dormant and which can create new life when given a chance.

Fresh

The third adjective is fresh. Fresh and Alive are almost the same since Alive food is necessarily fresh and food which is fresh has been recently alive. But there is a difference. Whole wheat bread which is fresh will be more nutritious than will be the same bread after it has been stored for a long time. With storage there is the problem of contamination with organisms which can destroy the nutrient value of the food and can also cause illness.

Varied

A natural diet is varied. By that I mean that since we are omnivores, we can best ensure getting the nutrients we need by consuming a wide variety of foods. The second advantage is that if the foods are varied from meal to meal, from day to day, and from season to season, there is much less danger of developing allergic reactions. In meats variety is introduced by eating more than just the muscles. This includes sweetbreads, liver, cartilage, even softer bones. In fish it may include whole fish like sardines. With fruit one can eat from a large variety depending more on the home grown types. The same applies to vegetables. One should consume the edible parts, including leaves, seeds, tubers, roots, and stems where feasible from as many kinds of vegetables as are available. The same applies to grains where one should use all the grains, not just a large number of products made from flour.

Non-toxic

The natural diet is non-toxic. It is obvious that our ancestors quickly eliminated those foods which were toxic, probably at first by trial and error. If they ate the food and remained well, this would become part of the diet. They did not have to worry about the addition of chemicals to the food to "enhance" flavor or to preserve it. The foods they ate were non-toxic, except when they tried to store food and it became contaminated with bacteria and their toxins.

Scarce

The food in a natural diet is scarce. By scarce I mean in comparison to the abundant food supply available today in high-tech societies. Our ancestors had to adapt to fluctuations in food supply by storing fat as a reserve energy source. During periods when food was abundant, their bodies would store more fat, and when food was scarce or when they were starving, their bodies would draw upon this energy reserve. Women had to bear a double burden when they were pregnant, and for this reason they adapted by storing even more fat before pregnancy and during pregnancy, in order to have enough food to provide milk for their babies. They alternated between having enough food and not having enough, but they did not have to contend with having poor nutritional quality food. Today in high-tech societies there is too much food and there are no periods of starvation or decreased supply. The fat which accumulates when too much is consumed is not taken off by any following period of food reduction or starvation.

Over-consumption is less likely with whole meat and fish, fruit and vegetables. It is more of a problem with the grains and nuts and seeds. Sugar is one of the major factors, as are the commercial fats and oils. Natural foods are more bulky, have to be chewed longer and cannot be eaten as quickly so it is less possible to overload the system. Prepared foods from ground and refined grains are usually combined with sugar, fat, and other additives. It is very easy to over-eat bakery goods. Many of my patients with eating disorders have told me that they would buy one dozen doughnuts and that they would be gone before they arrived home, or that they would eat a loaf of bread in one evening, or a pound box of candy in a few hours. Primitive societies did not have a surplus of food. They had to work for their food as well. Modern society does not demand as much calorie expenditure of its people while at the same time providing a huge surplus of attractive artifact foods which taste good and which can easily be eaten very quickly.

Endogenous

Natural food is endogenous. Foods before the dawn of agriculture and for thousands of years afterward were locally grown or harvested. Foods today may come from anywhere on the globe. There are both advantages and disadvantages to this. The advantages arise when the imported food is superior in quality to the home grown or endogenous foods. The advantage of home grown food of equal nutritive quality is that there is a better match between the essential fatty acid composition of the foods in local plants and animals and the fatty acids needed by the consumer of those foods. This is very important in northern and colder climates where the ratio of essential fatty acids to non-essential fats is important in developing cold tolerance. The colder the climate, the more important is it to both plants and animals to have more essential fatty acids. These are more unsaturated and therefore their freezing point is lower. They may be compared to the antifreeze one uses in cars. They are not needed in the tropics but very essential in northern Canada. If a native from Mexico is suddenly transposed to Saskatoon where it is minus 40⅓ F, he will be much more apt to freeze exposed parts of his body – his ears or the rolls of fat around his neck. If the same person moved to Saskatoon in the summer, his body would have time to adjust by laying down more unsaturated fatty acids and he would be much more cold tolerant by the time winter arrived. It is wise to depend as much as possible on endogenous foods but to supplement the diet with exogenous food which is known to be superior in quality.

Naturally Flavored

Natural food is naturally flavored. Ancient foods were not overly processed and no synthetic flavors were known. With more sophistication our ancestors began to flavor their foods with herbs. This became much more important when food which had gone bad had to be consumed. The herbs were used to cover the awful taste of these stale preparations. Fresh food for most people tastes pretty good, even without the addition of salt and sugar. Many people, however, cannot enjoy the taste of food unless it is saturated with the two substances salt and sugar because they have been so much a part of their diet for so many years.

Simple

The natural diet is simple. Our ancestors did not have our ability or our desire to compound food preparations. Many modern recipes call for over a dozen different items. In the past the foods were simple and therefore people eating them could know what it was they were eating. If they knew that rabbit meat made them sick, they did not have to worry that some rabbit meat might be present in other food preparations. Today we cannot be sure of the ingredients in food unless we make them ourselves. This is why people who know peanuts will kill them (anaphylactic shock) have died eating food they thought was safe because some person had added peanut oil to the preparation. One has to be very careful of all overly processed foods and to distrust even the labels on many prepared foods.

The Balanced Diet

In the perennial dance of the individual and the environment, time does not go backward. We cannot re-establish the world from which we have evolved. We cannot return to the dietary habitat of our prehistoric ancestors, nor do we need to. It is feasible to process our modern foods and to select from these foods the elements of what we had adapted to. Eventually everything that is done to our food from the farm to our kitchens will have to be treated so as to maximize its nutritional quality. I think we will one day have a public health law which will not permit the sale and distribution of any food preparation unless it is proven that these are as safe and as nourishing as the foods from which they were fashioned. This requires no new knowledge – just the will to do so. It would simply force all the food processors to perform animal feeding tests.

Our food should be processed and selected to fit the description of the diets to which we are adapted. We should be able to describe our foods as almost whole, alive, and fresh and distinguish them from the artifacts that are dead and stale. Visualize a scale or line which ranges from whole at one end (or alive or fresh) to artifact at the other end (or dead or stale). The objective is to move towards the healthy end of the scale as far as possible, knowing that this is an ideal most people won't reach. Nevertheless, it is better to be close to the healthy end than it is to be close to the disease end where we are today. Perhaps each item could be rated with a quality item or number starting with 100 and decreasing in value to the pathological end which would be 0. At the zero end life would be barely sustainable with maximum disease, while at the healthy end of the scale life would be sustainable with optimum good health.

I do not like the term "balanced" diet because it has been corrupted by dietitians and food processors who use it as a justification for allowing the many degradations in the food they make. For many years apologists for white bread maintained that since no one lived on bread alone, it did not matter if it was deficient in some nutrients. The rest of the nutrients needed to balance the diet, they maintained, would be provided by other food groups than grains. This is not true. If 90 percent of the diet was good, it would not matter too much if 10 percent was corrupted. But where 75 percent of the diet is corrupted, it really does matter. Ideally each food should contain its full share of nutrients required by the person. Whole foods are balanced already by nature. A diet consisting of natural foods is inherently balanced, provided enough variety is introduced. In the animal world monotonous foods are well balanced. An anteater eats a diet of live ants only and the koala bear eats only leaves from a few species of the euca-lyptus tree. The term "balanced" should apply only to combinations of natural foods -— only to the natural orthomolecular diet.

Nutrient Supplements

Nutrients as Medicine

The history of the use of food and vitamins for medicinal purposes has been divided into five ages by Dr L.J. Machlin. The first period ranges from about 1500 B.C. to 1880. Foods were used empirically to heal certain diseases. The second period ranges from 1880 to 1900. During this period deficiency diseases were produced in animals, and the vitamin hypothesis was developed. The third period ranges from 1900 to 1930. During this phase the vitamins were discovered, isolated, their structure determined, and their synthesis established. The fourth period begins about 1930 when biochemical functions of the body were studied, dietary requirements were introduced, and commercial production of vitamins became promi-nent. We are now into the fifth period which began in 1955 and is charac-terized by the recognition of therapeutic health effects beyond prevention of deficiency disease.

From 1880 to 1955, vitamins were limited in their application to the prevention of deficiency diseases such as beri beri (vitamin B-1 or thi-amine) and pellagra (vitamin B-3 or niacin). During this vitamin-as-pre-vention era, it was believed that the only role of vitamins was to prevent vitamin deficiency diseases, and they were needed in small amounts. This made sense since vitamins were catalysts of reactions in the body and cat-alysts are known to be needed only in small amounts as they are used over and over. Any dose above these small preventive doses was undesirable, wasteful, bad medical practice, and, to some, even criminal. Physicians have lost their medical licenses because of the unsubstantiated charges that they were prescribing large doses of vitamins that harmed their patients. Some hospitals still do not permit the use of intravenous ascorbic acid. These 'principles' make up the preventative vitamin or vitamin deficiency paradigm. They are still adhered to very vigorously by many dietitians, nutritionists, and physicians.

The old paradigm led to the creation of RDAs (recommended daily allowances) which have been like the holy writ for many years in spite of the fact they were designed to provide guidelines for only the healthy part of the population. They are of no value to individuals who are not average — not of value to 50 percent of the total population. Orthomolecular therapists have consistently argued against their use and have ignored them in their practices. Recently, Professor David Mark Hegsted, appointed to Harvard's New England Regional Primate Research Center in Southborough, Massachussets, recommended that RDAs be abolished, arguing that the system is unworkable because it was based on estimates using healthy young males — the group least likely in the population to have nutritional deficiencies. Dr J. Blumberg, Professor of Nutrition at Tufts Univer-sity, argues that "the RDA committee is locked into the old paradigm of nutrition — how much is needed to prevent deficiency disease. It has not shifted gears to where medicine is today."

In the middle 1930s just after it was recognized that niacin cured pellagra, the early pellagrologists found, I am certain to their great surprise, that the small doses of vitamin B-3 which prevented pellagra and which cured early (acute) pellagra did not help patients who had chronic pellagra. They required 600 mg per day, a huge quantity, compared to the tiny dose of less than 20 mg needed to prevent pellagra. This proved that the optimum dose even to prevent pellagra from recurring ranged from 20 to 600 mg daily. Chronic pellagra changed body chemistry (in humans and dogs) so that the small doses effective as a preventative measure were no longer adequate. Much larger amounts were needed, for they had developed a dependency on vitamin B-3. A deficiency is present when the diet is so bad that even the small preventive doses are not provided. A dependency is present when the needs of the body are so great that even the best diet cannot provide the right amount. The preventative vitamin paradigm does not recognize this therapeutic vitamin "law."

As such, the preventive vitamin paradigm as been very harmful to nutritional research. It inhibited the investigations of the therapeutic use of vitamins for at least 30 years. It is still harmful because it still has the medical school departments of nutrition in its sway. It is correct only for the very few classical deficiency diseases and is totally incorrect for the rest of medicine.

Our research published in 1955 proposed the therapeutic use of vitamins in large doses. The therapeutic vitamin paradigm is based on the following four observations. (1) We are all different and have different nutrient requirements. (2) Optimum amounts of vitamins are needed which range from smaller doses necessary to prevent deficiency disease to much larger doses to treat vitamin dependent conditions -— conditions like elevated cholesterol levels and too low levels of high density lipoprotein cholesterol. (3) The following variables determine the optimum need: age, sex, physical stress including pregnancy, psychological stress, lactation, diseases (whether acute or chronic), use of xenobiotic drugs. Thus there can never be one useful Optimal Daily Dose (ODD) schedule for everyone; there must be an Optimal Recommended Dose (ORD) specific for each condition and for each disease. (4) Vitamins can be taken safely for a life time.

The therapeutic vitamin paradigm opens up the use of vitamins for optimum health to everyone. In sharp contrast to drugs, which are very toxic and must be carefully controlled by trained professionals, vitamins are so safe they can be experimented with by any person secure in the knowledge that they are as safe as are any of the over-the counter medications readily available today. People can become their own therapists. Experimentation will not do them any harm, provided they have have taken a little time to examine the vitamin literature. With drugs too little is much safer than too much, but with vitamins a little more is much safer than too little if one wishes to obtain optimum health. If more than is needed is taken, there is no harm because the extra amount is not stored and is readily eliminated. There are very few exceptions. Thus one can try to find the optimum by taking increasing doses until it is reached. And if that dose is exceeded, the body can readily deal with it. If too little is taken, the desired therapeutic effect will not be obtained. The difference between optimum and less effective doses can be narrow. I have seen schizophrenic patients who did not respond to 3 grams per day of niacin, but when this was doubled, they began to improve very quickly. The same principle does not apply to minerals and may not apply to amino acids, even though they also have a wide tolerance range.

The Nutrient Regimen

After I have discussed the diet of the patient with the child and family and explained the principles of therapeutic use of nutrient supplements, I list for them an introductory vitamin program or regimen. The first vitamin I prescribe is B-3, which comes in two forms, niacin and niacinamide, 500 mg tid to start. The second vitamin to be prescribed is vitamin C or ascorbic acid, also 500 mg tid to start. Vitamin B-6 or pyroxidine, either 100 mg for smaller children or 250 mg daily, is also prescribed. As treatment proceeds the dosages for these vitamins may need to be adjusted and other vitamins, minerals, essential fatty acids, and amino acids may be prescribed.

Until it is clear the child is responding to the program, they are seen regularly every few weeks or every month. Once the trend toward recovery has been established, I leave it to the parents to determine how often the child should come to my office. Eventually the child need not be seen at all unless there is a relapse or change in their condition. On the average I see each child about three to four times before they can carry on without my intervention.

Generally children do not like to swallow pills, unless they are convinced they need them – that is, they feel better when they are taking them. Often this leads to a lot of arguments between parent and child and sometimes parents simply give up. The child and parents thus need to find the least difficult way for taking the vitamin tablets. When children realize the vitamins are important, there is usually no problem. Several children have called the vitamins their happiness pills and with them there was never any problem. Often the child would be convinced only after several relapses after not taking the pills. In each case one should find out why the child has a problem. Each child must be treated responsibly, like an adult patient. This means explaining the diagnosis, the nature of the condition, and the reason for the treatment. If the child understands and accepts the explanation, there is usually no problem. I have seen children as young as three and a half years old become responsible for taking their own pills. It is easier for the child if they have clearly recognizable symptoms such as hallucinations, nightmares, bed wetting, or not being able to read. It is more difficult if the main problem is behavioral, for many believe they are normal and that their parents are being unnecessarily difficult.

But even responsible children may have a problem swallowing. Niacinamide and pyridoxine taste very bitter. If the pills are too big or too rough they will taste them, especially if they swallow one at a time and hold them for awhile in their mouth. One should only use pills made by manufacturers who make smooth, smaller tablets, easier to swallow. The parents and children should be taught to swallow two or more pills each time, rather than one at a time. Surprising as it may seem it is easier to swallow more than one pill. There is a natural reflex which all mammals have of not swallowing little pebbles. But in nature there are seldom more than one in a mouthful so that if there are five, for example, there is less resistance of a reflex nature. Once children can master two, they can easily increase the number until they can take all of them with one gulp. This takes the chore out of taking vitamins. If the child takes the pills one by one using a half glass of liquid to swallow each, he is soon full of liquid. Pills are best taken after meals. The vitamins may be also ground and mixed with food, something like peanut butter and bananas, but the bitter taste of the niacinamide and pyridoxine will still be evident. Liquid preparations may be used but they generally do not contain enough of the B vitamins. Children should not take the pills to school to avoid embarrassment and teasing.

Parents have to be convinced that the vitamins are helpful. Parents motivated to come for this kind of treatment have already decided that the usual treatment for these children – that is, ritalin and some form of psychotherapy – has not helped or does not agree with their ideas. They still need an explanation of the whole treatment process. They may have to face the objections of their physicians who sometimes advise the parents not to give vitamins to their children, or the objections of separated spouses, or those of well-meaning relatives who have their own views of what is wrong. Too often children doing well have had to go to hospital for other reasons and they were promptly taken away from their program. They have often relapsed in a few days and the parents and child must start all over again. For many children, each relapse makes it harder for them to respond as quickly. What follows, then, is an explanation of the key nutrients used in orthomolecular treatment.

Vitamin B-3

The third water soluble vitamin to be discovered was called vitamin B-3 before it was shown to be nicotinic acid and its amide (also known medically as niacin and niacinamide). The name was changed to remove the similarity to nicotine, a poison. I had a chronic paranoid patient who refused to take nicotinic acid because he thought it was nicotine but who did not object to taking niacin.

The term vitamin B 3 was reintroduced by my friend Mr. Bill W. (Bill Wilson), co-founder of Alcoholics Anonymous. We met in New York in 1960, where my colleague Humphry Osmond and I introduced him to the concept of megavitamin therapy. We described the results we had seen with our schizophrenic patients, some of whom were also alcoholic. We also told him about its many other properties. It was therapeutic for arthritis, for some cases of senility, and it lowered cholesterol levels. Bill was very curious about it and began to take niacin, 3 g daily. Within a few weeks fatigue and depression which had plagued him for years were gone. He gave it to 30 of his close friends in AA and persuaded them to try it. Within six months he was convinced that it would be very helpful to alcoholics. Of the 30 friends, 10 were free of anxiety, tension, and depression in one month. Another 10 were well in two months. He decided that the chemical or medical terms for this vitamin were not appropriate. He wanted to persuade members of AA, especially the doctors in AA, that this would be a useful addition to treatment and he needed a term that could be more readily popularized. He asked me the names that had been used. Vitamin B-3 was the term Bill wanted. In his first report to physicians in AA he called it "The Vitamin B-3 Therapy." Thousands of copies of this extraordinary pamphlet were distributed. Eventually the name came back and today even the most conservative medical journals are using the term vitamin B-3.

Vitamin B-3 exists as the amide in nature, in nicotinamide adenine dinucleotide (NAD). Pure nicotinamide and niacin are synthetics. Niacin was known as a chemical for about 100 years before it was recognized to be vitamin B-3. It is made from nicotine, a poison produced in the tobacco plant to protect itself against its predators, but in the wonderful economy of nature which does not waste any structures, when the nicotine is simplified by cracking open one of the chemical rings, it becomes the immensely valuable vitamin B-3.

Vitamin B-3 is made in the body from the amino acid l-tryptophan. On the average 1 mg of vitamin B-3 is made from 60 mg of tryptophan, a 1.5 percent conversion rate. Since it is made in the body, it does not meet the strict definition of a vitamin, which is defined as a substance that cannot be made by the body. It should have been classified with the amino acids but long usage of the term vitamin has given it permanent status as a vitamin. I suspect that one day in the far distant future none of the tryptophan will be converted into vitamin B-3 and it then will truly be a vitamin.

The 1.5 percent conversion rate is a compromise based upon the conversion of tryptophan to N-methyl nicotinamide and its metabolites in human subjects. According to M.K. Horwitt, the amount converted is not inflexible but varies with patients and conditions. For example, women pregnant in their last three months convert tryptophan to niacin metabolites three times as efficiently as do non-pregnant females. The amino acid l-tryptophan provides some of the vitamin B-3. This amount ingested is converted into nicotinamide adenine dinucleotide (NAD), originally known as diphosphopyridine nucleotide (DPN) or coenzyme I. This reaction is catalyzed by pyridoxine, vitamin B-6. The reduced form is NADH. I will use NAD for the entire oxidation reduction system.

$$NAD \longleftrightarrow NADH$$

NAD is split by an enzyme called NADase which releases niacinamide, which in turn is converted into niacin, and this in turn is introduced into the pyridine nucleotide cycle into the NAD.

The body can make NAD from two sources, from l-tryptophan and from vitamin B-3. If therefore the food contains ample supplies of vitamin B-3, there will be less need to use tryptophan for a major source and it can be diverted into other uses – for example, to make serotonin and later melatonin. If the food is short of vitamin B-3, the body will have to use more energy to make as much NAD. Dr Linus Pauling has shown how the body could dispense with making its own vitamin C if adequate amounts were present in the food. This is why the mutation that prevented the body from converting glucose into ascorbic acid about 25 million years ago was genetically superior since there was enough in the diet. But when these ancient diets were supplanted by the modern diets, there was not enough ascorbic acid and the result has been world-wide sub-clinical and clinical scurvy. In the same way, I think, the body has begun to depend more and more on food-based vitamin B-3.

NAD and NADH are interconvertable in the body. This suggests that the active form is the reduced form, NADH, and that NAD is much less effective since it would first have to be reduced to NADH. The decreasing order of therapeutic efficacy would be NADH, NAD, and finally vitamin B-3. There would be no formation of NADH in the stomach from NAD, but there would be some made in the intestine. This potent coenzyme made from vitamin B-3 is available from Menuco Corporation, 350 Fifth Avenue, Suite 7509, New York, NY 10118.

The starting dose is 500 mg tid. It is then increased at subsequent visits until the full therapeutic effect is seen. This may take many months or several years. I usually start with niacinamide to spare the children the vasodilatation (flush) which accompanies the first use of niacin. If they can't stand the bitter taste of the amide, I will then start them on niacin, which is sour and preferred by some children. Patients should remain on the program for several, often many years after they have recovered. I advise the children to stay on until they are age 18. If they do go off after they are well, they may relapse, and if they do, they must immediately resume the program. Many children find that smaller doses are enough to keep them well. If the dose is too high, they will become nauseated and if the vitamin is not stopped will vomit. The dose must be reduced below this level.

I use the same dose range with niacinamide. It has no effect on cholesterol levels but when used for a long time may be just as beneficial to the vascular system. There is no flush with niacinamide in 99 percent of the people who take it. However, about 1 in 100 do flush with it; presumably they are able to convert it very quickly into niacin in their bodies. Many of these patients prefer the niacin flush which tends to be a bit more pleasant. I do not refer to patients who mistakenly took niacin thinking it was niacinamide or whose druggists gave them the wrong vitamin. There have been a few cases of mislabelling as well. Niacinamide tastes very bitter and niacin tastes very sour as does ascorbic acid. If you think the product is niacinamide and it tastes sour, you have the wrong preparation.

When the dose of either form exceeds what that person can tolerate, it will cause nausea, and if the dose is not reduced or stopped, this will proceed to vomiting. If nausea comes on, the vitamin should be stopped for a day or two and the resumed at a lower level. Usually it is possible to take more niacin than niacinamide and a few have taken enormous doses with no nausea. I think a few patients have been hurt by the nausea, vomiting, and dehydration because they did not stop it when they should have. Children will often not complain of nausea. They will simply lose their appetite. If a child on vitamin B-3 stops eating, one should immediately suspect this is a problem and proceed to a lower dose again after stopping it for a day or two.

Fortunately, patients who need it the most suffer the least discomfort with these recommended doses. The nauseant upper limit provides a remarkable safety valve against overdosing. I had one teen-age schizophrenic patient to whom I had given 200 tablets of niacin, 500 mg. The next day in a suicide gesture she swallowed the whole bottle. For the next two days she suffered mild abdominal pain. The number of side effects, as it is for all the vitamins, is remarkably low and vitamin B-3 is considered safe by the American Medical Association and approved by the FDA in the United States.

Vitamin C or Ascorbic Acid

Very few people knew about vitamin C until Professor Linus Pauling issued his first book on *Vitamin C and the Common Cold* in 1970. There was a marked increase in sales of vitamin C following that report. This was so disturbing to the medical community they began a major effort to discredit Dr Pauling, even to the point of calling him senile, trying to debunk his conclusion that vitamin C would be preventive and therapeutic for the common cold and for other conditions. A main complaint was that Dr Pauling, awarded Nobel Prizes for Biochemistry and Peace, was not a medical doctor and therefore should not be commenting on medical matters. One physician in Australia tried to link the resulting increased use of vitamin C to an equally dramatic rise in the incidence of kidney stones. He did not mention that the increase in kidney stones had begun long before Dr Pauling's book appeared and that after it appeared the incidence did not rise any further. A letter of rebuttal that I submitted to the journal which carried this report was rejected. Since then there has been a massive effort on the part of many doctors, dietitians, professors of biochemistry, and others to educate people against taking vitamin supplements because the average diet provided all that was needed. They linked vitamin C to every possible toxicity. Yet the public has its own way of dealing with medical ideas. It goes by how it feels. When a patient finds that he gets fewer colds after taking vitamin C, no amount of rhetoric will persuade him that his own convictions are unscientific. In any event the tide has turned and the once shrill voices against vitamin C have calmed down as more physicians have entered the megavitamin field. As an illustration of the increased demand, the price of ascorbic acid has gone up $3.75 per kilogram in the past year. The supply has not kept up with demand. The manufacturers will have to build new plants to match the increased demand.

Every human suffers from subclinical scurvy, from a deficiency of vitamin C or ascorbic acid. We cannot make any in our bodies, and the amount present in even the best possible diet will not provide more than 100 mg per day. This amount is totally inadequate for optimum health. There is no need to ask the question, do I need any vitamin C? The only question is how much is needed. There are many clues in nature. Of these the best is the amount of vitamin C which animals make in their body normally and also under severe stress. They are able to convert glucose into vitamin C. They make much more than we take in from our food. Thus a goat, weighing about as much as a man, will make 14 grams of vitamin C per day. Apparently all animals that make vitamin C make about the same amount per kilogram of body weight. Since we lost the capability of making vitamin C about 20 million years ago, our bodies have had to adapt to chronic deficiency after we moved away from a natural diet to a food supply that did not provide adequate amounts. We are still paying the price of this dietary change, but we no longer have to since synthetic ascorbic acid is very inexpensive. Every person should take ample quantities to replace what nature took away from us. Although we are not as sick as if we had scurvy, this is small consolation since scurvy is a terminal disease. I do not think we should be content with being just some distance away from death.

Vitamin C is therefore needed by everyone, not only to prevent diseases like scurvy but also to insure optimum health of the whole body. And in the presence of any pathology or stress, the amount needed increases very rapidly. It has been found that the more serious the condition the more vitamin C is needed. A good indicator of this is the ratio of ascorbic acid in its original reduced state to the amount of oxidized vitamin C, dehydroascorbic acid. Normally less than 5 percent of the total vitamin C in the body is in the oxidized state so that the ratio is better or higher than 20:1. However, when the individual is close to death almost all the vitamin C is in the oxidized state and the ratio is very small. For other diseases the amount of oxidized vitamin C decreases. In people who are very sick and begin to recover the amount of oxidized vitamin goes down quickly. It is apparent that the vitamin C must be in the reduced state since only then can it function as an antioxidant. The best way to ensure that the ratio is very low is to take ample quantities of the vitamin.

Vitamin C is indeed our chief antioxidant. We live in an atmosphere which contains about 20 percent oxygen. This is used in respiration to create energy. But excessive oxidation will be very harmful. Free radicals are formed which are very active and can damage cells and tissues. A free radical can pull another electron from another molecule and convert that into another free radical. This chain reaction will continue until the electron reacts with another electron, or is deactivated by an antioxidant, a scavenger, or an enzyme. The body has developed a system of antioxidants to protect itself against excessive oxidation. In the same way a potato will not turn brown until it is peeled and exposed to air. The brown pigment formed is the result of excessive oxidation in a tissue not protected by antioxidants. Vitamin C is the main water soluble antioxidant, but the body's defense system also includes other nutrients that work in conjunction with vitamin C, including antioxidant enzymes, superoxide dismutase(sod), catalase, glutathione peroxidase, vitamin E, beta carotene, non-enzymatic scavengers, uric acid, glutathione, and thiols in proteins.

These substances work together both within the cell and in the fluids outside the cells. They also reinforce each others activity: for example, vitamin E spares vitamin C. Vitamin C works mainly in the water medium, while vitamin E works primarily in the fat medium and on cell membranes. Free radicals are involved in a large number of processes in the body, including cancer, aging, Parkinson's disease, cardiovascular disease, cataracts, arthritis, and diabetes. By controlling these reactions antioxidants have a therapeutic role in all these conditions.

We had expected that this vitamin C would prevent the oxidation of adrenalin to adrenochrome. Vitamin C had been used to stabilize adrenalin solutions. But we found that it was not a very good inhibitor but instead had other useful properties. When adrenochrome and vitamin C are mixed in solution the red color almost instantaneously vanishes and the solution becomes slightly yellow. The yellow solution now contains adrenolutin and leukoadrenochrome. Adrenolutin is not as toxic as adrenochrome and is the indole which circulates in the blood and can be accurately measured. It is also an hallucinogen. The other compound is made in vitro and probably also circulates in the blood but no measure has been developed to test for its presence in the body. It has anti-tension and antidepressant properties. Thus, vitamin C does not prevent the formation of adrenochrome but its does convert half of the adrenochrome into the non-toxic leukoadrenochrome.

Vitamin C is therapeutic against schizophrenia. In 1952, at the Munro Wing, in Regina, Saskatchewan a middle aged women was admitted. She was diagnosed schizophrenic by her psychiatrist and he planned on starting her on ECT because she was so sick. She had received a total mastectomy for breast cancer, the surgical lesion became infected and ulcerated and then she became psychotic. I had decided to try large doses of vitamin C only on a few patients to test its efficacy. When I discovered she was in hospital I asked her psychiatrist whether he would delay ECT so that I could start her on vitamin C. He agreed to wait for three days only. I had planned on giving her 1 gram three times daily. But I knew that three days with such a small dose would be a waste of time. I therefore instructed the nursing staff to give her one gram each hour day and night. If she slept she would be given what she had missed during her sleep. Over the 48 hours she had received 45 grams. When her psychiatrist came in Monday to give her ECT she was normal and the treatment was cancelled. This immediately showed that large doses were safe and that it had been therapeutic for her psychosis. Her ulcerated lesion began to heal for the first time. She was discharged a few days later mentally normal. She died 6 months later from her cancer but had remained mentally normal. Since I then I have used ten grams or more daily for several patients to help control their anxiety and tension. I am convinced it is helpful for another reason. It decreases the frequency of viral attacks and colds and these are events which increase the possibility of relapse into schizophrenia.

Vitamin C is a weak organic acid, comparable to lemon juice. Compared to the strong acid present in the stomach, the addition of any amount of ascorbic acid makes a minor contribution to the stomach fluid acidity. Still, a number of people do not like the sour taste. For this reason it is fortunate that the salts of ascorbic acid are available. They are sodium ascorbate, potassium ascorbate, calcium ascorbate, etc. A few preparations on the market contain a variety of these salts of vitamin C. They are called mineral ascorbates. They do represent an improvement over the straight ascorbic acid which is never present in nature as the pure acid, as it is in tablets, but is associated with other nutrients. One such preparation I have been using for several years is Supergram Plus, non-acidic vitamin C. It contains calcium, magnesium, zinc, manganese, molybdenum, and chromium ascorbates, but most of the vitamin C there is sodium ascorbate. It is a good preparation containing other essential nutrients as well. The mineral ascorbates are more tolerable for many and are equivalent to taking the pure vitamin C (hydrogen ascorbate). A very small number of people, fewer than 20 seen over the past 30 years, cannot tolerate any amount of vitamin C. They have developed an allergy or idiosyncrasy to either the synthetic vitamin C or to some of the other ingredients of the preparations. They might try preparations made from other sugar sources. The common vitamin C is made from corn syrup. It is preferable to take the vitamin several times per day to decrease the amount lost in the urine.

Opponents of the use of vitamin C claim that taking more than a few milligrams per day is useless since the vitamin C is excreted into the urine. They cynically refer to urine rich in vitamin C. This, of course, is a foolish argument that only those ignorant of how vitamin C is absorbed and excreted could use. They ignore the fact that in most cases enough of any therapeutic compound must be given before it can be therapeutic and that this sometimes means allowing a major part to appear in the urine. If a person is given 50 grams per day of penicillin to save his life, most of that also appears in the urine. With vitamin C it has been shown that the more that is taken into the body, the greater is the amount retained and used by the body. In our early research we found we could inject chronic schizophrenics with 90 grams of vitamin C and could find none in the urine. If the dose is 1 gram, a fraction of that will be retained. If the dose is 10 grams, many grams will be excreted but many grams will also be retained. To increase the retention, the dose must be increased.

For children with brain dysfunctions and disorders, I start with 500 mg tid and may double or triple that depending upon the child's need. These low doses will not cure the condition but are enormously helpful. It decreases the frequency of colds and flu. According to Dr A. Kalokerinos, ascorbic acid protects children against the side effects of vaccination. I advise the parents to give their children at least one gram of vitamin C before they receive their injections. I have seen two children who began to convulse the same day they were given their vaccination and were left impaired. This might have been prevented by vitamin C.

The optimum dose is that amount which causes loose stools, too much gas, and some diarrhea. This is not dangerous but is unpleasant. This effect of vitamin C on bowel function can be turned to good advantage since the vitamin can be used as a laxative. Vitamin C is one of the best, natural, laxatives and ought to be used by everyone with this problem.

The maximum recommended oral dose of vitamin C is 75 grams each day, but very few can tolerate this extremely high dose because it exceeds the laxative dose. While the majority of people take under 12 grams per day, it is best to think in terms of the optimum tolerable dose. Each person can determine this for themselves or parents can help children to determine this. When more vitamin C is taken than that individual can absorb from the gastrointestinal tract, it causes increased formation of gas and the bowel contents become very fluid. If the dose greatly exceeds this level, diarrhea will develop. The ideal dose has optimum functions in the body without causing any effect on the bowel except to help regulate it. If the laxative level is 20 grams, for example, the optimum oral level will be around 18 grams. Dr R. Cathcart discovered that the more the body needs the vitamin, the more it can tolerate. I have observed the same, as have almost all orthomolecular physicians. My optimum dose has ranged between 30 and 3 grams daily depending on my state of health. If a lot more is needed, it is possible to train the body to accept more. Some AIDS cases in Australia have been trained to take 200 grams daily. If the higher doses cannot be reached, it may be necessary to take intravenous vitamin C. When given in IV drip, up to 200 grams can be given over several hours without any gastrointestinal effect.

Vitamin B-6 (Pyridoxine)

This vitamin is an integral part of many reactions in the body. One of these reactions is the conversion of some of the l-tryptophan into NAD. A deficiency of B-6 will therefore cause pellagra as much as a deficiency of vitamin B-3. But it has many other properties. These have made it useful in treating a number of psychiatric problems, including those present in children with learning and behavioral disorders. Dr Allan Cott, Dr Carl Pfeiffer, and Dr Bernard Rimland have pioneered use of pyridoxine for treating children. Dr Cott introduced it in his practice over 25 years ago, and about the same time Dr Rimland found that pyridoxine was more effective for autistic children than was vitamin B-3. Because of his interest in infantile autism, Rimland began to hear from many parents of these children who had on their own begun to experiment with various nutrients. "These unhappy people would write to me about the bitter disappointment and discouragement they had experienced with the usual treatment methods," Rimland explains. "They would then tell me they had read articles in the *New York Times* and elsewhere about the work of Dr Abram Hoffer and Humphry Osmond who were reporting good results when they used massive dosages of certain vitamins on adult schizophrenics. At first I was quite skeptical about the reports that some of the parents sent me about the improvement they saw in their sick children. . . . As the number of parent experimenters grew it began to include more parents whom I knew personally to be intelligent and reliable people. At that point I contacted a number of doctors in California and on the East Coast who I knew had been experimenting with vitamin therapy. The combined information from the doctors and parents convinced me I could not in good conscience fail to pursue this lead. I was, of course, aware that my working on the vitamin approach would create much hostility against me among many authorities in the medical world who were totally and irrevocably convinced that the use of vitamins would not be helpful."

After hearing from 57 parents and 7 physicians who responded in detail, Rimland developed a multiple-B vitamin tablet which was given with vitamin C, several grams daily. This preparation was made available to 200 parents of autistic children. This was a very careful study meticulously planned and evaluated. At the end of this investigation, Dr Rimland found that out of 191 placed on this regimen there was no response in 20, a slight response in 37, but 41 showed some improvement, and 86 showed definite improvement. Only 7 were made worse. Altogether 66 percent were clinically improved. For a short therapeutic study this is quite remarkable. In sharp contrast drugs given to 1591 children yielded a 27 percent improvement rate. Later Rimland initiated a large series of controlled studies which uniformly proved that these vitamins, especially pyridoxine, were therapeutic.

Rimland was a co-worker in the first double blind prospective controlled experiment which showed that pyridoxine was therapeutic for children who have infantile autism. As he reported, "there are now 17 published studies – all positive – showing that high dosages of vitamin B-6 and magnesium are a safe and often helpful treatment for autism. Thousands of parents are using B-6 and magnesium to help their children. Almost 50 percent show worthwhile improvement and the vitamins are immeasurably safer than any drug. . . . No studies have failed to show benefit and no significant adverse effects have been seen. No drug even comes close to vitamin B-6 in efficacy and safety."

Dr Pfeiffer and his co-workers discovered how to tell when extra amounts of vitamin B-6 are needed. His group followed up our work on the mauve factor, krytopyrrole (KP), and found that it combined with pyridoxine and zinc to produce a double deficiency. If the amount of KP in the urine was too high, this showed that these two nutrients would be needed. This applied to adults and children.

I add vitamin B-6 to the regimen if the child tests positive for pyrroluria or if it is indicated by physical examination and history. I ask about stretch marks on the body, white areas in the finger nails, pale skin. I start with 250 mg daily but may go to two or three times as much. Sometimes it will increase hyperactivity but this is corrected by giving the child magnesium. A calcium magnesium tablet providing about 375 mg calcium and half that amount of magnesium will prevent this increased irritability from pyridoxine. The beneficial effect much outweighs the potential minor side effect.

Vitamin B-Complex

The B complex should be added when the diet cannot be improved adequately or when there is additional evidence that they are needed. It is better to take slightly more than is needed rather than less. In sharp contrast, drugs are better used in slightly less quantities because of their toxicity. The B-complex 25s or 50s are suitable. They also contain other vitamins.

Vitamin E

This has been found in a few studies to be helpful in treating the hyperactive child.

Vitamin A and D

In northern countries where there is no ultraviolet light during the winter months the fish liver oils can be very helpful.

Essential Fatty Acids

There are two main classes of essential fatty acids. The omega "six" class and the more unsaturated omega "three" class. These essential fatty acids, omega-3 and omega-6 series, began to disappear from our diet about 75 years ago. Only 20 percent of our needs are available in the average diet today. Dr D. Rudin and Dr C. Felix call essential fatty acids the nutritional "missing link." They have presented convincing evidence that this missing nutrient is one of the main factors in producing much of the illness we have to contend with in our modern high-tech society. Omega-3 essential fatty acids are highly reactive fatty acids, some of which are converted in the body into the essential prostaglandins, but to do so they must be in balance with the omega-6 fatty acids. They are needed for growth, for many metabolic roles, for the integrity of the cell membranes, and to prevent skin drying and flaking. *Fats and Oils* by Udo Erasmus is one of the best simple books that describes the chemistry and biochemistry of the two series of essential fatty acids.

According to Dr Rudin, there is a rational explanation why both vitamins and minerals and essential fatty acids should all be therapeutic. The essential fatty acids are partially converted into prostaglandins. Therefore a deficiency of essential fatty acids will lead to a deficiency of prostaglandins. According to Rudin this is the cause of pellagra. But vitamin B-3 is also needed to assist in the conversion of essential fatty acids. Thus a deficiency of vitamin B-3 will lead again to a deficiency of prostaglandins and yield a somewhat similar end result. Pellagra is the vitamin B-3 deficiency syndrome but a deficiency of essential fatty acids is then a substrate deficiency form of pellagra. It seems then that hyperactivity in children is due to pellagra, a deficiency which may be caused by a lack of the substrate from which they are made or by a lack of essential nutrients which catalyze the reaction. The 1930s pellagrologists description of the children with subclinical pellagra could be used today to describe the modern children with hyperactivity and learning disorders.

Dr David F. Horrobin has been one of the foremost investigators who have brought these essential fatty acids to medical attention. EFAs assist the body in making gamma linolenic acid (GLA). It is made in the body by adding one double (unsaturated) bond to linoleic acid. It is found mainly in plant seeds, notably in evening primrose, borage, and black currant. As with all EFAs, the omega-6 series has two main functions: to provide flexibility to cell membranes and control behavior of membrane bound proteins; and to control a large number of rapid reactions in the body. Horrobin lists the following conditions which have been helped by GLA: atopic eczema, diabetic neuropathy, premenstrual syndrome, breast pain and prostatic hypertrophy, rheumatoid arthritis and other forms of inflammation, systemic sclerosis, Sjogren's syndrome, and dry eyes associated with contact lenses, gastrointestinal disorders, viral infection and post-viral fatigue syndrome, endometriosis, schizophrenia, alcoholism, cardiovascular disease, renal disease, cancer, and liver disease. It is clear that GLA is not a specific treatment for anything but that it has an enormous importance in the general health of the body. It helps repair biochemical problems which have helped create these pathological diseases. The simplest way of getting GLA is by taking evening primrose oil and other GLA rich oils. The dose range varies from under 1 gram per day to 10 grams for very serious conditions.

I. Colquhoun and S. Buondy have suggested that many of hyperactive children are deficient in essential fatty acids because they cannot metabolize linoleic acid normally, or because they cannot absorb EFAs normally from the gut, or because their EFA requirements are higher than normal. The evidence to support this hypothesis was five-fold. Most of the food constituents which caused trouble for these children are weak inhibitors of the conversion of these EFAs to prostaglandins. Boys in the study were more commonly affected than girls (about 5 times as common), corroborating other studies that show males need more EFAs than females. Many of the "hyperactive" children studied were very thirsty, often a symptom of EFA deficiency. Many had eczema and other evidence for allergies, often alleviated by EFAs. Many were deficient in zinc needed for the conversion of EFAs to prostaglandins. Some are adversely affected by wheat and dairy products which give rise to exorphins in the gut which can block the formation of prostaglandins. In a report in the *American Journal of Clinical Nutrition*, L.J. Stevens and colleagues also found decreased levels of essential fatty acids in hyperactive children.

The omega-6 type EFAs are less often lacking in the diet, but there may be difficulty in converting oleic acid to its first metabolite, linoleic acid. This is when oils rich in linoleic acid play a useful role, including evening primrose oil and borage oil. Evening primrose oil may be taken by mouth or can be applied to the skin, which is very useful for infants and children who cannot or will not swallow capsules. The dose varies between three to six capsules daily. Evening primrose oil has been helpful in treating hyperactive children. When Steven R. (age 6) was threatened with expulsion from school because of his impossible behavior, he was given evening primrose oil, 3 capsules rubbed onto his skin morning and evening. Five days later the change was remarkable. After three weeks the oil was stopped and his behavior became impossible again. Twenty-five children were treated and half of them responded. These results have been confirmed by M. Blackburn in a study published in the book *Omega-6 Esssential Fatty Acids: Pathophysiology and Roles in Clinical Medicine*.

The omega-3 essential fatty acids are present in fish oils and in flax seed. One of the best sources is linseed oil made from flax seed. Linseed oil used to be a very popular and widely consumed oil but now is mostly available in health food stores. It is very rich in omega-3 oils, up to 60 percent.

One to four tablespoonfuls per day are used. Also one may use ground flax seed as a meal, though it should be stored cold as it goes rancid very quickly. This can be added to cereal in the morning or to any food, for that matter. The common vegetable oils have a lot of the omega-6 fatty acid but are deficient in the omega-3 type. The omega-3 group are chemically more reactive, have lower melting points (they are more liquid at room temperature), and are made in cold climate plants to make them more resistant to freezing. Omega-3 fatty acids are also found in soybean oil, walnut oil, wheat germ oil, and in seafood.

Obtaining the correct oils is not that simple, however. John Finnegan in his book *The Facts about Fats* discusses some of the problems in the preparation of the commercial oils and fats. If we are to use these essential nutrients with skill and safety, it is important that we understand their chemistry and know how these oils are made. They are very unstable; they have double bonds in them which are avid for oxygen. This is why linseed oil is used to make a base for paint. For the same reason, once the oils have been extracted they will not store very well. During their deterioration or oxidation the oils are changed to products which are of no value and which may be harmful. Manufacturers have tried to avoid some of these changes by using what is called a 'cold' pressing process, which is supposed to avoid the use of heat. Heat increases oxidation and deterioration. But even when the oil is cold pressed, there is a lot of heat generated in the process, unless the oil is pressed so slowly that the heat has a chance to dissipate. This means that the cold pressed oils are little better than the heat treated oils. However, there are a few manufacturers who have produced oils that are very little deteriorated, and they store their oils under nitrogen until the bottle is opened.

Finnegan recommends that high quality oils must be produced by pressing at temperatures under 118⅓F. using light and oxygen excluding methods, then bottled in containers that prevent exposure to light that causes the oil to go rancid. He also recommends that the oils should be produced from third party, certified organically grown seed.

Amino Acids

Eight amino acids are considered essential supplements since they cannot be made in the body and adequate amounts must therefore be present in the food. These include l-tryptophan, phenyl-alanine, lysine, arginine, ornithine, and tyrosine. The other 14 amino acids are interconvertible in the body and for this reason have not been labeled "essential." These include glutamic acid, aspartic acid, cysteine, methionine, glycine, histidine, alanine, methionine, proline, serine, and threonine. They are all essential, however, and if there is a metabolic problem resulting in a deficiency of any of the 22, the results would be devastating to the body. There have been few systematic orthomolecular studies of the non-essential amino acids, but the eight essential amino acids have been examined more carefully and some have found a role in orthomolecular treatment. I will discuss l-tryptophan and tyrosine and phenylalanine from the essential group because they are so similar to each other and are therapeutic for the mental state.

L-tryptophan

Tryptophan is used clinically when it is thought that it will increase the production of serotonin in the brain. Serotonin is probably involved in controlling mood and sleep, with a deficiency causing depression and insomnia. It is also a precursor of vitamin B-3 in the form of nicotinamide adenine dinucleotide (NAD), as we have seen.

Tryptophan is used for treating depression as well for controlling manic depressive mood swings. It may be used alone or in combination with other antidepressants, such as the amine oxidase inhibitors, tyrosine and lithium. I have used tryptophan for at least the past 30 years but primarily for patients with insomnia. It is very helpful to 50 percent of the patients and they awaken in the morning without hangover. They much prefer it to hypnotics.

Tryptophan is used in doses of 500 mg to 12 grams daily. For insomnia, the dose is 1 to 3 grams taken before bed on an empty stomach. If it is taken with food, it has difficulty passing into the brain and therefore has no effect on the serotonin levels. When taken on an empty stomach, it does not have to compete with other amino acids. For depression I have been using 3 to 6 grams daily, as well as for manic depressives (the bipolar disease).

Phenylalanine and Tyrosine

Phenylalanine is partially converted into tyrosine. When the body cannot

make any, it causes a condition known as phenylketonuria. Untreated it
leads to mental retardation which may be very severe. These children have
to be on special phenylalanine free diets. Phenylalanine is used as a treatment for depression; the dl-form is helpful in controlling pain. Tyrosine is
a precursor to catecholamines (noradrenalin, etc.) and to thyroid hormone. It is also the precursor to melanin, a major pigment in the body. It
has antidepressant properties, probably because it acts in the same way in
the body as does phenylalanine.

Dr Priscilla Slagle, a psychiatrist, uses a combination of tryptophan
with phenylalanine and tyrosine as a treatment for depression. She was
depressed herself for many years, did not respond to the usual treatment,
but recovered on the program she developed, as she describes in her book
The Way Up From Down. She recommends that people suffering from
depression take tyrosine 500 to 3500 mg on rising in the morning and again
mid afternoon. These should be taken without high protein food. One
starts with 500 to 1000 mg daily for one week, then the dose is increased
gradually depending upon the response. After several weeks or months if
the response is not adequate, she adds phenylalanine to the program.

She also recommends l-tryptophan, 500 to 6000 mg at bed time, taken
on an empty stomach or with carbohydrate, not with protein; B complex
(50) at breakfast and again after dinner at night; ascorbic acid, to 4 grams
daily; and a good multimineral preparation providing calcium 250-1000
mg, magnesium 125-599 mg, manganese 10-30 mg, zinc 15-30 mg, selenium 50-200 mcg, and chromium 50-200 mcg. Dr Slagle also prescribes
dietary changes to improve this. Everyone who is depressed ought to read
her book. The results are probably as good if not better than the results
using antidepressant drugs. The program is more complicated than simply
taking a few pills each day but for many may be preferable.

Minerals

The body needs many minerals. Some like calcium and magnesium are
needed in substantial amounts, while others like selenium are needed in
trace amounts. It may well be that every mineral present in the oceans is

required. Every chemist knows how difficult it is to keep metallic impurities out of his purest of preparations or out of solutions. Producing pure chemicals requires an enormous amount of energy and time. It is likely that living matter had an equally difficult time in keeping out toxic elements. It would make good evolutionary sense for living cells to allow traces of these elements and to learn how to make use of them, making a virtue out of necessity. It would take too much energy to keep their composition absolutely pure. If this is true, every mineral would eventually find a useful role. There is an optimum amount needed. If it is high, it is needed in gram doses, if very low, in microgram quantities. In contrast to the vitamins there is a narrow range between optimum and toxic doses. Either too little or too much is dangerous. Luckily most of our foodstuffs do not contain excessive amounts of minerals. But they may be absorbed from the contaminants of our air, water and soil.

Trace elements make up a very small part of our diet but they are indispensable. They have been ignored by behavioral scientists and of course by physicians because of the belief our diets were adequate and trace element deficiencies rare. Since trace element deficiencies are widespread in domestic animals who often are better fed than humans it would be highly unlikely we are better off. Minerals are lost in washing and cooking foods. There is anther loss due to drugs. Many drugs are chelating agents. They bind with metal ions and sweep them out of the body. In his book *The Trace Elements and Man*, H.A. Schroeder was concerned about the number of patients on drugs who in time developed collagen disease, liver damage, arthritis, and blood disease. This has not been reported after treatment with naturally occurring substances such as digitalis, morphine, hormones, vitamins, and plant extractives in general. He thought these diseases may have resulted from a deficiency in trace elements.

Toxicity of minerals ranges from those that are toxic in microgram amounts to those toxic only when very large amounts are taken in. But the toxic elements are those who have no known biological function in the body and for whom no minimum need has been discovered. These include cadmium, lead, antimony, mercury, arsenic, and aluminum. Essential in small amounts but toxic in large amounts are selenium, germanium, tin, barium, fluorine, chromium, and copper.

Calcium and Phosphorus

Our bones hold 99 percent of the calcium and 80 percent of the phosphorus in our bodies. The smaller amounts in the rest of the body are vital. Calcium decreases neuromuscular excitability, normalizes nerve impulse transmission. Phosphorus is a key component of the high energy phosphate bonds and of enzymes such as the nucleotides. The amount absorbed from the gastro intestinal system depends upon what is present in the food, the acidity of the stomach and bowel, the ratio of calcium to phosphorus, and the presence of compounds such as iron, lead, and manganese which form insoluble phosphates. Phytic acid (inositol hexaphosphate) binds calcium and magnesium and impairs absorption. Lactic acid and a high protein diet increases absorption. Vitamin D-3 is essential for normal absorption and counteracts the effect of phytic acid. Blood plasma levels range from 8.5 to 11.5 mg 100 ml, while phosphorus levels range between 3 to 3.5 mg per 100 ml. Vitamins A, D-3, and C are all essential in the metabolism of bones.

Adults require 1 to 1.5 G of phosphorus daily and about 1 to 1.5 grams of calcium. The need increases to 1.5 G for nursing and pregnant women. Milk and dairy products are good sources if the individual is not allergic to them. Too much phosphorus, such as is provided by a high protein diet, will decrease retention of calcium by bones and is a main factor in osteoporosis.

Magnesium

The adult body contains about 25 grams of magnesium, half in the bones. Normally we eat 300 mg daily and absorb about one third from the small intestine. Blood levels are regulated by the amount absorbed, losses in sweat and in the urine. Absorption is controlled by the same factors which control calcium absorption. It is essential in about 100 different reactions. Large doses are narcotic and anticonvulsant. A deficiency causes tetany, seizures, ataxia, irritability, depression, and psychotic behavior or any combination. These are quickly reversed when the magnesium is replaced.

Under stress magnesium is lost. This occurs in surgical or traumatic stress, after severe burns, excessive sweating, infections. But short-lived deficiencies do not produce major symptoms. Still it is advisable to take extra magnesium during these stress related events. It can be given parentally. The usual tablets containing calcium and magnesium are about 25 percent absorbable.

Copper and Zinc

The body contains about 80 to 100 mg of copper bound with other substances. The average diet provides about 2 to 5 mg of which 1 mg is absorbed. Copper levels may be high due to copper plumbing, especially if the water is soft and slightly acidic. There is seldom a deficiency of copper in North America. It can occur in areas where soils are copper deficient.

Zinc and copper are inversely related in the blood. If copper levels are high, zinc levels tend to be low. The body has about 2 grams of zinc. Normal diets contain about 10 to 15 mg but one third is absorbed. It is a constituent of over 20 enzymes. It participates in protein synthesis, hormone release, and promotes healing after wounds or burns. A zinc deficiency retards growth, increases sensitivity to insulin, and causes changes in taste and smell.

Stress will quickly decrease zinc levels. Injured tissue needs a lot of zinc. Zinc is also lowered with contraceptive medication and in porphyrinuria and in pyrroluria. A zinc deficiency may lead to apathy, lethargy, decreased activity and difficulty in learning. Growth will be retarded. Some adolescent children grow more slowly because they are short of zinc. Because zinc and copper compete with each other in many reactions, a diet high in zinc will decrease the activity of ceruloplasmin, the copper containing enzyme. Adding copper restores its activity. Too much zinc is very rare but can produce anemia. Zinc decreases absorption of copper from the intestine and thus decreases levels in the blood. Zinc also protects against the harmful effects of cadmium.

Children with pyrroluria need extra zinc. I usually give about 15 to 25 mg daily for children and 50 mg per day for adults. Malnourished children are deficient in some of the minerals. This will be shown in their hair analyses. Hair zinc values were a good indicator of their nutritional state. Under 60 ug/g was associated with severe malnutrition. Normal children had over 100 ug/g.

Cadmium

This mineral accumulates in tissues with age, especially in smokers. Children who are exposed to smoking may have a problem but many children are already smoking by the time they are 11 years old. This decreases the amount of vitamin C in the blood. Vitamin C detoxifies cadmium. A high fiber diet does also. Cadmium is also present in car tire dust.

Thyroid

Soon after hypothyroidism was discovered over 100 years ago, an association was found between lack of thyroid and emotional and behavioral problems. But these patients had a very severe form of the disorder called myxedema which is quite rare today. It was due to a serious deficiency of iodine so that the thyroid gland could not make its hormone. In *Hypothyroidism: The Unsuspected Illness*, Dr Broda Barnes and L. Galton used basal body temperature as a measure of hypothyroidism. Body temperature is a functional test of thyroid hormone activity, for without thyroid the cells cannot maintain normal body temperature even if everything else is normal. Blood tests merely tell us how much hormone is circulating in the blood, not how well it is used. When these patients in this study were given supplementary dessicated thyroid, they became normal. Among the cases they described are children who had severe learning disorders and who became well with supplementation. Barnes's findings, corroborated by S.E. Langer and J.F. Scheer in *The Riddle of Illness*, have not been taken seriously by the medical profession but are used by many alternate practitioners. I have found it very valuable. I have seen many patients who tested normal on all blood tests for thyroid, who had low body temperatures and who became better with thyroid.

I think the main reason dessicated thyroid treatment fell from favor was that when the pure hormones T-4 and T-3 became available, drug supply companies stopped advertising the dried preparation and advertised their own product. Physicians were taught that only these pure hormones should be used because the dosage would be more precise. Desiccated thyroid contains combinations of T-3 and T-4. It is also taught that unless the blood levels indicate there is a deficiency it should not be used. Yet some of my patients with normal blood levels responded to thyroid and several patients with low levels who had not responded to the pure hormones were made well when they were given the dessicated thyroid instead.

Recently E.D. Wilson described "Wilson's syndrome," which is caused by a blockage in the conversion of T-4 to T-3. The levels of T-4 and T-3 and TSH are normal but the end receptors, the tissues, are not able to use T-3, the active hormone. T-4 must be converted into T-3. Using T-3 (Cytomel in Canada), Wilson has able to restore the ability of the body to make this conversion. This has cured many patients of a variety of obscure diseases which had not responded to other treatment. I have just started to use this treatment idea on adults and have already found it very helpful.

Vitamin vs Drug Therapy

Side Effects of Megavitamin Therapy

Every chemical, either made by nature or by mankind, will have both hazards and benefits when used in treatment. These must always be balanced. If the benefit is much greater than the hazard, even dangerous drugs will be used. There are very few drugs as dangerous as insulin, which in large doses can quickly lead to irreversible hypoglycemia and death. Yet the benefits are so manifest that millions of people can use it successfully once they are trained how to avoid the dangers. If the benefit is great, a good deal of toxicity can be tolerated. If the benefit is very slight, then even minor toxicity should be avoided. In medical compendiums where drugs are described in extensive detail, the measure of the relative benefit may be estimated by the number of words used to describe the indications and uses and the number of words used to describe the contra indications, the side effects and the toxicities. With drugs, the number of words used to describe dangers are much greater than those used to detail their uses. With natural substances commonly found in the body, the reverse is true. The number of words needed to describe dangers is much less.

In pharmacology, in the study of drugs, each drug is assessed for its therapeutic effect and for its toxicity. This is mandatory. The drug will not be released for general patient use unless the government agencies are convinced that the drugs are effective and relatively safe. These studies are done by feeding the drugs first to a variety of animals for a long enough period of time. Since animals used in the laboratory are short lived, they are on the drugs for a substantial proportion of their life span. The animals are examined for any pathological changes in their organs, for the effect the drugs have on growth rate, on their ability to reproduce, and of course for the LD_{50}, the measure of the ability of drugs to kill.

A positive side effect is a beneficial effect arising from medication for the treatment of a specific condition above and beyond what one would expect. For example, if a patient with cardiovascular disease, with high blood cholesterol and triglycerides is given niacin to lower his fat levels and if he then feels less depressed, more energetic and healthier, this would be a positive side effect. This would not be observed with drugs such as the new statins whose only action is to lower blood fat levels. Conversely, if a patient with schizophrenia is given niacin to treat his disease and also has a beneficial lowering of his blood fat level, this would be a positive side effect. This would not be achieved with tranquilizers.

Nevertheless, megavitamins potentially can cause negative side effects and even toxicity. Since they may occur, it is necessary for the patient and physician to be aware of them and to know what to do a if they should occur. None of the children I have ever treated, however, has been damaged by the use of vitamins. When we first began to use megadoses in 1951 we were aware of this and therefore carried out very careful studies of the vitamins we were using. The vitamin literature at that time was reassuring. Toxicity trials had been conducted on animals which showed there was a wide margin of safety. Smaller animals, including dogs could take up to 4 g of niacin per kg of body weight for many months. This is equivalent to about 280 g, over one half a pound, of vitamin B-3 for a 70 kg person. Since no human has died from this vitamin, there was no way of telling how much would be needed to kill someone. I mentioned before one patient who, in a suicidal rage, swallowed the whole bottle of niacin, 500 mg tablets. The 200 tablets made her stomach sore for about three days. I have known patients who took 50 g daily for many months with no discomfort.

As such, vitamin B-3 is considered non-toxic. Since it is very effective for a large number of diseases, it has a very wide therapeutic index – that is, the ratio of the toxic dose to the effective dose is enormous. The same applies to vitamin C and all other water soluble vitamins.

A toxic reaction is one which if allowed to continue will lead to serious injury or death. Fortunately, the water soluble vitamins are so safe. There have been no deaths from vitamin C or from pyridoxine. There have been two from slow release forms of niacin, none from niacinamide. With a phenomenon as rare as this it is almost impossible to assign blame to any particular nutrient. For the average adult, taking vitamin B-3 is safer than not taking it. In other words, there is an increased risk of death when off the vitamin. This is because niacin prolongs high quality life and decreases mortality.

The water soluble vitamins are so safe because they are readily excreted and therefore can not build up to toxic levels in the body. They have probably been present before life itself began to develop and life has had millions of years to use and adapt to them. They are so bulky that it would be impossible to commit suicide by taking niacin or vitamin C. The body would reject them by vomiting long before there would be any harm done. The major toxic reaction, very rare, is jaundice.

Vitamin B-3

These are the common beneficial side effects of vitamin B-3 treatment but there are others: (1) an anti-arthritic effect of both forms of vitamin B-3; (2) beneficial blood fat effects, decrease in total cholesterol, decrease in triglycerides, elevation of HDL, and decrease in the ratio of total cholesterol over HDL; (3) an anti-senility effect; (4) a general healing effect on all tissues, including burns and wounds; (5) an anti-cancer effect.

The most striking negative effect is the pronounced flush which occurs in most people when they first take niacin. It usually begins in the forehead and gradually works its way down the body. It usually stops somewhere in the abdomen but on rare occasions may affect the whole body. The flushed areas feel hot and prickly. The flush is over within about three hours, then slowly fades. Thereafter, each time the niacin is taken the flush is less intense and in most people will be of little consequence in a few weeks. Patients must be forewarned this will happen for it can be very frightening. A small number of patients do not adapt in the same way, and if they still flush excessively after a few weeks, will have to stop taking the same dose. The extent and rapidity of the flush depends upon the amount taken and whether or not there is food in the stomach. This flush (vasodilatation) is not a direct effect of the niacin but is due to the release of histamine from the mast cells because of an effect on the prostaglandins.

Any factor which quickly elevates blood niacin will quickly cause the maximum flush. Injections intra venously will produce an almost immediate reaction. The niacin is absorbed most rapidly in the stomach. A solution of niacin in a hot drink would probably cause a very intense flush. Conversely, anything which slows down the release of niacin and its absorption in the stomach will reduce the intensity of the flush. Thus a cold drink taken after a large meal will moderate the flush. Some patients enjoy the flush. These are usually patients with arthritis who find the effect on their joints soothing. Most patients do not object to this side effect.

The flush can be moderated by by-passing the stomach with sustained release preparations. I generally do not like these preparations even though some patients cannot tolerate any other form. The three or so patients who have been damaged by niacin used a slow release preparation. Many years ago I tested an aluminum nicotinate for a drug company. It was a terrible product and caused extreme abdominal discomfort. A better way is to combine the niacin with another substance which then releases the vitamin slowly. The best are esters such as inositol niacinate. This is one inositol molecule surrounded and bound to 6 niacin molecules. It is hydrolyzed slowly in the body and the niacin is not released fast enough to cause sufficient histamine release to produce the flush. A patient discovered that if he took 250 mg of inositol just five minutes before he took the niacin, most of the flush reaction was alleviated. I have passed this tip on to others and they have found the inositol similarly helpful.

Antihistamines will also moderate the flush. They can be taken before or during. They can do so because the flush is caused by the histamine which is released. But the best anti-flush substance is niacin because when one takes it regularly it prevents any flushing. The niacin empties the histamine storage sites and there is no time between doses for the build up to recur. Patients may only flush in the morning after an overnight fast. This means there has been enough time for the histamine to build up in the storage sites. When this happens, I advise the patient to take the last dose just before bed. Niacin probably decreases heparin content of the mast cells as well. This may be advantageous since the heparin molecules are remarkable scavenger molecules. They tend to bind all sorts of toxic molecules and help remove them from the body. One or two aspirins taken a few days before starting the niacin can also moderate the flush.

If the flush is too intense or if it is feared, this may be the case a lower starting dose should be used. If the flush is contraindicated for any reason including cosmetic ones – for example, flushing at unexpected times – then niacinamide should be used. Only 1 percent of the people who take niacinamide flush. The second side effect is nausea, and if the vitamin dosage is not adjusted, vomiting. If one increases the dose of either form, eventually that person will develop nausea. Niacinamide has a lower nauseant dose than niacin. Dr D. Hawkins has suggested this could be used to determine the optimum dose. One would increase the dose slowly until the patient began to have nausea, then the dose would be decreased by 1 g. Thus if the patient became nauseated on 7 g daily, the optimum dose would be 6 g.

If the nauseant dose for either form is too low, the patient can still get sufficient B-3 by using both, each at its optimum level. If the nauseant dose is 3 g daily for both, one could use 2 g of each daily and not have nausea. Sometimes the nausea can be controlled by tranquilizers. If the nausea is severe, the vitamin should be stopped because it may lead to vomiting and this could lead to dehydration.

Medicine inherited a false fear of niacin long before we began to use it in megadoses. In the 1950s a wave of interest developed for a disease caused by depletion of methyl groups. Methyl group deficiency, it was believed, produced fatty livers in a few animal experiments using rats. Niacin is one of the few methyl acceptors. It was logical to think that a large dose of niacin would remove too many of these methyl groups and that this would lead to fatty degeneration of the liver. In these early animal experiments, the proportion of fat in these livers from these animals increased from about 3 percent to 11 percent. The idea of the hepatic toxicity of niacin arose from this single experiment on these rats. However, a few years ago

Professor R. Altschul repeated the experiment using the same type of animals and found no increase in fat content of the liver, nor were there any histological pathological changes when liver sections were examined under the microscope. Professor Altschul concluded that the early results were fallacious because the laboratory used infected animals. Before 1950 it was very difficult to maintain disease free animals.

Even though the original experiment could not be repeated, this fear of vitamin B-3 toxicity has not died. The idea of hepato toxicity was bolstered by the observation that liver function tests indicated there was something wrong. However, when the niacin was stopped the tests became normal within five days, long before any damaged liver could have repaired itself. Furthermore, patients on niacin a long time were found not to have damaged livers by any other tests, nor was there any clinical indication of this. In a major niacin study by Dr William B. Parsons Junior, liver toxicity did not occur. The best evidence was the fact that the only patients in this comprehensive study that lived longer with a lower mortality rate were the patients on niacin. This beneficial effect continued long after the niacin was discontinued.

Still, I have seen a few patients become jaundiced on niacin. It was an obstructive type jaundice which cleared rapidly when the niacin was stopped. In some of these patients I resumed the niacin and the jaundice did not recur. I have estimated that about 1 patient out of 1000 may get jaundice. This is so infrequent that it is difficult to show cause and effect since out of a thousand some will get jaundice for other reasons. A large proportion of the patients I started on niacin were schizophrenic and alcoholic. A physician in Saskatoon, who saw very few schizophrenics and alcoholics, treated over 600 patients without a single case of jaundice. These two groups of patients are more prone to developing jaundice in any event. One 7-year-old child needed vitamin B-3 very badly, but on either form he would turn yellow in a couple of days, even though his liver function tests remained normal. On inositol niacinate he did not turn yellow over a five year period of observation. I am still puzzled by this finding. It has been recommended that liver function tests be done at regular intervals. In my opinion this is not necessary. If jaundice does develop there, is ample time to stop the vitamin.

Niacinamide has no effect on carbohydrate metabolism as measured on the sugar tolerance curve, though niacin has a variable effect. In one third of the subjects I tested, it increased glucose tolerance, in one third it had no effect, and in the last third it decreased it. For this reason no glucose tolerance test should be run unless the patient has been off the niacin for at least five days. Diabetics may have to adjust their insulin requirement up or down but the adjustment in doses is usually slight. I do recommend it be given to diabetics since it protects them from developing the vascular side effects of this disease. It lowers their triglycerides and total cholesterol and elevates the HDL. Niacinamide decreases the chance that children genetically predisposed will develop juvenile diabetes.

Niacin increases blood uric acid levels slightly but it does not increase the tendency to gout and can be given to gouty patients. I have treated several with niacin for other conditions. One of my patients had both gout and arthritis. On niacin his arthritis came under control but he continued to have his episodes of gout at the same rate as before he had started to take the vitamin. Blood levels of uric acid are positively correlated with a species life span. Uric acid is an efficient antioxidant, a scavenger of free radicals. It is about as efficient as ascorbic acid. Humans cannot break it down. Perhaps this is a partial replacement for vitamin C which we cannot make. Part of the beneficial action of niacin may therefore come from the slight elevation of uric acid.

Because niacin is an organic acid it has been feared that it would make people with peptic ulcer worse. However, niacin is such a weak acid that when it is dumped into the stomach it has a minor effect on the acidity of the stomach. One study showed that it bound more hydrogen ions than it released – that it decreased the acidity slightly. However, niacin releases histamine and in a few subjects the histamine has greatly increased the secretion of acid in the stomach. Most of the patients with peptic ulcer find not only that niacin is no problem in causing pain, but that it facilitates the healing of the ulcer. The worst part about the niacin is its name, nicotinic acid. It is the term acid which frightens patients.

Rarely adults develop edema in their ankles, especially in very hot weather. It is a benign dependent edema which usually clears by morning. It can be removed by lowering the dose of niacin. Over the past two years I have found that adding folic acid, 5 mg per gram of niacin, will be of great help in removing this peripheral edema. Very rarely the flush and itch is so great it is intolerable. One patient had a rash over her whole body and it cleared when the niacin was stopped. Antihistamines will help remove this rash and may also prevent it from occurring. Sometimes niacin drys the skin.

The thalidomide affair is still not forgotten. Many women are concerned about the possible effect of what they take during their pregnancies and many doctors still warn their pregnant patients that they may harm their babies by taking vitamins. Many of my patients who have been on vitamin B-3 for years will call because their doctor has told them they must stop taking their vitamin when they are pregnant. They then risk becoming sick themselves. There is no evidence any baby has been damaged by taking these vitamins, however. On the contrary, I have now given this vitamin to over 5,000 patients and I cannot recall a single instance where any of the women have given birth to any child with a defect. Their children have been healthy. Since many of my population of patients were schizophrenic, more prone to have birth defect babies (about 3 percent compared to 1 percent for non schizophrenic women), it is possible that the use of the vitamin prevents birth defect. This should not be surprising since if the vitamin helps the mother become and stay well, it will certainly do the same for their babies who have similar genes. In addition, vitamin B-3 has been shown to protect animals against the teratogenic effect of thalidomide. Had the women who were given this drug had ample amounts of this vitamin in their diet they might have given birth to normal children. I do not consider pregnancy a contraindication for vitamin B-3. On the contrary I think they should all take extra B-vitamins, including vitamin B-3.

The best way to consider toxicity is to compare the toxicity of a compound against the toxicity of medication which has been released for therapeutic use. I have selected clozapine to compare with niacin as an example of one of the most toxic drugs which is recommended for the treatment of schizophrenia. Clozapine was announced with great fanfare and some of our most eminent schizophrenia research psychiatrists jumped on the bandwagon stating this was a major contribution to the treatment. They have consistently ignored the use of vitamin B-3. To make this comparison I have compared niacin against clozapine by the number of lines of writing used to describe them in the *Compendium of Pharmaceuticals and Specialties*, 30 edition, 1995.

	Niacin	Clozapine
Indications	13 lines	2 lines
Contra indications	6	over 400
Precautions	34	about 110
Adverse effects	0	about 360
Total warnings	70	870
Ratio T/I*	5.4	27.2

T = total warnings, I = indications.

It is obvious which compound is the most dangerous.

Vitamin C

Every physician who has studied the medical literature and has used vitamin C or ascorbic acid knows not only that it is safe but remarkably beneficial with only minor and transient side effects. I can best describe how safe and beneficial it is by quoting from a report prepared by Dr John Marks, Fellow, Tutor and Director of Medical Studies, Girton College, Cambridge: "This is a vitamin that has been consistently administered in high dosages for very prolonged periods. Quantities in excess of 1 gram are being ingested by many people as a prophylactic against the common cold, in various cancers, in the detoxification of drug addicts, in schizophrenias, for wound healing and for the prevention of the formation of nitrosamines in the stomach. Some critics of high dose vitamin C administration have alleged that the substance causes kidney stones through the increased excretion of oxalate: interference with vitamin B-12 metabolism; rebound scurvy upon sudden cessation of therapy; excessive iron absorption and a mutagenic effect. . . . An extensive and very thorough analysis of the data during the past years has disproved all the serious allegations. Some patients, particularly in the early days of high-dose administration, do experience a laxative effect. Even this mild and harmless adverse effect is not found consistently."

Vitamin C is remarkably safe but this has not prevented the formation of a delusional system about it initiated by Dr V. Herbert, who published the first suggestion that vitamin C could cause kidney stones and soon followed this with indications that the "could" had been changed to "would." Yet there has been not a single scientific account of this ever happening and all the recent investigators working with vitamin C have ignored this pseudo-finding. I have never seen vitamin C cause this reaction in over 40 years of using it in large doses. Dr R. Cathcart has had an amazing experience with vitamin C on huge numbers of his patients. He told me that the incidence of kidney stones in his practice is much less than one would expect, not the contrary. Neither does vitamin C cause kidney or liver damage, also ideas put forward by opponents of megadoses vitamin therapy. They tried to scare people away by these erroneous claims and succeeded in scaring doctors away from giving it to their patients. Perhaps one day someone will work out the cost of this pernicious attempt to deprive people of the good health they could have had by taking vitamin C.

A few of my patients were allergic to vitamin C and could not tolerate even small doses such as 50 mg. This is probably due to their extreme sensitivity to trace amounts of chemicals still present in the crystalline product derived from the source or by the chemical process used in converting glucose into ascorbic acid. They could not be allergic to the vitamin C present in food or else they would have been dead long ago. No one can live without vitamin C.

The most common negative side effect with vitamin C is a loosening of the bowels which in the extreme may lead to diarrhea. This is dose related. According to Dr Cathcart, this can be used to determine the optimum dose. One increases the amount until this occurs and then decreases it one or two grams daily. It varies enormously from a few to over 50 g daily. I have not given children more than 3 g daily and have seldom run into this problem. It is a useful laxative, especially for the elderly constipated individual.

Vitamin B-6

Pyridoxine in the doses I have used, up to 750 mg daily, has not caused any serious side effects. It may increase irritability and should be combined with magnesium to prevent this from happening. I do not always need to add magnesium.

Pyridoxine is receiving increasing attention as a nutrient involved in the protection against arteriosclerosis, heart disease, and strokes. It is one of the nutrients essential in the conversion of homocysteine to the non-toxic cystathionine. I have discussed this under folic acid, another of these essential nutrients. J.G. Hattersley has provided us with a comprehensive outline of the relation between pyridoxine and the development of ather-osclerosis. His interest was aroused when he heard about the pioneer work being done by a physician practicing in Johannesburg, South Africa. Dr Moses M. Suzman, an internist, had theorized that atherosclerosis was a vitamin deficiency disease. He suspected multiple vitamin and mineral deficiencies, primarily vitamin B-6. He published an abstract of his work using pyridoxine 200 mg, folic acid 5 mg and vitamin E 100 to 600 iu, all daily. He also used other nutrients in smaller amounts. Of 62 typical heart patients followed for an average of 52 months there were four reinfarcts (two were fatal). Dr J.M. Ellis has been using pyridoxine for a long time to treat carpal tunnel syndrome with great success. He too observed that few of his patients on this vitamin had heart attacks.

There are very few side effects and the ones that do occur are minor and transient. Much has been made of the few patients collected from several medical schools who took between 2,000 and 6,000 mg per day. The paper describing these results was quite inadequate because it did not describe whether they were taking any other nutrients and what type of diet they were on. These patients developed a peripheral neuropathy which cleared after a year. But based on this report the idea became current that vitamin B-6 was toxic. Dr Marks, however, counters this myth: "It has been claimed that high doses of pyridoxine can lead to liver damage, interference with the normal functions of riboflavin, and a dependency state. With the possible exception of the dependency states, these suggestions are not substantiated by scientific data. The dependency states were very transient."

Tryptophan

In the United States, tryptophan is not available because many fear it is toxic. Although it has been shown that the toxicity was caused by a contaminant, not by pure amino acid, this amino acid still has not been released and is now the center of a major controversy between the FDA and the health food industry and physicians who had been using it very successfully. In Canada it was available from health food stores and also on prescription. The health food store preparation has been withdrawn but the prescription products called Tryptan have not and have been freely available throughout that controversy.

Here is what happened. In October 1989 several people in New Mexico became very tired with sore muscles. Their white blood cells were increased. All had taken the amino acid. This condition was later called eosinophilia-myalgia syndrome (EMS) and was reported in Europe and elsewhere in America. Symptoms included pain, swelling of the extremities, and severe muscle symptoms involving nerve damage. The eosinophil count went high. By August 1990 more than 1500 cases had been reported with 27 deaths. In November 1989 tryptophan supplements were recalled, and a few months later all products containing tryptophan were also recalled.

The Center for Disease Control suggested, however, that the problem was caused by a contaminant. Six companies in Japan made all the tryptophan used in the United States. In October 1990, K. Sakimoto isolated and identified an impurity from tryptophan which, in acid fluid, like in the stomach, broke down into tryptophan and a toxic chemical. Even though tryptophan was thus proven safe and effective, the FDA has still not removed the ban on its use. The health food industry believes that this is a political decision, not based upon scientific data, and is fighting back.

Tyrosine and Phenylalanine

In Canada tyrosine and phenylalanine are not readily available. The Food and Drug Division of Health and Welfare appears to want to prevent people from looking after their own health by placing a number of unwarranted restrictions on the sale of amino acids. In 1989 their expert advisory committee on amino acids submitted the results of their deliberations: "Low daily doses of the amino acids, such as 500 mg in capsule form, were perceived as not being harmful for the healthy individual, with the possible exception of tryptophan. There was no evidence that consumption of free-form amino acids in amounts equivalent to the daily intake would be unsafe if added to the daily diet and consumed throughout the day." However, the committee saw no rationale for the use of the amino acids as nutritional supplements and worried about the long term side effects: "There would appear to be no convincing rationale for having amino acids generally available to the public. If amino acids exert the pharmacological effects claimed, they are unsafe if not taken under medical supervision for a specific benefit; if they do not exert these effects, then there is no reason for marketing them. Furthermore, all of these amino acids were considered to have the potential for producing certain toxic effects in susceptible individuals or if consumed in large amounts for an extended duration." The key word is potential. There is nothing which is not potentially dangerous, even water. They did not discuss the actual toxic reactions and harm done to people who had taken these amino acids without medical supervision, or even with it.

On the one hand, the committee concluded these amino acids were safe. On the other hand, they concluded they might be dangerous. The FDA is tied to its pet scheme that anything for which claims are made, except for food, must be dispensed by prescription to protect the public. Since the use of amino acids, like vitamins, cannot be patented, there is no incentive for any company to spend the immense sums of money required to convince the FDA that they should not interfere in the sale of these safe products. If they were to be consistent, all the vitamins must be taken off the market. This, I think, they are afraid to do because of the enormous backlash from the public and even from the medical profession which would be inundated with huge number of patients demanding prescriptions. It would be similar to the experience in the Canadian Maritime provinces long ago when people could buy liquor only on prescription. There have been rumors that they are thinking of such a move, but I was advised by one of the ministers of health, when I inquired, that they would never do so. But as few people are aware of the value of the amino acid, they can with impunity introduce regulations which, in my opinion, are totally unwarranted. They hope that the public remains generally ignorant and that people will never develop the same enthusiasm and affection for amino acids that they now have for vitamins and minerals. They are trying to forestall a problem they see developing which would go against their policies. The FDA should be restricted to making sure that all products sold are non-toxic (that is, less toxic than are the over-the-counter drugs they allow all drug stores to dispense so freely) and that the label requirements are met. I would be happier if they would put aspirin on prescription. Many people die from aspirin each year, while no one has died from the use of pure vitamin and amino acid supplements.

In my opinion, Dr D. Rowland, Canadian Institute of Nutrition, made the most sensible recommendation. He argued that the consumer should be allowed access to these nutrients because amino acids are similar to vitamins and hence are non-toxic; there are more hazardous substances available, such as cigarettes and alcohol. All of the over-the-counter non-prescription items such as antihistamines, analgesics, and cough medicines are much more dangerous than any of the nutrients. The consumer should be helped to make informed choices. If no benefit is derived from a product, the consumer will not buy it.

Toximolecular Treatments

The three key vitamins (B-3, B-6, and C) in the orthomolecular treatment of children with brain dysfunctions and behavioral disorders are non-toxic and relatively free of side effects, unlike the drugs used in "toximolecular" treatments.

The following orthomolecular (vitamins) vs toximolecular (drugs) table created by Dr Bernard Rimland in consultation with Dr Humphry Osmond outlines in more detail the relative toxicity of vitamins and drugs as used in treating children.

When Dr Osmond read Dr Rimland's megavitamin study on a large series of sick children, it occurred to him that this data lent itself to an examination of the efficacy as against the toxicity of drugs and vitamins. Efficacy is the improvement due to the drug while toxicity is applied to any worsening of the condition. Relative efficacy will be the ratio of the first over the second. Thus if a drug helped 50 percent of the treated population and made 10 percent worse, the relative efficacy ratio (RE) would be 5. If it helped 25 percent and made 25 percent worse, it would be 1. If it helped 10 percent and made 50 percent worse, RE would be 0.20. Obviously the best drugs will have high RE ratios. To make these estimates I have added the number of children who were definitely helped or showed improvement over the number made a little worse or much worse.

Medication	Total	Helped	Worsened	Ratio (RE)
Dexedrine	172	44	80	0.55
Benadril	151	34	25	1.36
Deanol	73	17	10	1.70
Dilantin	204	57	43	1.33
Stelazine	120	40	28	1.43
Valium	106	31	31	1.00
Ritalin	66	22	27	0.81
Mysoline	10	4	4	1.00
Mellaril	277	101	55	1.84
All drugs	1591	440	425	1.00
Vitamins	191	127	7	18.14

It is clear that the vitamin program is much more effective with a very high RE. The best drug, mellaril, has an RE of 1.84.

Where change occurs, mellaril and the vitamins apart, it is as likely to be for the *worse* as for the *better*. This applies to both categories of improvement and worsening. With mellaril the chances are 2:1 in favor of improvement. I am a poor statistician but go by Sir Ronald Fisher's rule, as told to me by Leonide Goldstein, that in medicine the kind of statistics you need are those that don't require statistics. Mellaril looks better to me than the assembled drugs. However, when we come to the vitamins, the chances of being definitely helped are three times that of mellaril, while the chance of being made much worse are less than 1:25. If one concentrates on the definitely helped/much worse figures, compares mellaril and vitamins, and uses the product of these two categories, by my reckoning the vitamins are 12 times as effective as mellaril because they are (roughly) three times more likely to produce *definite help* and four times less likely to do harm. I do not know what medicines have ever been assessed in this way before, but it seems to me that an examination of this and other medical procedures in these terms would be possible and might throw a very different light on drug and other treatment effectiveness.

I do not doubt that there are more elegant and efficient ways than those which I have suggested here to inform patients and parents about the relative benefits and risks of vitamin vs drug therapy, but since at this moment so far as I know no method of this kind is in general use, mine can stand until superseded. It has much bearing when it comes to measuring the nature and extent of improvements in medicine, surgery, and health care over the years. In my experience medical matters are rarely presented in this manner. Were this done so it might be easier for us to discriminate among the various treatments available and allow doctors, patients, and their families to chart realistically the best course of treatment. This approach would also draw our attention to those illnesses in which the current natural history has been insufficiently investigated for us to be able to make a reasoned and reasonable decision regarding the changes that treatment will help rather than hinder.

One can argue that Rimland's data applies to a special group of children who had failed to respond to drugs and that they were therefore not representative of these children at large, but not for very long. Rather, the data reinforces the conclusion that the megavitamin approach is superior since it improves a large proportion of children who have failed to respond to standard drugs and with very few side effects. If all the children had been started on megavitamins, not just the failures, it is highly probable the treatment results would have been much superior. Also most of these children were autistic or schizophrenic, the sickest and most difficult of all children to treat.

Megavitamins thus fit the "Millichap" definition of the ideal drug much better than do any of the other drugs tested by Rimland. Dr Millichap defined the ideal drug as follows: "The ideal drug for the treatment of children with minimal brain dysfunction should control hyperactivity, increase the span of attention, reduce impulsive and aggressive behavior and have measurable beneficial effects on visual and auditory perception, reading ability and coordination without inducing insomnia, anorexia, drowsiness or other more serious toxic effects." What Millichap demands is not available in any of the standard chemotherapies but this would not be an argument against drugs if no better treatment were available. His treatment of choice is ritalin, methyl phenidate, even though it does not meet his own criteria. However, he was not aware of the therapeutic efficacy of megavitamin therapy. He reported that out of 367 children treated 84 percent were improved and 14 percent suffered side effects. We do not know his definition of improved. Certainly ritalin decreases hyperactive behavior, and if this is all that is needed, but it has been unsuccessful in helping the children I have seen who are "failures" on ritalin treatment.

The usual dose for ritalin is 10 to 30 mg daily. Parents give it in the morning and at noon. By the time their children are home from school, they are becoming very restless again. The main side effects are nervousness, insomnia, anorexia, and interference with normal growth (weight gain and height), stomachache and rashes. A glimpse of the usual description of ritalin in any compendium will illustrate the number of potential side effects as compared to the therapeutic effect.

I am amazed that ritalin with an RE of 0.81 should be so popular compared to mellaril. Credit must be given to the two companies selling these products, to the manufacturer of ritalin for promoting it so well and to the maker of mellaril for not promoting it at all for this purpose. This is probably due to the FDA which would demand large scale studies before any claim could be made for mellaril. Thus the most popular drug which is much inferior to vitamins is the one in current use, not because it is better for the children, it is in fact not as good as mellaril, but because it has been promoted far more efficiently. I have found mellaril better than ritalin but use it very rarely.

Nevertheless, in carefully controlled dosages, drugs to play a role in the treatment of children with learning disabilities and behavioral disorders. Rarely the child does not respond fast enough to the above regimen and both child and family need relief from the continuing pressure of the illness on everyone in that family. I use the antidepressant imipramine 25 to 50 mg before bed. Often there is relief within a few days. The child sleeps better, awakens refreshed, and will stop wetting the bed. The drug is discontinued eventually. This is determined by trial. There are very few side effects. I have not tried any of the modern antidepressants. Even more rarely I use thioridazine, the phenothiazine with the greatest benefit and least side effects of any of these drugs. I use a dose range between 10 and 75 mg daily. However, I avoid using the more popular ritalin (methyl phenidate) because of the serious side effects unless the children referred to me are already using it. I will maintain it until the orthomolecular program described here becomes effective. Nearly all of my patients are able to come off ritalin. I remove the ritalin slowly, allowing the child to adapt to each new dose before making another adjustment downward. Many of my patients have already failed to respond to stimulant drugs and they and their familiar find the side effects very worrying. I am, therefore, opposed to their use, unless they are used to achieve a very rapid response which will provide some relief to the family until the vitamin program has started to work. The track record for ritalin is not very good unless one assumes it is the only treatment available.

Since parents who are pleased with the effect of this drug on their children will not have them referred to me, I cannot judge from personal observations what effect it has had on them. The children brought to me have not responded well to ritalin or have had serious side effects or their parents could not tolerate the idea of using such an active drug which covers the symptoms but does not get at the root of the problem. According to *Newsweek* (18 March 1996), more than one million children in the United States are on ritalin, an increase of 250 percent since 1990. Professional opinion of its value ranges from considering it one of the "raving successes in psychiatry" by Dr Laurence Greenhill at Columbia University Medical School to the view that it is both over-prescribed and dangerous. Dr Peter S. Jennings, Chief of the Child and Adolescent Disorders Research Branch of NIMH, USA, comments, "I fear that ADHD is suffering from the 'disease of the month' syndrome. The use of ritalin varies tremendously by states. Thus Georgia in the southeast, and Michigan near the Great Lakes consumed over 2 grams per 100 people in 1994 while California consumed 0.58 and Hawaii only 0.25. This does suggest that the use of this drug, classified as a Schedule 2 controlled substance as are cocaine, methadone and methamphetamine, is determined more by the popular prescribing habits of physicians than it is by the incidence of hyperactivity."

I have found imipramine more effective and freer of side effects than ritalin. It is taken once in the evening and works all day. Ritalin must be given several times daily and the effect wears off within a few hours. Many of the children controlled by ritalin during school hours come home almost freed of its sedative like effects and display the full force of their hyperactive behavior to their parents. This is one of the reasons parents have been bringing their children to see me for nutritional, megavitamin, or orthomolecular treatment.

Prevention

Prevention begins before fertilization. Both parents should ensure they are in good health before pregnancy is started. A healthy man is more apt to have healthy sperms. The woman should ensure that she is adequately nourished, that she is taking in ample amounts of the essential nutrients. She should ensure that throughout her pregnancy every illness is promptly attended to, that she continues to take the supplements, and that she does not smoke, drink alcohol, take street drugs, or any other drug which may be damaging to her baby. The last cautionary statement does not apply to vitamins and minerals used as described because the only effect they have on the baby is positive. They help ensure that the baby will be freer of birth and congenital defects. Folic acid and vitamin B-12 are especially important in preventing spinal column deformities.

The baby should be breastfed unless there are very powerful reasons why this cannot be done. Baby food should be free of added sugar and other additives. Allergies must be investigated if the baby has many colds, earaches, and so on. Dairy products are the most common food allergies in children. Each child should be given supplemental vitamin C since no one can make any and many will need to supplement their diet with B-complex vitamins as well. That will be adequate unless the child does not develop properly or develops learning and behavioral disturbances. This then becomes a treatment problem, not a question of prevention, except that early and effective treatment will prevent major disturbances and illness later on in life.

Vulnerable families are families where one or more members have had learning or behavioral disorders or have been schizophrenic. In these families it would be wise to give all the children a B-complex preparation, and if this is not adequate, to supplement it with vitamin B-3 using at least 100 mg daily.

If one parent has schizophrenia, there is a probability that it will also occur in about 10 percent of their children. But over the past 40 years I have observed that children from schizophrenic parents may develop behavioral and learning problems even though they do not become schizophrenic. The genetics of this disease is not clear, nor is it known whether more than one gene is involved, although it is likely that there are two or more genes. These children with a gene from their parents which does not express itself as schizophrenia will respond to vitamin B-3. Many of the children described in this book fall within this group. If both parents are schizophrenic the odds are about 50 percent that their children will also become ill. That is why I recommend that all children of schizophrenic parents should be watched very carefully, supplemented with vitamin C and with at least 100 mg daily of vitamin B-3. If there is clear evidence of a problem they will need more, 500 to 3,000 milligrams daily. Parents with schizophrenia do not have to have any schizophrenic children.

I have recommended several times in the past that enough niacinamide should be added to our daily food, perhaps in the flour, which already contains small amounts of this vitamin. There would be a major decrease in the incidence and prevalence of disturbed children and the incidence of schizophrenia would be significantly decreased within the next ten years.

Parents who have had learning and behavioral disorders should follow the same principles. If they have responded to vitamin therapy, they should ensure that their children are also given the benefit of the same treatment. First order relatives of people who have responded to vitamin B-3 therapy can test themselves by taking the vitamin, even if they feel they are normal in every aspect. They may be surprised to find out how much better they feel. Here is one example. Many years ago I did a survey of identical schizophrenic twins. I saw one member of a twin pair who was schizophrenic, while his identical brother considered himself completely well. The normal twin was a high school principal, his sick brother was not working. The schizophrenic twin recovered on vitamin treatment. His brother, who always came with him to my office, then asked me whether he could also take the same vitamins. He was so impressed with what they had done for his brother he wanted to take them himself, even though he felt he was normal. A month later when they came back again he told me that after starting the same vitamins he began to feel much better, that on looking back from his new state of wellness he realized that he had not been as well as he thought but he had not known anything else and had assumed this was what normality was like. I have seen this so frequently I have no doubt that first order relatives of these patients would be wise to try the vitamins on themselves. They must have some of the same genes, but not enough to make them ill. These genes need extra amounts of vitamin B-3. I expect that when the schizophrenic genes are identified, they will have a lot to do with vitamin B-3 and its coenzyme, the oxidized and reduced form of nicotinamide adenine dinucleotide (NAD/NADH).

Prevention means using the same program which helps patients recover, but starting before they are ill, and if they become ill, starting as soon as possible.

3 | CORROBORATION

Orthomolecular Pediatric Research

Every investigator has found the same therapeutic response when they have used the correct doses for a long enough period of time. Megavitamin therapy does not usually cause rapid responses as do drugs. The therapist has to be patient and wait for the results. In addition they may have to use other therapeutic adjuncts during the recovery process. There have been no negative reports from physicians who have tried seriously to repeat this work. There have been a few botched attempts using inadequate amounts for too little time followed by claims totally unjustified by the evidence they were able to obtain. Following their procedure, I could easily repeat their test and confirm the fact they were not able to see any response. I will, therefore, not waste time referring to these botched inadequate studies. There is no need to refer to studies that do not follow the basic rule of all investigation — i.e., repeat the study the way the original investigator described it was done.

The first doctor to adapt our megavitamin research to his practice of medicine was Dr L. Silverman, the best known and popular pediatrician in North Dakota, practicing in Grand Forks. He heard about our studies in 1972. He visited me for several days, visited other orthomolecular practitioners, observed our results and began to treat. By April 1974 he had treated a large number of patients. The results were so impressive that he rapidly expanded the series and added another 250 patients. When families in North Dakota heard of his success, they began to flock to him, even adults. One day he told me his definition of a pediatric case. He said in his practice they were anyone under 30. He began to treat them because there was no other doctor in his area familiar with megavitamin therapy.

As he observed, vitamin therapy quickly supplanted drugs in his treatment of children. "Since beginning the orthomolecular approach, however, we find that in many cases the need for such drugs has been markedly decreased, if not entirely eliminated. In a number of children, including many in whom all other current accepted methods of therapy have been used for an extended period with minimal or no success, not only have the parents reported lessened hyperactivity, improved behavior and attention span, better motivation, but also a remarkable improvement in reading and other academic skills. There has also occurred in a few children such a rapid and total improvement in all areas of functioning including coordination, that it not only suggests that it may be more appropriate physiological treatment, but probably also enhances metabolic functioning in related areas of the nervous system rather than by merely acting as a suppressive agent."

"A striking example is that of a 9-year, 8-month boy who was first seen in July of 1972. His depressed mother was distraught because he announced that he would not return to school the following term. He had repeated kindergarten and was retained in the first grade. He had had extensive psychological studies in 1970 and in early 1972 where testing suggested borderline intelligence with perceptual defect. His mother also described his writing as sloppy. He had been tutored extensively and the family had been counseled. He had also received a course of visual exercises in an attempt to improve his reading skills. Despite the efforts described above, which also included medications, he had remained extremely hyperactive and distractible and his teacher had complained that his behavior was extremely disruptive in the class for the fall term. The physical examination was non-contributory, but a five-hour glucose tolerance test revealed a flat curve indicating some impairment of intestinal absorption. His bone age was delayed about two to three years and the only other finding in the medical study was a mildly abnormal electroencephalogram. His dietary proteins were increased and he was placed on an orthomolecular regime.

"In September he returned to special education first grade and after several weeks his teacher stated that his attention span, responsiveness and cooperation were excellent. His reading improved so that he brought books home which he had never done before and his writing became more legible. His teacher at the time also stated that she could not understand why he had been failed before. In January of 1973 (about five and one half months after beginning orthomolecular treatment) the mother called and said he had been transferred from the first grade special education class directly into the third grade regular class where to this date he is functioning acceptably and is proud of his academic accomplishments. This was checked with the school authorities and was confirmed by the school social worker assigned to the special education department."

Dr Silverman concluded that, on the basis of a rather concentrated experience, the orthomolecular treatment was the first and safest treatment of choice in children with perceptual and behavioral problems associated with minimal neurological difficulties. Silverman stressed that three basis conditions were essential for optimum recovery: (1) the child must receive proper analysis and diagnosis; (2) the patient must be educable with no major structural defect, severe malformation or progressive neurologic disease; (3) the patient must relate on a sustained basis with at least one person who is in contact with reality. That person must be stable, concerned, and devoted to the handicapped person's welfare. He observed several favorable by-products or positive side effects. Many of the children experience increased vigor and a sense of well being. In addition many families lost their sense of guilt and made it possible for them to be more adequate in solving management problems that presented themselves. Finally, because families were alerted to the biological and genetic aspects and were alerted to any problem which appeared in other members of the family.

Dr Bernard Rimland, author of *Infantile Autism*, has had more intimate experience with a variety of treatment approaches for children with autism than most other specialists in this field. In 1973 he reviewed how he had come to be interested in megavitamin treatment and the results he had seen arising from his large scale experiments. He first became interested when he read the literature which described the use of large doses of vitamin B-3 for the treatment of schizophrenia. Because he had become dissatisfied with the results of psychiatric treatment for children with severe mental disorders, he established the Institute of Child Behavior Research. He quickly established contacts with a large number of parents or children who had not been appreciably helped by modern psychiatry. His institute received communications from professional workers and parents in virtually every state in the USA as well as from Canada, England, and nearly a score of other foreign countries. He became aware of an enormous range of innovative treatments. The treatments included the talking typewriter, computer approaches, patterning, play and music, rage reduction, sensory deprivation, visual and motor training, tactile stimulation, LSD and other hallucinogenic drugs, steroid injections, spine adjustments and colonic purges, to name a few.

As he observed, "Exposure to this diversity of approaches, most of which are presented as breakthroughs by enthusiastic proponents citing dramatic clinical material, naturally engenders a certain skepticism. Despite my initial skepticism one method of treatment was reported to us to be effective so frequently by both physicians and parents that I decided to evaluate it in a carefully designed study." That method was orthomolecular treatment.

Rimland was persuaded by the following evidence. Many of the cases represented individual reports conducted on a trial and error method independently of each other, but there was a surprising consistency converging toward the two main vitamins. The children were so ill they presented gross behavioral disturbances with improvement so marked there was no mistake in evaluating that it had occurred. Most of the children had already failed to respond to the usual psychoactive drugs. Their parents had already become extremely skeptical that any medication could effect any improvement. Out of a 57 child sample only 2 out of 9 given Mellaril had shown significant improvement. Mothers reported that when the vitamin was discontinued either by design or by error there was a prompt relapse to the original condition. Some mothers reported that there was a dose relationship with a positive response showing only with higher doses.

He was particularly intrigued by the fact that the majority of psychiatrists who were violently opposed to the megavitamin approach were themselves using psychotherapy and psychoanalysis. Both these forms of talking therapy (in classical analysis the psychiatrist does not talk) have been shown to be entirely ineffective for both children and adults. Rimland then designed a study in which about 200 psychotic children from all parts of the USA and Canada participated, each one under the supervision of his own physician. He used vitamin B-3 (niacinamide), pyridoxine, pantothenic acid, and vitamin C. These vitamins were given for a three month period followed by a one month no-treatment period during which the children were re-evaluated. A computer was used which grouped children on the basis of certain similarity in their history and symptomatology. This was done before they were started on the vitamins. Some of the children improved markedly and it was not randomly distributed. Previously the best response had been to Mellaril which helped 36 percent of 277 children and worsened behavior in 20 percent. This compares with 66.5 percent helped by the vitamin program and 3.7 percent impaired. Autistic children, as a group, showed the best response, primarily to pyridoxine.

As Rimland concluded, "It seems quiet clear from both the statistical analysis of our data and the clinical response of those who have observed the children that there is indeed a substantial proportion of psychotic children who can be expected to benefit from treatment with high dosages of the vitamins used in this study. Other vitamins and minerals may also be effective for a further proportion of such children and would to seem to warrant investigation on a priority basis." In a report to the annual meeting of the National Society for Autistic Children in 1975, entitled "Where Does Research Lead from Here?" Rimland answered, "It continues to lead very strongly in the direction of orthomolecular psychiatry. The vitamins were not only found to be of benefit in a absolute sense, but were also of benefit to a far greater percentage of the children in the study than were the drugs which had been previously used. Furthermore, we found the vitamins to only rarely produce side effects, in sharp contrast to the drugs."

Dr Allan Cott, a New York psychoanalyst, was one of the first psychiatrists to treat children with orthomolecular methods. After many years of practicing psychiatry he had gotten fed up with his practice. He was ready to give it up and turn to other activities. We met many years ago through his good friend Dr Jack Ward in New Jersey. After looking into the use of vitamins for schizophrenics, he became very interested and within a few years had a large and successful orthomolecular practice. He found his new way of treating patients so exciting because he saw recoveries he had not seen before. He gave up any idea of leaving psychiatry. He became a major player in the orthomolecular field, a teacher, lecturer, author, and treated many children from the New York area and elsewhere. To honor his work a school for sick children in Birmingham, Alabama was named the Allan Cott school. By 1973 he had treated 500 children.

Based upon this extensive and wide experience he concluded that the majority of the children who persisted in the regimen of orthomolecular treatment achieved significant improvement in many areas of functioning. "Most significant," he concluded "was the decreased hyperactivity and the improvement in concentration and attention span which led to improved capacities for learning. In those children who had been unable to learn at all, a desire to learn became apparent. . . . With the vitamin treatment results are frequently quick in starting and dramatic in nature, but in most instances six months is the usual time in which significant changes are seen. The child begins to understand and obey commands, exhibiting a willingness to cooperate with his parents and teachers. Gaze aversion ceases – the hyperactivity which is one of the cardinal symptoms of the childhood psychoses subsides slowly."

Cott was such a good psychiatrist because as an analyst he had learned patience. Analysts do not expect rapid responses. Their training conditions them to watch for slight changes patiently for years, if necessary. There is no quick fix with vitamins as there is with ritalin. Most modern psychiatrists are so accustomed to the rapid response to drugs that they have no patience with slow treatments. They are willing to accept the short term gain even though there is no long term benefit. Vitamin therapy does not promise short term gain. It promises recovery if the parents, patients, and therapist are patient and persevere with the treatment.

In a special issue of the *Journal of Orthomolecular Psychiatry*, Dr Cott summarized his wide research and treatment experience. "There is rapidly accumulating evidence that a child's ability to learn can be improved by the use of large doses of certain vitamins, or mineral supplements, and by improvement of his general nutritional status through removing 'junk' foods from his daily diet. . . . With orthomolecular treatment, results are frequently quick in starting and the reduction in hyperactivity often can be dramatic but in most cases several months elapse before significant changes are seen. The child exhibits a willingness to cooperate with his parents and teachers. These changes are seen in the majority of children who failed to improve with the use of the stimulant drugs or tranquilizer medication. The majority of children I see have been exposed to every form of treatment and every known tranquilizer and sedative with little or no success even in controlling hyperactivity. Concentration and attention span increase and the child is able to work productively for increasingly longer periods of time. He ceases to be an irritant to his teachers and classmates. Early intervention is of the utmost importance, not only for the child, but for the whole family since the child suffering from minimal brain dysfunction is such a devastating influence on the family constellation. He is the matrix of emotional storms which envelop every member of the household and disrupt both their relationship to him and to each other. . . . Control of the child's diet is an integral part of the total treatment and failure to improve the child's nutritional status can be responsible for achieving minimal results. Greater concern must be shown for the quality of the child's internal environment in which his cells and tissues function if we are to help him attain optimum performance. The removal of offending foods from the diet of disturbed children can result in dramatic improvement in behavior, attention span and concentration. Since many disturbed and learning disabled children are found to have either hypoglycemia, hyperinsulinism or dysinsulinism, cane sugar and rapidly absorbed carbohydrate foods should be eliminated from their diets. It has been the universal observation of those investigators who assess the child's nutritional status that they eat a diet which is richest in sugar, candy, sweets and in foods made with sugar, The removal of these foods results in a dramatic decrease in hyperactivity. The appalling fact about the constant consumption of these 'junk' foods is the parents' belief that these foods are good for their children.

"Neither improved nutrition, vitamin and mineral supplementation, enriched educational opportunities or visual and perceptual motor training alone can be successful in fully helping the child with learning disabilities. All must be used in a co-ordinated program to develop each child's potential. Because research can not at this at this time give unequivocal or full answer to the question of what effect malnutrition or malnourishment has on intellectual development is not a valid reason to delay programs for improving the nutritional status and eating practices of mothers and infants. Information demonstrating the benefits of good nutrition in improved health, physical growth and improved learning already justifies such efforts. We can not afford the luxury of waiting until causes can be unquestionably established by techniques yet to be developed. We can not postpone managing as effectively and honestly as possible the five million or more children who desperately need help now."

Cott continued, "It seems quite clear from the clinical reports of parents, teachers and others who have observed the children I've treated that there is indeed a large number of disturbed children and children with learning disabilities who can be expected to benefit from orthomolecular treatment. . . . Investigation of this treatment modality by controlled studies should be given the highest priority, for we are dealing with a patient population of 20 million children." This was a modest proposal from a very good clinician and researcher, and when he wrote this I agreed with him. Today, 20 years later, I am not in agreement with his suggestion. We do not need any controlled double blind studies. We do need a large number of clinicians to use the treatment so that they can themselves be convinced of its efficacy and in this way convince their skeptical colleagues. We need demonstration studies not because the data are inconclusive and inadequate but merely to satisfy the skeptics' resistance against action.

Many years ago in Saskatchewan when the College of Agri-culture, University of Saskatchewan, wanted to introduce a new variety of wheat, it ran across the same skeptical reaction from the farmers. The College then approached farmers in many areas and asked them to plant the grain in a few small demonstration plots. As the crops grew farmers driving by could see for themselves what the new variety looked like in comparison to the grain they themselves had planted. In this way the new variety soon became popular and was introduced. We need something like this in medicine. We need enterprising doctors who will not be afraid to use the treatment, who will allow the people to see the results. In this way the treatment could be introduced in a few years instead of having to wait for 40 years. I have referred to the enormous cost of having delayed the introduction of folic acids to prevent spina bifida. The cost to society is enormous. Thousands of lives will have been ruined simply because of the skepticism of the profession.

Dr Elizabeth Rees, another pioneer using orthomolecular treatment, was a pediatrician specializing in allergies. To this she added the megavitamin approach. Following her studies she concluded, "Many hyperactive and schizophrenic children can be diagnosed and treated in the routine office. The most important part of the examination is a detailed history which includes family history, the birth development and feeding of the child, as well as the present problem. Megavitamins, while very important, are sometimes better prescribed after the general nutrition and allergies of the child have been treated so that the parent does not rely upon pills alone to solve the child's problems. Children must have access to education, habit and character training, psychological care as well as correction of physical defects in addition to specific therapies for problems."

At the New York Institute of Child Development, Dr Krippner and Dr Fischer divided students into four groups. Group one (28 boys and 8 girls) received only neurological organization (NO) procedures. Group two (6 boys and 8 girls) were assigned randomly and also received only NO treatment. Group three (10 boys and 4 girls) were similar to group two but received megavitamin therapy as well. Group four (18 boys and 6 girls) were given megavitamin therapy four months after the original visit and diagnosis. All the children were evaluated using the Doman-Delacato Developmental Profile. In group one and two there was no significant improvement in the neurological quotient, whereas in group three and four after six months there was a significant improvement. A factorial analysis of variance was done for the entire sample. Of 93 students, improvement in each of six evaluated categories (competence in mobility, competence in speech, manual competence. visual competence, auditory competence and tactile competence) reached high levels of significance – i.e., the probability these improvement were due to chance is less than one in a thousand.

A series of other studies corroborate the effectiveness of orthomolecular treatment. Dr Paul Cutler found that out of 62 children with learning disabilities 40 percent were positive for KP and another 20 percent were suffering from trace mineral imbalances. They responded very well to treatment with pyridoxine and zinc and manganese solutions. G. von Hilsheimer and colleagues concluded that the megavitamin treatment program was more helpful than was placebo in treating children with severe behavioral disorders, alcoholics, addicts and schizophrenics. They ruled out any placebo response. Dr Brenner concluded that hyperactivity was multifactorial, and that a significant number are caused by vitamin deficiency or dependencies. He treated 100 children. They were given a preliminary treatment trial with thiamin 400 mg qid, placebo, calcium pantothenate 218 mg, and finally pyridoxine 100 mg tid each for three to four days in this order. Thirty-eight did not respond, 26 improved on thiamin but 22 deteriorated, 23 improved with pantothenate with 9 getting worse, and 18 got better on pyridoxine with 16 being worse. The remaining children showed no response in this short time to any of the treatments.

The children who showed improvement were then started on a second trial of vitamin for seven days followed by placebo for seven days. Out of 21 given thiamin, 11 showed a dramatic response. Four of these needed it only for a few months. Four needed it after more than three years. From 15 on pantothenate only 2 showed a better response than had ritalin. From 18 treated with pyridoxine 9 responded and needed long term treatment. Six became refractory until zinc was added. Five needed from 500 to 2000 mg daily. By trying various additions and subtractions of these B vitamins, they were able to determine which vitamin or combination of vitamins was best for each child.

General practitioners have also found the orthomolecular treatment approach practical and valuable in their practice. These include Dr Max Vogel, Calgary, Alberta, who over the past 30 years has treated large numbers of adults and children, as well as Dr Glen Green, Prince Albert, Saskatchewan. As we have seen, Dr Green has proposed the term subclinical pellagra, first used in 1938, to describe behavioral disorders. This term accurately described the syndrome present in children and adults which is responsive to vitamin B-3. In one of his early reports, Dr Green observed, "In a seven month period since November 1968 I have diagnosed well over 100 cases of subclinical pellagra; 65 percent of the cases were under 16 years of age. They all responded to vitamin B-3, which is niacin or its amide within a few days or weeks. The chief criterion for diagnosis of this disease is the presence or absence of perceptual changes. All the senses are involved in these dysperceptions to a greater or lesser degree. The other symptoms which are common to almost any disease are fatigue, depression, anorexia, headache, dizziness and various aches and pains. A disinclination to work was common. None of these patients had a symmetrical skin rash involving the exposed parts, although a few did have a chronic dermatitis of one kind or another. Stomatitis, esophagitis, diarrhea, etc. were not of any consequence. Poverty and pellagra are hand maidens and ignorance is their boon companion. The exception to this is the teenager who won't eat properly."

The combined experiences of Dr Vogel and Dr Green lead to the conclusion that every general practitioner will find many cases of subclinical pellagra once they start looking and start using perceptual tests. I expect that some of their most difficult patients will turn out to have unrecognized subclinical pellagra and that they will not respond to drugs until their vitamin B-3 needs are met – and then they may not need them. Although Dr Green and Dr Vogel did not have sufficient time to analyze all their cases, lacking the benefit of research grants, institutional support, and grants from drug companies, their clinical experience was great and in my opinion was sound, confirming what I had seen many years ago and still continue to see.

The literature on orthomolecular treatment is now quite extensive. When the vitamins-as-prevention paradigm was the only one around, few doctors and parents had any interest in this new form of treatment. This new vitamins-as-treatment paradigm is now entering medicine very quickly, though not nearly as rapidly into psychiatry, and these corroborating studies have a new relevance for health-care professionals, parents, and children with learning disabilities and behavioral disorders.

Clinical Trials

First Clinical Trials

In 1967 I gave up my jobs as Associate Professor of Psychiatry, University of Saskatchewan at Saskatoon and Director of Psychiatric Research, Province of Saskatchewan. By then I had treated a fair number of children with vitamin B-3 and vitamin C. The clinical evidence showed that this treatment was helpful to children, but I did not have enough data to determine what type of problem would respond best.

In 1954 I had treated a small number of children considered mentally retarded from a school for the mentally retarded. It was a double blind experiment using one gram of niacin or one gram of placebo per 50 pounds of body weight over a three-month period. I had assumed that since adults required this dose, children would need the same amount. Later I found that children need larger doses than adults, and I used double that amount accordingly. I made no attempt to cover the flush produced by the niacin so that it was a controlled placebo experiment but was not double blind. Because of this flush, it is impossible to double blind niacin for any experiment. It was, however, as blind as were the Montreal studies of Professor H. Lehmann and Dr T. Ban or those of Dr Wittenborn in New Jersey – and these were used to attack the work we had done in Saskatchewan. This is not a major flaw when testing children since they do not react to placebos in the same way adults do. Most of them did not like the pills and would have been much happier without having to take anything.

At the end of the three month trial the parents were asked to report what they had seen. Out of 11 on placebo, 3 were found to be improved compared to 7 children of the 8 that had been given niacin. This difference is statistically significant at the 0.01 level. I did not report this study because it was not double blind and would have been ignored by the purist in psychiatric research. It also included a large number of different conditions such as retardation, schizophrenia, Down syndrome, and organic cases.

Later I completed another controlled study on 24 retarded children with the cooperation of the local school for the retarded. They were all tested for the mauve factor (KP) and were then started on niacinamide 1 G pr 50 pounds weight. The vitamin was provided free to their parents for as long as they wanted to keep their children on the program. I assumed that parents of retarded children who were getting better would want to continue and that parents who saw no improvement would not. After one year of treatment the children were evaluated. Out of the 16 children who were KP negative, only 5 were still taking the vitamin. Out of 8 that had been KP positive, all were still on the vitamin. Their parents were optimistic and believed that their children were better – that is, quicker, quieter, less aggressive, and able to learn more easily. By chance this kind of difference would have occurred only once in 500 trials. It suggested that KP positive children were much more responsive to niacinamide treatment.

My last experiment was a double blind prospective controlled study using niacinamide and placebo in 1967. All the seriously disturbed children referred to me who were age 13 or less were taken into the study, provided the parents agreed. They were all supplied free vitamin tablets for the three years of the study. Diagnostically, they fit into the group of children with learning and behavioral disorders. I wanted to determine which kind of condition would be most responsive to vitamin B-3. I hoped to find a group of children homogenous with respect to their response to the vitamin. This I would then use to describe the typical vitamin B-3 responsive child.

They were all started on a sugar-free diet, niacinamide 1.5 to 3 G daily, with the same amount of ascorbic acid. Drugs were hardly ever used and these children were not given any form of psychotherapy. I advised the parents that as a condition of the study I would place them on placebo to replace the niacinamide after they had recovered. The placebo would be continued as long as the child remained well. But if they became convinced that they were relapsing, they could return them to the niacinamide, recording when and why they had done so. The children were evaluated every three months.

The results of this clinical trial are shown in this table:

Subject	Sex	Age	Diagnosis	Stand	Vitamin	Placebo	Condition
AB	M	8	Down	None	None		Unknown
WF	F	10	Anx		Well	Rel	Normal
BF	M	8	Learn	None	Well	Rel	Normal
TF	M	6	Learn		Well	Rel	Normal
DG	M	6	Learn		Imp	Rel	Unknown
RG	M	13	Beh		M.I.	Rel	Unknown
DaG	M	10	Beh		Imp	Rel	Unknown
DR	M	6	Schiz	None	M.I	Rel	M.I.
DRu	M	5	Schiz	None	Well	Rel	Normal
TH	M	12	Schiz	None	Well	Rel	Normal
KD	F	8	Schiz		Well	Rel	Normal

Subject	Sex	Age	Diagnosis	Stand	Vitamin	Placebo	Condition
PS	M	9	Schiz		Well	Rel	Normal
BS	F	8	Schiz	None	M.I.		M.I.
MA	M	12	Schiz	None	Well	Rel	Normal
JB	M	13	Beh		M.I.		Unknown
WW	F	8	Beh		M.I.		Very ill
RW	M	6	Learn		Well		Normal
SW	F	6	Beh		M.I.		M.I.
KB	M	10	Schiz		Well	Rel	Normal
RA	F	4	Schiz		Well	Rel	Normal
PC	F	6	Schiz		Well	Rel	Normal
BF	F	11	Schiz		Imp		Unknown
BI	M	8	Schiz		Well	Rel	M.I.
EY	M	8	Schiz		Well		M.I.
RD	M	7	Schiz		Well	REI	Normal
RoD	F	10	Schiz		Well	Rel	Normal
JN	M	7	Schiz		Well		Normal
MV	M	10	Schiz	None	Well	Rel	Normal
RV	M	7	Schiz		Well		Normal
RL	M	7	Schiz	None	M.I.		Unknown
EJ	M	8	Schiz	None	None		Not imp
WT	M	10	Schiz		M.I.		Unknown
CH	M	5	Schiz	None	Well		Normal
EC	M	7	Schiz		Well		Normal
MD	M	11	Schiz	None	Imp		Unknown
MT	M	7	Learn	None	M.I.		M.I.
HW	M	9	Schiz	None	Imp		Not Imp

Learn: a learning disability   Schiz: schizophrenia;
Beh: behavioral disorder   Down: Down syndrome
Anx: anxiety state   M.I.: much improved
Imp: improved   Rel: relapsed
Stand: standard treatment   Vitamin: niacinamide and vitamin C
None: no improvement

Of the 37 children started on this study, 21 were normal and 14 were improved or much improved. Two did not respond. Of these AB was a Down syndrome child and EJ a severely retarded autistic child who had not developed any speech when I first saw him at age 8.

Only 19 patients were placed on placebo. They were not all switched because they were lost to the study before they became normal, or more rarely because the parents thought it would have been harmful to their child because the initial recovery had been so slow and difficult. I agreed with this since I had seen that in previous cases children taken off the vitamin often required a lot more intensive work with the program to get them back to their original normal state. All the children placed on placebo relapsed within four weeks, most within two weeks. One child was promoted by his school to his normal grade after he had recovered. The school was not aware of the study. He was then placed on placebo. Two weeks later the teacher told his parents they had made a mistake in promoting him and were sending him back. On renewing the vitamin he recovered and has remained well. Ascorbic acid did not prevent relapses.

At last contact in 1974, 19 out of the 37 were normal, 6 much improved. The outcome for 9 was unknown and 3 remained unimproved. Thus 25 out of 37 or 68 percent were much improved or normal. The children not improved included AB with Down syndrome; these children require a much more elaborate and sophisticated approach before they will respond. DG, REG, and DaG were all improving, but their mother, a chronic schizophrenic, was not able to cooperate, and their father, an alcoholic schizophrenic, killed himself. JB was improving, but later refused to cooperate and left home. WW was much improved but eventually refused to take any medication, and when last evaluated, was a chronic schizophrenic, a ward of social welfare. BF was improving but stopped taking vitamins and was lost to the study. RL was improving but failed to keep appointments and was removed from the study. EJ showed no response and had no speech by age 8. WT, while improving, eventually refused to continue on vitamins. MD would not take vitamins. HW was unable to swallow any pills.

The chief reason for failure was thus the inability of the child to remain on the vitamins prescribed. They did not want to swallow or could not swallow the tablets and their parents did not know how to cope with this problem. These children would have been helped if it had been possible to get the vitamin into them. BS, for example, was a failure on six grams of niacinamide daily. She was then seen by several other psychiatrists who all found her untreatable. In desperation she was brought back to me again, and after one year on 12 G of niacin she was much better and after that made steady improvement.

The "100" Study

Between July 1, 1967 and June 30, 1973 I had seen over 100 children under the age of 14. During July and August 1973, John Hoffer, my son, then a medical student at McGill University, surveyed all the children 13 years old and younger who could be reached from Saskatoon and its surrounding district within a radius of 50 miles. If they could not come to my office, John would visit their homes and talk to the patients and to their parents. John prepared a report outlining the information he had obtained and summarizing each case. This population of children represents about 60 percent of the children I had seen from Saskatoon and its surrounding district between July 1, 1967 and July 1, 1973. It does not differ from the 400 children I had seen from the rest of Saskatchewan, and is similar to the children I have seen since moving to Victoria in 1976.

I was interested in the response to orthomolecular treatment. This was judged by the results on the behavioral rating scale (hyperactivity scale) and using a four-point improvement index.

The clinical response is shown by this four number code. The first number represents the presence or absence of symptoms, the second number represents whether behavior at home was normal, the third number represents whether behavior was normal at school, and the last number the social behavior in general. Thus a score of 1111 means the child was normal in all areas. A score of 0000 shows he was abnormal in all areas. A score of 0101 indicates he was normal in behavior at school and in general but still was not well in the symptoms area and still behaved badly at home. A score of 4 (adding up the individual points) recognizes a normal child, a score of 3 a child much improved, a score of 2, improved and the other two scores are given to children who have not improved.

I (A.H.) saw many of the children about the same time John Hoffer (J.H.) made his final assessment and I was in agreement with his conclusions. Whenever possible, we also compared the hyperactivity scale score for these children at first visit with the score at the follow-up visit. The following table summarizes the results of treatment for these 110 cases.

Code	Name	Age	Sex	Clinical Evaluation J.H.	A.H.	Hyperactivity Initial	Score Last
(1)	JRA	7	M	0101	0111	97	61
(2)	RA	4	F	1111		81	29
(3)	BA	4	M	0111		95	45
(4)	TA	11	M	1,0.5,0.5,0		85	51
(5)	Bar.A	10	F	0111	0111	97	47
(6)	Ter.A	7	M	1000		61	39
(7)	Rob.A	11	M	0111		65	45
(8)	CB	13	F	1111	1111	87	55
(9)	KB	7.5	M	0100		75	47
(10)	SB	2.5	F	1111		81	29
(11)	LB	5	F	0111		77	37
(12)	EB	11	M	0110	0111	106	51
(13)	PB	8	M	1111		95	33
(14)	AC	8	M	0111	0111	85	55
(15)	TC	8	M	0111	0111	79	41
(16)	BC	9	M	1111		69	47
(17)	CC	8.5	M	1111		57	55
(18)	And.C	10	M	0110		87	51
(19)	RD	7	M	0000			81
(20)	Ros.D	10	F	1111		87	31
(21)	AE	7.5	M	1010		84	73
(22)	MF	14	F	1111	1111		
(23)	DF	9.5	M	1111		45	
(24)	BF	6	M	1111			29
(25)	TF	6	M	1111			
(26)	WF	10	F	1111			

Code	Name	Age	Sex	Clinical Evaluation		Hyperactivity	Score
				J.H.	A.H.	Initial	Last
(27)	CF	9	M	1101			61
(28)	VF	4	M	0110		75	31
(29)	MDB	9	M	0100		71	59
(30)	PC	6	F	1111			33
(31)	GC	11	M	0110		93	51
(32)	LF	10	M	1,.5,.5,0	1101	43	49
(33)	Br.C	12	M	1111		55	35
(34)	SG	14	M	1011		109	62
(35)	NG	8	M	Improved		51	41
(36)	RG	9	5M	0011		37	40
(37)	MH	11	F	1111			
(38)	CH	5.5	M	0000	1111	107	37
(39)	Our.H	5	M	1111		113	29
(40)	PH	4	F	Improved		63	51
(41)	JH	11	M	1011		47	31
(42)	BI	8	M	0001		93	59
(43)	RJ	5	M	0001		79	71
(44)	SJ	8	M	1111		63	52
(45)	EJ	8.5	M	0000		65	70
(46)	DK	9.5	F	1001		79	51
(47)	BK	9.5	M	0.5,1,0.5,0		57	51
(48)	SK	10	F	0001		97	49
(49)	Ben.K	11	M	1111		43	34
(50)	LL	10	F	1111		77	35
(51)	BL	7	M	1111			
(52)	SL	7	M	0111		79	33
(53)	KL	3	M	0000	0111	74	50
(54)	ML	7.5	M	0000	0111	95	40
(55)	DM	1	M	1111		67	45
(56)	TM	7.5	M	1111		89	35
(57)	RM	4	M	0010		85	
(58)	JN	7	M	0100	1111	92	27

Code	Name	Age	Sex	Clinical Evaluation J.H.	A.H.	Hyperactivity Initial	Score Last
(59)	DP	9	M	1111			31
(60)	SP	3.5	M	0101		105	69
(61)	LP	9	M	1110		79	37
(62)	CP	7	M	0000			102
(63)	LAP	12.5	F	0001		79	43
(64)	PR	9	M	0001		75	61
(65)	CR	11	M	1111		79	43
(66)	LR	11	F	1111		67	55
(67)	GR	6	M	0000			
(68)	GR	9	M	0010		77	55
(69)	NR	7	F	0111		7	35
(70)	DR	6	M	0,0.5,1,0.5		47	
(71)	WR	6	M	1111			
(72)	CS	8	F	1111		85	39
(73)	GS	13	M	1110		99	45
(74)	Gus.S	14	M	0000		101	65
(75)	YS	14	F	1111			
(76)	TS	13	M	0100	0111		
(77)	ES	14	M	1111		41	27
(78)	MAS	7	F	0111		84	39
(79)	RS	4.5	M	0100		109	89
(80)	KS	14	F	1,1,.5,.5	1111		
(81)	LS	6	F	1111		91	47
(82)	KS	7	F	0011	0111	101	47
(83)	DT	10	M	0000	1111	91	67
(84)	PT	11	M	1000	1111	93	77
(85)	AU	9	M	0.5,1,0.5,1		45	49
(86)	RU	8	M	0101		59	49
(87)	FU	11	F	1111		95	
(88)	Alb.U	11	M	1001	1101	83	37
(89)	MV	10	M	1111		59	27
(90)	GV	14	M	1111		95	

| Code | Name | Age | Sex | Clinical Evaluation | | Hyperactivity | Score |
				J.H.	A.H.	Initial	Last
(91)	RV	7	M	0111		101	9
(92)	JV	14	M	1000		41	
(93)	DV	8	M	1,0.5,0.5,0		51	53
(94)	CW	12	M	0011	0111	53	29
(95)	KW	8	M	1111		51	33
(96)	Ca.W	12	F	0.5,0.5,0.5,0	71	55	
(97)	DW	9	F	Normal			
(98)	FW	14	F	Normal			
(99)	TW	14	M	1111		59	
(100)	MW	13	M	0,0.5,0.5,1		75	35
(101)	LW	12	M	1000	1111	97	83
(102)	MW	10	F	1110			39
(103)	SW	14	F	1111			
(104)	KY	6	M	0111		59	43
(105)	EY	7	M	1111			29
(106)	VY	8	M	Normal			
(107)	RY	8	M	1111		43	55
(108)	SV	5	M	0.5,0.5,0,1		72	49
(109)	RW	6	M	0111			37
(110)	CW	6	F	1000			75

Case history accounts for each child are provided in the next section, but several general observations and conclusions can be made first to aid in understanding these cases.

Age

There is the usual preponderance of boys over girls in this series – 80 boys to 30 girls. No study has shown why this should be the case as it was for this series and for other published series. I have now seen over 1,500 children and again the ratio of male to female runs about 4 to 1. It does suggest that males have a greater need for supplementation with either vitamin B-3, vitamin B-6, or both than females. This idea is supported by the finding in this series that more females respond to vitamin therapy. Out of 30 females, 17 (57 percent) were normal at the last evaluation, while out of 80 males, only 26 (33 percent) were well. Being female not only protects against the development of learning and behavioral disorders, but when it does occur it is not as severe and responds better to megavitamin therapy.

Genetics

These children came from 91 families. Both parents were ill and vitamin B-3 dependent in 3 families, the mother only in 16 families, the father only in 13 families, and siblings in 2 families. Out of 91 families, a second child was vitamin B-3 dependent in 34 families. Both parents were equally dependent. However, of the 18 children who did not improve, 5 had a schizophrenic mother, not one had a schizophrenic father. It is likely that having a schizophrenic mother is a detrimental factor probably because it is more difficult for a sick mother to properly look after her children and to enforce the diet and supplementation. The most important single variable is a firm parent who can ensure supplementation will be taken. If this does not occur the child will not recover. In 15 families, 2 or more children had been treated.

Children Who Did Not Respond

The response is clearly related to duration of treatment. This is shown in the table below.

	Clinical Rating				
	0	1	2	3	4
August 1973	9	17	23	20	41
Last seen	5	13	18	26	48

There was a shift toward recovery as treatment continued. The percentage of the children who were much improved and well increased from 61 percent in August 1973 to 74 when last evaluated. There were several reasons why some of the children did not improve. The most frequent was too low a dose of niacinamide or niacin.

I gave some of the children placebo. These were single blind in that the mother knew and agreed to the procedure. Most of them relapsed either within a few days, a few weeks, or sometimes after several months. When the vitamins were resumed, they recovered, but some children took twice as long to regain the earlier normal condition and needed more vitamin. For some, relapse induced by placebo can be very serious. I have not followed this procedure for the last 20 years as I do not consider it ethical to expose children and their families to this procedure.

Children on treatment and well for long periods are able to go off the vitamins without the same danger of relapse, and if they have been well many years, may never have to go back on, or if they do can take them as needed. Parents often took their children off during the summer as a test. Others would not give it to them on weekends. But they were observant and at the earliest indication of relapse would place them back on the program again. I advised parents to tell their children once a year why they are taking the vitamins. If they start early, they may have forgotten they ever saw the doctors who started them. I have had several teenagers who have suddenly asked their parents why they are taking vitamins and some of them have refused to continue. After it has been explained to them they are less reluctant.

Some of the non-responders had other conditions. From this series 3 had serious other conditions – hydrocephalus, severe epilepsy, and spina bifida. Some failed because I was not experienced enough and used too little vitamin, or did not pay enough attention to food allergies. Some needed pyridoxine as well as niacinamide. The need of children with KP in their urine to get pyridoxine was not then clearly established. Thus RJ was given both. When his mother ran out of B-6, he relapsed. On B-6 alone he did not recover. He had to have both. This is an example of a double dependency.

A few children will need much larger doses. Children are more tolerant of high doses of vitamin B-3 than are adults. One of my patients, not described in this series, had failed to respond to 6 G of niacinamide and treatment was stopped. I was not surprised as she had the appearance of a Down syndrome child. Over the following two years she was taken from clinic to clinic and given every possible treatment without success. The family was very disturbed and brought her back for me to try again. Her older brother had recovered from childhood schizophrenia on mega-vitamin therapy as had her father from his depression. When I saw her for the second attempt at treatment, she suffered from constant harassment from visions and voices which ordered her to attack her mother. She was very restless, agitated, and practically was out of control. As a last resort I started her on niacin 4 G three times daily and dilantin 150 mg. She had never convulsed but I thought this drug might provide additional support. A month later she was more relaxed. Her parents took 12 hour shifts with her to nurse her and hold her because she was so fearful of being alone. She was more relaxed, more at ease, and was able to sit quietly while she spoke about her hallucinations. One year later she was normal and had been well three years when I saw her last. Perhaps similar dosages might have helped some of my failures. Not many children are willing to take so much medication or might develop nausea. Luckily this patient was so disturbed and fearful of her symptoms that she would have taken anything I recommended and she could swallow pills by the handful.

Another patient, RS, who was better but still rated unimproved, did not make any major improvement until foods to which he was allergic were removed from his diet. Over the past 20 years, I have routinely investigated for the presence of allergies and place all my patients on an elimination diet, eliminating sugar and junk even if they have no specific food allergies.

Thus, when a child does not respond quickly enough, one should immediately check for the following factors: (1) Is the dose adequate; (2) Are there other organic reasons such as epilepsy, hydrocephalus, hypothyroidism, other vitamin deficiencies; (3) Are other vitamin and mineral dependencies present; (4) Are there mineral toxicities, such as lead or copper; (5) Are there food allergies. These must all be taken into account and treated.

Response by Age When Treatment Started

There was a trend for children over age 5 to respond better compared to children under age 5. The earlier age group showed a 50 percent response, the age 5 to 9 group a 66 percent response, and for the over 9 group a 73 percent response (much improved and well). This suggests the prognosis is better when the illness comes on later in life. Perhaps early appearance is a measure of the degree of genetic vitamin B-3 dependency. The earlier it appears the greater the genetic component. This may also account for a peculiar finding which has puzzled me for a long time. The usual effective starting dose for adults is 1 G per 50 pounds body weight. This was the dose originally used with children but with more study it soon became apparent that for most children this was not adequate. They needed two to three times as much and before long I started all children, even those under 50 pounds on 1G tid. The need for higher doses may also be a measure of the genetic need. The earlier the illness expresses itself the stronger is the genetic component and the higher the dose required relative to weight. It suggests the earlier the disease appears the more intensive the treatment must be.

Relation of Behavioral Scores to Clinical Evaluation

There is a slight curvilinear relationship between the hyperactivity scores and the improvement rating, as shown in this table:

	Clinical Evaluation Score	Hyperactivity Mean Scores	Number
Before treatment		76	84
Unimproved	0	78	8
Unimproved	1	60	18
Improved	2	50	17
Much improved	3	44	24
Well	4	37	29

The normal hyperactivity score is 45 or less. Ratings from 0 to 1 yielded the greatest decreases in hyperactivity scores – 18 units – while the change from 3 to 4 corresponded with the least decrease – 7 units. Parents were generally content with a much improved (3) or well (4) rating and a few were pleased with a 1 (unimproved) rating because they had not seen even these minimal responses with any other treatment. Of course, they did not remain pleased very long if the child did not improve further.

The hyperactivity score can be used to estimate the clinical improvement. Scores under 40 indicate the patients are well, between 40 and 46 indicate they are much improved, and scores of 47 to 55 indicate they are improved. Higher scores show they are not improved. Out of 33 who scored 39 or less, 18 (54 percent) were well and 12 (36 percent) much improved – i.e., 90 percent were in this category. Out of 12 who scored between 40 and 46, 2 were well, 7 much improved, 2 improved and 1 not improved. The hyperactivity scale thus correlated quite closely with clinical assessment. Since the hyperactivity scale can be used by any adult familiar with the child, parents can thus use the scale to measure progress and to test for relapse.

The Response to Orthomolecular Treatment

Out of 110 children, 74 were much improved or well at final evaluation. It is likely this number would have increased with continuing treatment. Another 16 were improved. Altogether 84 percent showed improvement. This data is similar to results reported by Dr Bernard Rimland in his studies. Psychiatric diagnosis was not closely related to outcome. What is more important than the descriptive diagnosis is an etiological diagnosis – i.e., whether allergies are involved and which nutrients are needed in above normal amounts. The children in this series responded equally well whether they were clinically schizophrenic, hyperactive, or dyslexic. Today they might have received any one of 50 different diagnoses. The poorest responders were children from mothers ill with schizophrenia, children with organic complications, children who had been sick for a long time, children who did not start speaking by age 5, and children who had behavioral disorders with no striking symptoms such as hallucinations, etc.

That this response was not due to orthomolecular treatment seems improbable for several reasons. The four double blind prospective experiments completed in Saskatchewan between 1952 and 1960, the first in psychiatry and the first in North American medicine, proved that vitamin B-3 is effective in the treatment of schizophrenia. Using vitamin B-3 treatment alone (without sugar-free, allergy-free diets) doubled the two-year recovery rates from the usual placebo 35 percent to 75 percent. Since then every clinical study using this treatment has confirmed these results. Chronic patients require much longer treatment periods, but they too respond to a combined nutritional supplement approach of which vitamins B-3 and B-6 remain the most important components.

The children switched over to placebo to replace the vitamin B-3 all relapsed, even when the ascorbic acid was not discontinued. Since all the tablets looked alike these children were not aware of any change. Their parents did know. but it is highly unlikely that their attitudes had any effect. The same attitude which might have been therapeutic because of the faith of the parents had not worked for long periods of time before they were started on the vitamins. Even if the faith of these children in the vitamin had played the major role, then if they relapsed on placebo, they should have responded almost immediately as soon as they went back on the vitamins. But usually after any relapse it took much longer for the same therapeutic response to reappear. Besides, very few children like to swallow pills and almost everyone had a negative outlook and no faith whatever in the tablets they were forced to take. They were big, rough, and tasted awful. The ones who did develop faith were the ones who became aware of the beneficial effect, like the children who called niacinamide their "happiness" pills because they felt happy when they were taking them. Finally, these children had not responded to medication, the colored tablets, easier to swallow and smaller, which they had taken in the past without any improvement. One would have to conclude that the placebo response was highly specific to vitamins only. No one has yet shown that placebo responses are that specific.

The placebo response is not dose related, yet the vitamin response is. Many children did not get well until the dose had been doubled or tripled.

Older children responded more quickly than the younger children. Female children responded better than male children. I know of no evidence the placebo response is age and sex related. There was a negative relationship between frequency of interviews and response. A placebo response depends on the relationship between therapist and patient. Many of these children had had close and frequent relationships with the mental health personnel who were treating them, often for years with very little response. Yet on the vitamins with a minimum of visits to my office they did respond. Very seldom do I see these patients for any form of psychotherapy except for the interviews when the treatment is explained to them and for follow up visits to find out how they are getting along.

The individual case studies of these 110 children related in the next chapter provide the anecdotal complement to these clinical trials.

Case Histories

During the course of my career, I have treated over 1,500 children with learning disabilities, behavioral disorders, and brain dysfunctions. For many of these children, I have created case studies. I have described these patients, some more carefully and in greater detail than others, in order to illustrate the kind of child treated, the response to treatment, and the difficulties which will arise from continuing treatment. There is enough detail so that physicians can use the protocols here as a guide to treatment. Parents will profit from reading these case histories for they will certainly find among these cases children whose problems may be similar to the ones they are experiencing. And this will encourage them to continue with treatment, no matter how sick their children are or have been. They are similar to children seen by other psychiatrists; I am sure of this for many of these children had been diagnosed and treated by other psychiatrists before they were referred to me.

The 110 numbered cases recorded here correspond with the 110 patients interviewed by John Hoffer in the clinical follow-up study described in the previous chapter.

(1) J.R.A.: Born October 1966, first seen April 1973. John was hyperactive from the moment he came into my office with his mother. This behavior began when he was 6 months old, after which time he slept very little and demanded a lot of attention. The marital situation became difficult and his parents separated. He remained hyperactive in school, got along very well with a good scholastic performance, but could not get along with the other children. At home he frequently suffered nightmares, saw ghosts and monsters coming at him, and would run from his room. He had been given ritalin 30 mg daily, which settled him a little. I started him on niacinamide 1 G after each meal, three times per day, or after breakfast, after supper, and before bed; on pyridoxine 250 mg twice daily, after breakfast and after supper; and on a sugar-free diet. One month later he was better. He resented swallowing pills and was instead given a powdered mixture which contained less niacinamide. After another month he no longer had his nightmares. His teacher, not knowing he was taking vitamins, reported, "John has made excellent progress in all subjects this year. He has devel-

oped good work habits and always tries to do his best. I am pleased to see him working and playing and cooperating with other boys and girls. I can see a real improvement in this area. With his ability and good attitude toward school I am sure he will do well in year two." At the same time the home situation improved. His mother began to live with a man who was sympathetic and liked John. His mother decreased the ritalin to 20 mg each day.

John Hoffer interviewed him July 4, 1973. He was still restless, had fewer nightmares, but got on well with his family and had made friends. He still reversed many numbers. He was rated 0101 – i.e., improved. By the end of July, he wanted to start back on the pills. By the end of September his ritalin was decreased to 10 mg daily. I stopped all the vitamins and gave him complamin instead, 300 mg three times daily. This is an ester of niacin and xanthine. He continued to get better, learned to play chess, but was still too impulsive and hyperactive. By mid-November there was a dramatic change. He was now well without any of the sedative effect of the ritalin, which had left him devoid of emotion. His parents preferred the complamin. The nightmares were all gone and he was doing well at school. His mother still gave him ritalin, 10 mg two or three times each month. His hyperactivity score went down from 97 on April 6, 1973 to 61 on November 14, 1973. His final rating was 0111 (total 3), or much improved.

(2) R.A.: Born November 1964, R.A. was first seen April 1968. Her mother reported that R.A. had been ill for three years, but had been much worse over the previous three months. She was very restless, kept on wandering away from home, suffered frequent temper tantrums. She was obsessed with being ill and with medicine. She lived in a world of pretense. She could not play with children and had begun to wet herself during the day. I started her on niacinamide 1 G od and vitamin C 1 G od plus a sugar-free diet. Three weeks later she was much better, and after three months was nearly well except for some residual irritability. On July 22, 1968 I started her on placebo to replace the niacinamide but not the ascorbic acid. Three weeks later her behavior had deteriorated so much she was almost out of control. The niacinamide was resumed. This time she responded more slowly, and on October 2 the dose was doubled. By February 1969 she was normal.

When examined by John Hoffer in July 1973, she was still well. She found mathematics hard but led the class in all the other subjects. She especially enjoyed reading and art. Her hyperactivity score had decreased from 81 in April 1968 to 29 July 4, 1973. The final evaluation was 1111 (total 4) – normal.

(3) B.A.: Born June 1967, B.A. was first seen in May 1971. He was well behaved and quiet but was too shy to speak to me. He had developed quickly, began to walk by age 9 months, and had been hyperactive ever since. He was a chronic fidgeter and could not sit still even during meals. His parents had started him on a multivitamin preparation which contained 25 mg of niacinamide. After one week he was a little better and then showed no further improvement. I started him on niacinamide 1 G three times daily (hereafter tid) and later had to reduce it to 1 G twice daily, hereafter bid. One month later he was better. He had wet the bed only twice in the month compared to every night before then. In September 1971 he was normal but then had a slight relapse. He was given niacin 1 g od plus the niacinamide, and in December, because he liked the niacin so much better, was given 1 G tid and the other B-3 was stopped. On July 3, 1973 he was normal. He had finished kindergarten. He still had a few nightmares with a fear of monsters in his closet. The niacin was increased to 4 G daily. His hyperactivity score decreased from 95 on May 21, 1971 to 45 on July 3, 1971. His final evaluation was 0111 (total score 3) – much improved.

(4) T.A.: Born January 1960 (adopted), T.A. was first seen in May 1971. When he was 2 years old, he suffered one grand mal convulsion. He was adopted by age 4, had begun to speak early, was brilliant in Grades 1 and 2, but then deteriorated. He became hostile, ambivalent, and no longer responded to positive or negative sanctions. He could read but could not write legibly and was very restless. He was found to be allergic to dairy products, pork, peas, carrots, and grasses. One year of therapy at a child mental clinic produced no improvement.

When he was 6, during a bout of pneumonia, he saw a skeleton, heard his name called and had responded to it. When I saw him he could hear himself think (this is a classical schizophrenic symptom). It sounded like a voice which spoke of war and ordered him to throw pins, which he did sometimes. He felt unreal, had many daytime fantasies of war and of killing people. He was convinced people were talking about him in a nasty way, suffered interruptions in his flow of thought, and his memory was poor. I started him on niacinamide 1 G tid, ascorbic acid 1 G tid, and the sugar-free diet. One month later he was better, but I increased the niacinamide to 2 G tid. After five months he was much better, more cooperative, more agreeable, and enjoyed school more. By June 1973 he was nearly well. He still had difficulty relating to his classmates. On August 24, 1973 he still had a few problems at home, resisted taking the vitamins, and argued a lot with his family. His allergies were worse, but his last school report was the best he had ever had. I decreased his niacinamide to 1 G bid. In June he was started on a preparation containing nicotinic acid 1 G, ascorbic acid 1 G, thiamin 150 mg, and pyridoxine 200 mg per teaspoon, tid. His hyperactivity score decreased from 85 in May 1971 to 51 in August 1973. His final evaluation was 1.5, 0.5, 0.5, 0 (total 2.5) – improved.

(5) Bar.A.: Born December 1962, Bar.A. was first seen in June 1972. She was very irritable and could not get along with other children at school. Her grades at school had dropped form Bs to Cs and Ds. Reading was a problem in the first two grades. Her parents started her on niacinamide 500 mg tid but saw no improvement after two months. She told me she saw her nightclothes turn into animals and often felt there were animals in her closet so she kept the door closed always. She saw large ghosts in her room, larger than men, but knew they were not real. Words jiggled about on the page, she suffered from nightmares, and heard herself think. Her thinking was paranoid, believing people were talking about her, laughing at her. There was blocking, comprehension was poor, as was her memory and concentration. She was, not surprisingly, very tired, depressed, and irritable. I started her on niacinamide 500 mg tid, pyridoxine 250 mg bid, periactin 4 mg tid, ritalin 20 mg od, and the sugar-free diet. On September 5, I increased the niacinamide to 1 G bid. By then most of the perceptual symptoms were gone. By October 13, 1972 she was well. On April 13, 1973 she had deteriorated a little, and I added niacin 500 mg tid. In August 1973 I started her on inositol niacinate 1 G tid because she was having some nausea from her niacin. On November 7, 1973 she was making steady progress. By February 8, 1974 she was normal. Her hyperactivity score decreased from

97 in June 1972 to 47 in June 1973. Her improvement rating was 1111 (4) – normal.

(6) Ter. A.: Born February 1966, Ter. A. was first seen in December 1972. He was was B.A.'s brother. He could not read, could not understand words nor remember them. All letters appeared upside down, and when he tried to write, the words appeared funny. Early in 1972 he had surgery for a constriction of his aorta which had cut off circulation to his legs. Following that his problems became worse, and he became easily upset and harder to discipline. He told me he was afraid of the dark because he saw monsters in the shadows and often saw a big face staring down at him from the ceiling. He knew these images were not real but was still afraid of them. Often he heard footsteps in the attic and insisted his mother search the house. In school he believed his classmates were making fun of him. He was occasionally depressed and tired. I started him on niacinamide 1 G tid and pyridoxine 250 mg od. One month later he was less paranoid and less disturbed by his visual illusions but he continued to see double. Three months later the diplopia was gone, he was free of perceptual symptoms, but he was very restless. I decreased the niacinamide to 500 mg tid, added niacin 500 mg tid, and ritalin 10 mg od. By June 1973, although still having a problems with reading and spelling, his marks in school had gone up from fair (the teacher's rating) to between good and very good. John Hoffer saw him and found him not improved, scoring 1000. In August niacin was stopped because it took away his appetite, and he was restarted on niacinamide 1 G od. In November 1973 inositol niacinate was added 2 G od. His behavior improved, but reading still remained a problem. In February 1974 this was increased to 3 G od, pyridoxine was added 250 mg od, and ritalin was stopped and replaced by imipramine 25 mg before bed. His hyperactivity score decreased from 61 in December 1972 to 39 in June 1973. His final evaluation was 1000 (1) – not improved.

(7) Rob. A.: Born September 1961, Rob. A. was first seen in October 1972. One year before I saw him, he had been in the emergency ward of a hospital where he had seen several severe accident victims. After that he became seclusive, fearful, began to suffer severe nightmares, and eventually refused to go to school because he could not think. He became very paranoid. He

told me he felt rotten, nervous, and could not sleep. He was started on a diet and a moderate vitamin program by a chiropractor and began to improve. After they moved to Saskatoon he was off his vitamins for one week and quickly relapsed. On examination he reported that people were watching him all the time so he kept his curtains closed. In his nightmares he saw an invasion from other planets, and if he awakened the dream would stay with him. In the shadows he saw men and other living beings. He was afraid to go to the bathroom at night. He heard himself think and talked back to these thoughts and often felt unreal. In school he thought other boys were plotting against him. He could not think without interruptions, his concentration was poor. Numbers confused him. As a result he was depressed, nervous, tired, and had been suicidal. I started him on niacinamide 1 G tid, ascorbic acid 1 G tid, pyridoxine 250 mg od, and the sugar-free diet. In December 1972 he was better, the rotten feeling was nearly gone, school was easier, all symptoms were less intense. I then added a compound containing amitriptylene 25 mg and perphenazine 2 mg at bedtime. In March 1973 he was a lot better. In May he came through red measles with no relapse. In August John Hoffer found he still had a few visual illusions, had had one hallucination, and was still nervous. On the hyperactivity test his score decreased from 65 in October 1972 to 45 in August 1973. His improvement score was 0111 (3) i.e. much improved. His HOD scores decreased from very high to normal or near normal levels. Total score decreased from 123 to 32, perceptual score from 10 to 2, paranoid score from 10 to 2, depression score from 11 to 5.

(8) C.B.: Born April 1959, C.B. was first seen in February 1972. She had been getting progressively more nervous for four years with fatigue and nervousness at school and overactivity at home. She told her mother all the children were against her and hated her and her parents. She was very fond of junk food. To me she complained only of intermittent pain in her abdomen. I started her on niacinamide 1 G tid, pyridoxine 250 mg od, and the sugar-free diet. One month later she was well. On July 23, 1973 John Hoffer found she was not following her diet and had stopped taking her vitamins because she did not like swallowing pills. According to her parents had relapsed to her previous condition. She had failed grade 7. She was rated 0000 – i.e., not improved. Because she did not like the taste of

niacinamide, I started her on capsules instead and again she was well one month later. She no longer objected to taking these capsules. Her hyperactivity score decreased from 87 in February 1972 to 40 in April 1972, then increased to 55 in July 1973. Her final evaluation was 1111 (4) – well.

(9) K.B.: Born March 1962, K.B. was first seen in August 1969. He was brought in by his mother who was recovering from chronic schizophrenia on megavitamin treatment and she was worried her son was becoming sick. She complained that at times he was unaware of what was going on, unresponsive and sluggish. His memory was very poor, he was repetitive and slow. At times he appeared normal. I did not think he had schizophrenia, but because it was possible it could be starting gave him niacinamide 500 mg tid. In February 1971 he was no better. There was a complication. The school nurse advised his mother she was not giving him enough love. I increased the vitamin to 1 G tid and started him on parnate 10 mg in the morning. He had to stop the drug in four days. By August 1971 he was better at school but not at home. On November 8 I added ascorbic acid 1 G bid and pyridoxine 250 mg od. In February 1972 I added ritalin 20 mg od and two months later increased this to 40 mg. That summer I stopped the ritalin. In September 1972 he was nearly normal, but he did not like taking vitamin pills. By November 26, 1973 he remained only on niacinamide and was not doing as well. He had trouble modulating his voice, especially when excited, but had made a B average at school. John Hoffer in July found he still had visual illusions, was forgetful and depressed. He was not on the sugar-free diet. J.H. concluded that his schizophrenic mother had difficulty coping with her son and did not supervise his treatment well. His hyperactivity score went from 75 in February 1971 to 47 July 1973. He was rated 0100 (1) – not improved.

(10) S.B.: Born November 1970, S.B. was first seen in May 1973. For 6 weeks before she saw me she had hardly any sleep. After she was born, she had severe colic and was found to be dairy allergic. She was hyperactive from birth, walking and running from 11 months. She began to speak at 1½ years. She was then put back on milk. I advised her parents to eliminate both dairy products and sugar and added niacinamide 1 G od, ascorbic acid 1 G od, 150 mg thiamin od, and 200 mg pyridoxine od. Three days later she

terrorized her mother by her demands for sweets, her temper tantrums and hyperactivity. I added ritalin 10 mg od and allowed small amounts of sweets. But each time she took ritalin she was worse for two hours. On July 5, 1973 I started her on niacin 1 G tid and pyridoxine 250 mg od. By October 11, 1973 she was normal but had many colds. I added ascorbic acid 2 G od and halibut liver oil 1 capsule od. Her hyperactivity score decreased from 81 on May 23, 1973 to 29 on October 11, 1973. Her improvement score was 1111 (4) – normal.

(11) L.B.: Born February 1967, L.B. was first seen in February 1972. When she was 3½ years old she found some pills containing LSD which had been hidden in the back lane. Within a few hours she was very disturbed, bizarre, ataxic, and could not speak clearly. Her pupils were widely dilated and she was very hyperactive. She was admitted to hospital for two days and heavily sedated. The hospital was unaware of the findings I had published several years before that niacin was an excellent antidote against LSD. She appeared to be hallucinating. From then on she remained hyperactive, irritable, could not get along with other children, and became a discipline problem. She told me she was seeing ghosts and black monsters. Objects were distorted, the tip of a pencil looked like a face, and when she took off her jacket her arm appeared hairy and manlike. She heard voices. Any one having experienced the effect of this hallucinogen can sympathize with her. I started her on niacinamide 1 G tid and pyridoxine 250 mg od. Five weeks later she was better, most of the visions were gone, and she had not heard voices for ten days. The niacinamide caused nausea and she had been able to take only half the dose. I then started her on niacin 1 G tid. Four months later she was nearly well. She was restless occasionally and sometimes slightly paranoid. After another two months she was well. John Hoffer in July 1973 found visual illusions were still present. When she closed her eyes, she could visualize cities, witches, and frightening images. Her mother had stopped all the vitamins two months before, thinking her daughter was well and was not aware that she still had these illusions. Her hyperactivity score decreased from 77 February 20, 1972 to 37 August 7, 1973. Her improvement rating was 0111 (3) – much improved.

(12) E.B.: Born April 1960, E.B. was first seen in April 1971. In March 1966

he was taken to an outpatient clinic for children because of a speech defect. He was in the low normal intelligence range and a little restless. After a year the clinic concluded there was nothing wrong with him and blamed his mother, because, they said, she was unable to tolerate a normal noisy youngster and failed to show him any affection. Not surprisingly, his mother refused to go back to the clinic. In April, Eric complained he could not get along with other students, that they teased him too much, and he was bored at home. His mother was worried about the deterioration of school performance, about his lying, and his temper outbursts. He gave a good account of his own mental state:

Perception: He suffered recurrent fearful nightmares, prophetic dreams, heard his name called frequently, especially when he played his guitar, heard people chattering about him that they were going to kill him, talked to himself, and felt unreal. He often felt there was another person in his head.

Thought: He often believed he was a skeleton dreaming about what had happened to him when he was alive. Children were talking about him, laughing at him, making fun of him, and spying on him. His memory and concentration were poor and he blocked.

Mood: He was sad, often wishing he had never been born.

I started him on niacinamide 1 G tid, ascorbic acid 1 G bid. One month later he was better. I wanted to increase the amount of vitamin B-3 to accelerate improvement and added niacin 1 G tid but later had to change this to inositol niacinate. He continued to improve slowly, and in April 1973 I increased his niacin to 3 G tid and started him on parenteral B vitamins, once each week. By July 1973 he was much better. John Hoffer interviewed him on July 9, 1973. His mother described his as normal and ascribed the major improvement to the injections. His family doctor was very surprised and impressed by his remarkable improvement. He had fewer mood swings, got on much better with others, was happier. He still had headaches in the morning and was still paranoid but there were no behavioral problems. On October 4, 1973 he was normal. His hyperactivity score decreased from 106 on April 28, 1971 to 51 on October 4, 1973. His improvement rating was 0110 (2) – improved. His mother thought he was 0111 (3).

(13) P.B.: Born May 1964, P.B. was first seen in July 1972. He began to walk at 12 months and was immediately hyperactive. His mother was able to cope with his activity until she was informed by a social worker that he was hyperactive. At 4½ years he was examined by a psychologist who reassured the parents that he was normal but overactive. In grade one he had great difficulty, he learned slowly, and could not relate to the other children. He was promoted to grade 2 anyway and began to suffer fearful dreams. He hallucinated monsters at night and became afraid other children would beat him up. By now it was clear he could not read and was dyslexic. From November 1971 to March 1972 he was treated by an educational consultant under the supervision of a child psychiatrist who believed that all these children were the product of difficult child-parent relationships. There was no improvement. He told me about his visual illusions he had seen before and how he could get rid of them by turning the light on. His memory and concentration were poor. In the office he could not sit still, constantly jiggling in his chair and looking all around the room without pause. I started him on niacinamide 1 G tid and pyridoxine 250 mg od. On September 5, 1972 reading was easier and more fun. He could now read a page in 5 minutes. It had taken 30 minutes before that. On February 27, 1973 he was normal. He was learning so quickly he was taking classes in both grades two and three, and his teachers fully expected him to reach his peer level. He was active in sports, hockey, swimming. John Hoffer found him normal on August 1, 1973. His mother told John that a few months before he had refused to take his pills and he quickly began to regress. If he missed the vitamins for two days, he regressed. His hyperactivity score decreased from 95 on July 25, 1972 to 33 on August 1, 1973. His improvement evaluation was 1111 (4) – normal.

On February 27, 1973 P.B.'s father came to see me. After seeing his son's dramatic recovery on the vitamins, he remembered that as a child he too had been hyperactive, aggressive, and had a violent temper. He had been very self-conscious, had paranoid ideas, and could not concentrate. His mood was down, with depression and irritability. He had started to take niacinamide 1 G tid and in a few weeks was much better. He completed the hyperactivity test as if he were back into his childhood and scored 85. On August 1, 1973 he was well. He and P.B. were teaching each other how to spell.

(14) A.C.: Born March 1965, A.C. was first seen in April 1973. A.C. came to see me because he could not read and was hyperactive, compared to his identical twin. He had to read slowly, had trouble understanding the meaning of the words. Words moved back and forth on the page, dots ran together, and four dots looked like five. In his dreams he saw himself kicking people around. When his name was called, it reverberated through his head. He was started on niacinamide 1 G tid, pyridoxine 250 mg od, and the sugar-free diet. Two months later he was better, and by August 22, 1973 he was well. John Hoffer found him almost well. On October 23, 1973 he had impetigo, became more restless, and again could not get on in school. But by November 13, 1973 he was again much improved. His hyperactivity score decreased from 85 on April 12, 1973 to 55, October 23, 1973. His improvement score was 0111 (3) – much improved.

(15) T.C.: Born 1965, T.C. was first seen in April 1973. A.C.'s twin brother, T.C., also was learning disabled, could not understand words, and did not like math. He had received remedial reading instruction the previous summer with little improvement. At times he drifted into a world of his own. His behavior at home was bad. Often in the morning he could hear yelling, which he said was his brain calling him. It was the same sound he heard before falling asleep the previous day. He was started on the same program as his twin. On June 12, 1973 he was better, could read easily, and found this so exciting he could hardly put down the books. John Hoffer on August 22, 1973 found he had a few visual illusions. His teacher found his improvement astounding. His final evaluation was 0111 (3) – much improved. His hyperactivity score changed from 79, April 12, 1973 to 41, October 23, 1973.

The father of these twins had been depressed for 23 years, hearing voices, feeling unreal, with blocking, paranoid ideas, poor memory and concentration. He was started on treatment as well. When last seen he was free of perceptual symptoms but was still depressed.

(16) B.C.: Born May 1961, B.C. was first seen in September 1970. B.C. was overactive by age 3, as well as inattentive, unresponsive to punishment, defiant and troublesome. By age 9 he was worse. At school he was an average student. He tended to stare at lot into space. He believed people were watching him at night in his room and was very fearful of a far corner of his room where he sensed a presence. He had prophetic dreams which often came true. He was started on niacinamide 1 G tid and neuleptil 5 mg after supper. Between September and January 1971 his appetite improved, he became less fearful, less irritable, and he gained 5 pounds. August 1972 he developed abdominal pain. In December I decreased the vitamin and added pyridoxine 250 mg od. He was off drugs for four months. Instead he took niacin 1 G tid. On August 29, 1972 he still suffered abdominal pain every two weeks. He was now on imipramine 25 mg before bed and periactin 4 mg od as needed. Later that fall he became jaundiced and itchy and passed clay-colored stools and dark urine. The vitamin B-3 was stopped and his jaundice cleared. When the niacin was resumed his jaundice came back. His mother was advised to give him inositol niacinate if he should deteriorate while continuing him on pyridoxine 250 mg od. He remained well. His hyperactivity score decreased from 69, September 1970 to 47, July 1973. His improvement evaluation was 1111 (4) – normal.

I have seen only two cases of jaundice in children on niacin or niacinamide but never with the inositol ester. One child who became jaundiced on both forms was well on inositol niacinate. Both children recovered completely when the vitamin was stopped. Perhaps too rapid a release of vitamin into the blood stream was responsible, swamping the liver enzymes. A product which releases it very slowly, as does the inositol ester, will probably not produce this side effect.

(17) C.C.: Born June 1964, C.C. was first seen in December 1972. C.C. walked by age 16 months, began to speak at age 3, and was soon after a little overly active. He did not speak clearly, and received speech therapy. When I saw him, he still had a speech defect and he could not read. Words looked funny. I started him on niacinamide 1 G tid, ascorbic acid 1 G bid, and pyridoxine 250 mg od. One month later he was more relaxed but still moody in the morning. His visual illusions were gone, he slept dry, was more inquisitive, and his memory had improved. Three months later he remained

at the same level. I asked his mother to stop the vitamins as a test. John Hoffer saw him July 10, 1973 after he had been off vitamins for ten days. He was well, 1111 (4). His mother felt he was close to normal and he had shown marked improvement in school. His hyperactivity score, which was 57 on December 9, 1972, remained about the same at 55 on July 10, 1973.

(18) And.C.: Born April 1962, And.C. was first seen in July 1972. His mother began to worry when he was 2½ years old because he could not complete puzzles his younger brother had no difficulty with. He could not tell a triangle apart from a square. He had started walking at age 19 months. When he was 3 years old, his physician concluded he was too dependent on his mother. At age 4 he was evaluated by a mental health clinic and diagnosed as minimally brain damaged (a term no longer used). His I.Q. was tested at 50. When I first saw him, he had been on ritalin 20 mg for two years with minimal response. I started him on niacinamide 1 G tid and pyridoxine 250 mg od. One month later he was better. He was more independent and had learned to fish over the summer. By November he was much improved. Socially he was so much better that his brothers and sisters invited him to go along with them to play. They had never done this before. In February 1973 he was normal three weeks out of four. John Hoffer on July 5, 1973 found him the same. The dose of niacinamide had to be reduced because it caused some nausea, but as the dose decreased, the hyperactivity increased. His clinical evaluation was 0110 (2) – improved. On October 24, 1973 he was worse again as he was not able to take the vitamin. He was very restless but still did well at school. He was therefore started on niacin 1 G tid. On December 31, 1973 he was on ritalin 10 mg and a smaller dose of niacin but remained well. His hyperactivity score decreased from 87 on July 31, 1972 to 51 on July 5, 1972.

(19) Ri.D.: Born May 1961, Ri.D. was first seen in October 1968. He was a pale, sick-looking child who complained he was very nervous. He had failed grade one and was repeating it. He did not join in any activities, his attention span was brief, he was always in trouble, and behaved foolishly. Coordination was poor, reading was slow, and when he wrote, he reversed words and wrote mirror writing. He was perceptually disturbed, convinced people were always watching him, had horrible nightmares of

people's heads being chopped off, and hallucinated little men the size of footballs who spoke to him. He often had told his mother about these. Sometimes he saw visions on the floor and tried to get rid of them by stamping upon them. He was also paranoid, believing his hallucinations were real. Learning was very difficult. He was entered on a placebo controlled study and happened to get niacinamide 1 G od and ascorbic acid 1 G od. After one month his nightmares vanished as did his hallucinations; he was better in school but his behavior remained unchanged. His niacinamide was changed to 500 mg tid. On January 7, 1969 he was well according to his mother, but over the following month was worse again. The niacinamide was increased to 1 G tid, but the hallucinations had recurred. On January 7, 1969 I added mellaril 25 mg at bedtime and in June 4, 1973 increased it to 50 mg. From December 31, 1970 to September 24, 1970 he continued to improve, except for a time in June when he hid his pills and began to regress. On September 24, 1979 he was started on placebo, and after three days rapidly relapsed to a frightening degree. He was quickly placed back on the vitamin. By the end of 1970 his behavior was normal but he still could not speak clearly and coordination was poor. I increased the niacinamide to 5 G od. In April, 1972 his mother thought he was almost well, but by March 1973 he was again a discipline problem and doing badly at school. John Hoffer saw him on July 4, 1973 and found him not improved. He could bring back his visual illusions at will, was paranoid, had difficulty with reading and concentration. He was just getting by in school. Whenever he did not follow the regimen, he behaved foolishly. On September 5, 1973 he was enrolled in a special class for emotionally disturbed children. His hyperactivity score was 81. By December 26, 1973 he had gained more confidence, was free of perceptual symptoms, but was still socially inept and had difficulty getting along with people. He was now given niacin 1 G tid, pyridoxine 500 mg tid, and zinc manganese supplement. It was about this time that orthomolecular psychiatrists became aware that for children with kryptopyrrole in their urine pyridoxine and zinc were very important. When tested in October 1971, he excreted a lot of KP in his urine.

(20) Ro.D.: Born December 1959, Ro.D. was first seen in March 1969. She was Ri.D.'s sister. Her mother, a recovered schizophrenic patient of mine,

brought her in after she told her she was having visual hallucinations. She told me about her nightmares, her visual illusions and hallucinations seeing animals in her room, a monkey hanging by his tail looking down at her, and she heard her name being called. She once felt something bite her. Math was a problem and she could not concentrate. She was miserable and depressed. Her mother had started her on vitamins before I saw her, which in a few weeks stopped the hallucinations. I kept her on niacinamide 500 mg tid and ascorbic acid 500 mg tid. She had kryptopyrrole in her urine. By December 31, 1969 she was well. On September 12, 1970 I started her on placebo, stopping the vitamin. A few weeks later she began to complain of headache, insomnia, visual illusions. The niacinamide was resumed and she recovered. She remained on her vitamins until March, 1972. John Hoffer saw her on July 4, 1973 and found her normal. She remembered her previous symptoms. On December 26, 1973 she was still well, her urine was free of KP. Her hyperactivity score decreased from 87 on March 1969 to 31 on July 4, 1973. Her clinical evaluation was 1111 (4) – well.

(21) A.E.: Born August 1965, A.E. was first seen in March 1973. His mother had recovered on megavitamin therapy after many years of depression. She brought her son in because of his extreme hyperactivity. He suffered many visual illusions. Shadows appeared to be people, words moved up and down the page, letters were reversed or were upside down, and he could hear and see monsters. He believed children were making fun of him, did not like him, and on several occasions thought a boy had tried to kill him. He was depressed with suicidal ideas. I started him on niaci-namide 1 g tid, pyridoxine 250 mg bid, and the sugar-free diet. Two months later he was much better. On August 2 he was examined by John Hoffer who found him free of perceptual symptoms but still paranoid and having difficulty with children. In school his performance oscillated from good to bad every few days. When ever he went off his vitamins he quickly relapsed. He was evaluated 1010 (2) – improved. On September 25, 1973 I added niacin 1 G tid. His hyperactivity score on Feb 26, 1973 was 84, on May 31, 53, on August 2, 67, and on September 25, 1973, 73.

(22) M.F.: Born May 1959, M.F. was first seen in April 1973. Her mother was a chronic schizophrenic who had recovered on megavitamin therapy with

a series of ECT and a diet free of red meat. M.F. became very nervous about three months before I saw her, about schools and other things, with no apparent reason. The nervousness would come and go accompanied by excessive perspiration. She was worse before her period. She had become less active socially and was always depressed. Her main complaint was that she felt unreal. I started her on niacinamide 1 G tid, pyridoxine 250 mg bid, and diet. By June 4, 1973 she was much better, but the feeling of unreality had not gone. On August 16, 1973 John Hoffer found her well (1111). She still felt slightly unreal but had no other problems. In school she was excellent. Her parents had noted the major change came after starting the program. In September she had two bad weeks. She stopped eating red meat and in a few days was well again. In November I added ascorbic acid 1 G bid. She remained well.

(23) D.F.: Born May 1961, D.F. was first seen in October 1970. D.F.'s only complaint was that his eyes were sore when he read for a while. Words would jump up and down on the page and he would get a headache. His mother found him irritable, hard to handle, and slow in school. As a baby he had a speech defect. He told me faces appeared blurry, that his pink desk often looked blue, and his floor shimmered. I started him on niacinamide 1 G tid. By January 14, 1971 he was much better. Most of his symptoms were gone. On April 12, 1972 he was well, and when John Hoffer saw him on July 10, 1973 he was still well, 1111 (4). His original hyperactivity score had been 45.

(24) B.F.: Born July 1959, B.F. was first seen in October 1967. From age 2 onward, B.F. was irritable and whiny. At age 3 he began to wet the bed. When he was 6, his parents started him on niacinamide and he stopped wetting his bed soon after that. At that time he was also receiving remedial reading for a disability. After a few visits to the speech clinic, he was discharged. I increased his niacinamide to 1 G bid, adding ascorbic acid 1 G bid. In November 1967 he got mumps with pancreatitis and high fever. During this he relapsed, his grades at school dropped, his speech became garbled, and he developed panic attacks. On February 11, 1968 he was placed back on his vitamins because he was very anxious, irritable, could not stop crying, could not study, and his spelling and printing deteriorated. On May 29, 1968 he made his first A ever in spelling. In July 1968 he

was paranoid about his schoolmates but was doing well at school and was at the top of grade 4. Before treatment he was at the bottom of his grade. In February, 1969 he was still irritable at times and his grades had dropped but he had more friends. On May 15, 1969 I started him on ritalin 10 mg od with no improvement. On March 2, 1970 I added neuleptil 5 mg, and by December 23, 1970 he was in grade 6 with a high B average. John Hoffer found him well on July 11, 1973. I found he was allergic to milk, and dairy products were withdrawn. His improvement score was 1111 (4).

(25) T.F.: Born August 1961, T.F. was first seen in October 1967. T.F. was two years younger than his brother B.F. He was a small, overly active boy who was normal but began to wet the bed when he was 6. His parents started him on niacinamide 1 G od and he began to sleep dry. In October 1967 he again started to wet and was tired all the time. On November 13, 1967 I doubled his niacinamide and his ascorbic acid to 1 G bid. On January 11, 1968 he was normal. I then started him on placebo to replace the vitamin B-3. Just before I did so his teacher had advanced him into a higher grade because he was doing so well. She did not know he was on this treatment trial. A few weeks on placebo his teacher found he was falling behind again and returned him to his previous grade. He began to wet again. His niacinamide was restored but he responded more slowly, and March and April were very bad for him. I increased his vitamins to 1 G tid, and by April 29, 1968 he was better, sulked less, and had a better appetite. On July 5, 1968 his vision was no longer blurred, bedwetting was very rare, and he had his best academic year. On June 1, 1970 he was normal. He called his niacinamide his happiness pills. On December 23, 1970 when still well he went off his vitamins. John Hoffer found him well July 11, 1973. His final evaluation was 1111 (4).

(26) W.F.: Born May 1857, W.F. was first seen in October 1967. W.F. and her two younger brothers B.F. and T.F. were the three siblings from four who came to me for treatment. Their father had been treated for schizophrenia in 1954 and was part of our original double blind controlled study. He was on placebo and did not respond. Later he was given niacin and became well. He remained well until one of his doctors ordered him to stop taking niacin. After awhile he relapsed. During this relapse, his wife also became schizophrenic. The problem for the community was so great they were

banished to Saskatoon where they arrived in 1960 on welfare. I saw them both and they both recovered on the megavitamin regimen. They have been well ever since. The mother has become a responsible, highly educated professional and the father has worked steadily. Three of their children were ill and are today normal. The fourth child did not need treatment.

When she was nine, her parents started W.F. on niacinamide 500 mg tid because she was so nervous, irritable, and difficult. Within a few weeks she was much better and her school grades increased from a low C to a mid B average. Two months before I saw her, she again was not doing well. She complained of headaches and she was more irritable. I doubled the vitamin dose and, on November 13, 1967 increased it to 1 G tid. By the end of the year she was well, cheerful, and had more self confidence. On January 11, 1968 she was started on placebo and soon began to deteriorate. Back on the vitamin she recovered and by July 1968 was well. During the summer of 1972 she went off her vitamins. John Hoffer in July 11, 1973 found her well. Her final assessment was 1111 (4).

(27) C.F.: Born October 1961, C.F. was first seen in March 1970. Both his parents were early schizophrenics. C.F. had been different from the time he was born. He did not respond to discipline, was very sensitive, easily hurt. At the mental health clinic he was diagnosed reading disabled. During the summer of 1969, his mother started him on niacinamide for one month. He was better but after the vitamin was stopped he reverted back. Three weeks before he came to see me they resumed the vitamin and he had started to improve. He was still very self-conscious, reversed words when he read, forgot very quickly what he had learned. He had never been affectionate or cuddly. I increased his niacinamide to 1 G bid with ascorbic acid 1 G bid. On April 6, 1970 he was better, words were easier to see, he no longer heard voices, but he was still reluctant to go to school. On July 6, 1970 he started grade 3. He felt well but had had some difficulty relating to the other children. John Hoffer on July 10, 1973 found him well. He did not follow his regimen carefully but as soon as he felt low would resume taking the vitamins. He was evaluated 1101 (3) – much improved.

(28) V.F.: Born July 1964, V.F. was first seen in June 1968. By age 3 he had temper tantrums, but he had been difficult from his birth, had matured

very slowly, and did not speak intelligibly by age 4. He appeared to understand. He spoke better to himself or to an imaginary playmate. He began to walk at 18 months but could not run by age 4. His father, a recovered schizophrenic, told me his son had suffered many nightmares and that he lived in a world of his own. I started him on niacinamide 1 G od and ascorbic acid 1 G od. One month later he was better with few temper outbursts, was more cheerful, began to explore more, and slept better. By October 22, 1968 he was much better. In January 1969 his father made up a new vitamin mixture for him which he did not like and refused. He quickly got worse. Back on his vitamin regimen, he again began to improve. On November 27, 1969 I started him on niacin 4 G od with mellaril 30 mg od. His parents had separated but V.F. was much improved, the best he had ever been according to his mother. He was nearly well until the summer of 1971 when he went off all pills for the summer. The regimen was resumed and by December he was well. His parents divorced in June 1972. He was seen by John Hoffer on July 17, 1973 and evaluated 0110 (2) – improved. His hyperactivity score decreased from 89 at age 3 to 27 at age 7, in 1971. But during his relapse the score increased to 75 on September 1972. His final score was 31 on July 17, 1973.

(29) M.D.B.: Born July 1962, M.D.B. was first seen in August 1971. He was slow to develop, began to speak by age 3, but his speech was very jumbled and indistinct, and he could not read. From age 3 he remained backward and immature, learning very slowly, and playing only with younger children. He received a lot of remedial reading. He had visual illusions, including the feeling people were looking at him, words moved up and down the printed page or they would momentarily disappear, and had visions of a dark man with a flashlight. He sometimes heard his name called and footsteps walking behind him. All his friends hated him, there was blocking, and he could not concentrate. I started him on niacinamide 1 G tid, ascorbic acid 1 G bid, and pyridoxine 250 mg bid plus sugar-free diet. In September the dose of niacinamide was reduced to 500 mg tid. He was only slightly better by October 1971 so I doubled his niacinamide and added niacin the same dose. He could not tolerate the niacin. At school he was better, but at home they saw no change. John Hoffer saw him August 2, 1973 after he had been off vitamins for 1½ years. He had the same visual

illusions and hallucinations, was still very paranoid and sad. He was promoted to grade 6 so he could stay with his peers and did not have the
capacity to do this grade. His final evaluation was 0100 (1) – not improved.
His hyperactivity score decreased from 71 on August 31, 1971 to 59 on
August 2, 1973.

(30) P.C.: Born June 1962, P.C. was first seen in April 1968. She had to be
removed from kindergarten because she cried all the time. She was not
able to work at school, being afraid she would do everything wrong. She
had nightmares and was very afraid because she heard people walking
around the house. Her mother was worried she was becoming schizophrenic and had started her on niacinamide 1 G bid and ascorbic acid 1 G
bid four weeks before I saw her. Her mother had one sister and two brothers, all schizophrenic. After taking these two vitamins for two weeks she
was much more cheerful and called them her happiness pills. By the time
I saw her she was not as good. She had many visual illusions and hallucinations of ghosts dressed in black clothes whose faces were distorted. She
could even see them in my office if she let herself. She also heard voices
talking to her. She was very much afraid of the hallucinations and was
depressed. On April 28, 1968 to September 4 she took 1 G of each of the
vitamins. But there was little improvement. In grade 1 she cried all day,
could not learn, and refused to have breakfast. After that I doubled both
vitamins. By March 19, 1969 she was much better, became fussy about
cleanliness, had no more hallucinations, played well with other children,
and her reading was improving. Her teacher did not think she would pass
grade 1. By July 15, 1969 her mother thought her normal. On March 19, 1970
she had deteriorated. Over Christ-mas she had started to eat more sugar.
Her performance at school got worse, she complained of stomachache,
nightmares returned, and words moved on the page. She had not been
taking her vitamins as recommended. I increased her niacinamide to 1 G
tid. By July 3, 1970 she was normal unless she ate sweets when she became
much worse. On October 1, 1970 she had been taken off the program for
July and August and had relapsed. After resuming the program she was
well in 7 days. August 24, 1973 J.H. found her normal. She was getting on
well in school in grade 6. Her evaluation was 1111 (4) – normal. Her hyperactivity score when seen by John Hoffer was 33.

(31) G.C.: Born February 1957, G.C. was first seen in May 1968. He was adopted at age 7 months and had been a difficult baby to rear. He was always very tense and on the verge of exploding. At school he was slow, could not read, and could not do math. He denied having any problems. He had perceptual illusions, hearing his name called, was paranoid, and suffered thought blocking. He did not excrete kryptopyrrole. I started him on niacinamide 500 mg tid, ascorbic acid 500 mg tid and pyridoxine 300 mg od. Five months later on October 25, 1968 he was better, the voices were gone, and he did better at school. Over the summer months he had deteriorated. This is not unusual since parents have less control over their children's eating habits over the summer when they are more on their own. I increased his niacin-amide to 1 G tid, ascorbic acid 1 G od, pyridoxine 100 od, added mellaril 20 mg od, and eliminated gluten from his diet. One month later he was better again. On January 14, 1969 there was no additional improvement, and I increased his mellaril to 25 mg. On April 11, 1969 there was no further change, and I stopped the tranquilizer and added ritalin 10 mg. By October 31, 1969 he was better again and made more progress in school. It became apparent that he deteriorated every summer when he cheated on his diet and ate more sweets. I increased his niacinamide to 2 G tid. On May 28, 1970 he was a bit better. I decreased the niacinamide to 4 G od and again placed him on mellaril, 100 mg. In August he had again relapsed and had started wetting the bed. His behavior had deteriorated so much I gave him a series of 6 ECT in mid September and after that he was better. On October 11, 1972 he was much better, a C student. On July 5, 1973 he was on 1 G of niacin-amide. Any more caused nausea. He was still hyperactive but his mood was good, his school report was very good, and he had made a few friends. He was evaluated 0110 (2) – improved. His hyperactivity score decreased from 93 retrospective for age 7, to 51 on July 5, 1973.

(32) L.F.: Born October 1961, he was first seen in July 1971. He began to speak at 18 months and to walk by 19 months. When 3 his speech remained unintelligible, but when I saw him he was speaking normally. He had a learning disorder for the previous two years. He told me letters sometimes reversed, lines wobbled, and comprehension was difficult. Remedial reading had helped a little. At night he often saw a large black ghost-like object

which filled the door and stayed until morning. He knew there were no ghosts and was not fearful of his apparition. At times he felt his hands were getting bigger and smaller. He was paranoid, blocked, found it hard to concentrate, and tested low on intelligence tests. His mood was down, sad and nervous. I started him on niacinamide 1 G tid, ascorbic acid 1 G bid. One month later he found it easier to learn but was still restless and on occasion still saw the ghost. His parents found him a lot better. In February 1972 improvement was sustained. He was free of perceptual changes and his self confidence was going up. On August 8, 1973 John Hoffer saw him. His mother reported he had done very well the first year on vitamins but had deteriorated during the second year. He still found it hard to concentrate, was a little suspicious, and was a slow reader. He was evaluated as 1, 0.5, 0, 0.5 (2) – improved. On September 10, 1973 I added pyridoxine 250 mg with a slow release niacin. He could not take the niacin. On November 29 that year he still had difficulty reading and was a little depressed. On February 28, 1974 he was well, 1111 (4), on niacinamide 1 G tid, ascorbic acid 1 G tid, and pyridoxine 250 mg od. His hyperactivity score was 43 on July 26, 1971, 35 on September 17, 1971, 61 on August 8, 1973 and 49 on November 29, 1973.

(33) Br.C.: Born December 1959, Br.C. was first seen in August 1971. For four years he had suffered continuous pain over his entire head and face most days. Rarely it was gone by mid-morning. Any excitement made it worse. He began to talk by age 14 months but needed speech therapy. When I saw him, he was speaking well. His school record was good, but he was easily hurt and lacked confidence. He complained of visual and auditory illusions and felt unreal. In school he was certain the students were talking about him and spying on him. He blocked, his memory and concentration were poor. When angry, he would think about killing the person he was angry at. He was sad, and when pain was severe, thought about killing himself. I started him on niacinamide 1 G tid, ascorbic acid 1 G tid, and pyridoxine 250 mg od. He remained on the program until the end of 1971, free of headaches. In April 1973 he experienced headaches every two weeks. In August 21, 1973 John Hoffer found him well. His mother was convinced the megavitamin program had made him well since nothing over four years before he started had been helpful. He was evaluated 1111 (4) – well. His

hyperactivity score decreased from 55 on August 27, 1971 to 35 on August 21, 1973.

(34) S.G.: Born December 1959, S.G. was first seen in May 1973. His father had become my patient in November 1972, and his response to megavitamin therapy had been marked. This interested him in having his son come as well. He had been worried about his son for a long time because he stuttered, would not associate with other children, and would cling to his father. S.G. felt he had no sense of personal space and could not get out of people's way. His father stated that when he looked at S.G. it reminded him of his own childhood. S.G. was being treated by a psychiatrist with tranquilizers. This made him worse. Under pressure from his father, the psychiatrist agreed to start him on niacinamide 500 mg tid and pyridoxine 250 mg od and the sugar-free diet. After a few months his stutter was gone, he was much better at school making Cs and Ds, an increase from Ds the previous year. S.G.'s parents felt the psychiatrist blamed them for their son's illness and asked to be referred to me. He was still irritable and easily aroused to anger. His father had taken him off the vitamins for several weeks before so that I could see what he was like without treatment. I increased the niacinamide to 1 G tid and pyridoxine to 250 mg bid. John Hoffer on July 27, 1973 found him free of symptoms, in grade 7. His father felt he was very much better. S.G.'s mother was a sullen, irritable, quiet woman who did not believe in medicine or diet and refused to cooperate. This threw the entire burden of care on his father. On November 13, 1973 S.G. complained he could not swallow pills and a liquid preparation was given him. He was still much improved. A younger sister was hyperactive but refused to follow any program and remained no better. S.G.'s HOD scores February 1973 were total 42, perceptual 5, paranoid 0, and depression 12. In May 1973 they were 3, 0, 0, 0. His hyperactivity score decreased from 109 in February 1973 to 62 in July 1973.

(35) N.G.: Born December 1965, N.G. was first seen in March 1973. He was referred because he had a reading problem and was making slow progress in school. He had been well until one year earlier when he became hyperactive, distractible, and slow. At the children's mental health center he was placed on bedtime sedation and remedial reading was recommended. I

found he could not read because of his visual illusions. Words moved about on the page, colliding with each other, and lines touched each other. He also suffered fearful nightmares which did not leave him when he awakened. In the semi-dark, clothes looked like bears. He could never sleep until he closed the closet doors. Voices called him and told him what to do. I started him on niacinamide 1 G tid and pyridoxine 250 mg od. Two months later he had started to get better. He was able to concentrate more, the perceptual symptoms were less troublesome, and he was able to read better since words were now quiet. He found it hard to swallow pills and only took ⅔ of the recommended dose. On August 27 he was much better and so evaluated by the clinic where he had first been evaluated. Instead of needing to repeat grade 2, he was functioning well in grade 3. John Hoffer found him improved. On December 24, 1973 his mother was worried he was becoming a behavioral problem. He was able to swallow pills, and his niacinamide was increased to 1.5 G tid, pyridoxine 250 mg od, and a pill containing amitriptyline 10 mg and perphenazine 2 mg at bed time. His hyperactivity score decreased from 51 on March 30, 1973 to 41 on September 27, 1973.

(36) R.G.: Born August 1963, R.G. was first seen in November 1972. He was asthmatic until age 2 but then discovered which foods made him worse. He became a very fussy eater, but his asthma disappeared. He remained a slow learner and was able to keep up only because he received special tutoring. He had to repeat grade 1. He was seen by a professor of Child Psychiatry who found him normal. His foster mother remained concerned about his lack of progress and his poor writing. Often in the dark he had visual illusions, seeing a man without a head pointing a gun all around. He was paranoid about other children, thought very slowly, had poor concentration and memory, and felt different from other children. He ate a very poor diet because he did not like the smell of many foods. I started him on niacinamide 1 G tid, pyridoxine 250 mg bid, and a multivitamin-multimineral preparation. He could not swallow pills. I therefore changed the program to niacin 1 G tid dissolved in juice plus a liquid multivitamin preparation. On February 28, 1973 he was more relaxed and could read for up to 1½ hours. He still refused medication and took his niacin powder mixed in his cream of wheat. On May 31, 1973 he was irritable but doing

better at school. John Hoffer saw him August 7, 1973 and found he had only one perceptual problem: he heard his name called rarely. He was still slow in his thinking and hesitant in speech and his language was sometimes bizarre. His diet was still too low in protein due to his many food dislikes. He was evaluated 0011 (2) – improved. On November 6, 1973 he was doing well at school. He had started bedwetting when he had started drinking milk. When this was eliminated he became well. His hyperactivity score was normal – 37 in November 1972 and also on August 7, 1973 it was 40.

(37) M.H.: Born June 1958, M.H. was first seen in February 1969. Her parents had separated in 1962. Her older sister lived with the father but rejoined her mother in 1967. From this time there was continuous bickering and fighting because her sister ignored M.H. but not a younger brother. She felt very badly about this. Her sister was schizophrenic who recovered on megavitamin therapy. M.H. had been a good student with a B average, but her marks at year end before I saw her had deteriorated to a C average. She always felt homely, sad, and that no one liked her. Her mother was very worried about these changes in her personality, even though the situation at home had improved a lot as her sister became well. I started her on niacinamide 1 G bid and ascorbic acid 12 G bid. On May 5, 1969 everything was better. She could concentrate better, no longer believed she was ugly, and her freckles had started to fade. On December 31, 1970 she was back to her usual B average at school but still felt the other students were against her. She was seen again in August 1973. Her mother had in the meantime married an alcoholic who was abusive to M.H. and had threatened her. She was disturbed by this as she tried very hard to get along. This marriage was also on the verge of disintegrating. She had been off all her vitamins for two years but had remained well. Her older sister had married and invited her to live with her. I advised her to take a moderate multivitamin mineral preparation. Her final evaluation was 1111 (4) – well.

(38) C.H.: Born May 1964, C.H. was first seen in December 1969. His mother became my patient in February of 1969. She had been drinking excessively for three years to control headaches, depression and irritability. She complained of visual illusions, voices, and was very paranoid. I diagnosed her schizophrenic and started her on niacinamide 1 G tid. By the

end of 1969 she was well. She gave birth to a girl in April 1970. She was taking niacin 4 G od and ascorbic acid 2 G od. She gradually became more depressed and in October 1970 I gave her 6 ECT as an outpatient. By March 1971 she was normal. In December 1972 she was admitted to hospital for a tonsillectomy, and because she could not swallow, was off all pills for ten days. Her voices came back, she became irritable and depressed, and on January 5, 1973 was admitted to hospital where she was given 5 more ECT. By April 1973 she was well.

C.H. was her first child. As a baby he had rocked a lot and later ran around in circles. In May 1969 he began to demand more attention, clung to his mother, became disobedient. Often he could not understand her. In school he had severe temper tantrums, would scream at the teacher and threaten to kill her. As his behavior in school deteriorated he became worse at home. A child psychiatrist saw him and concluded he was not sick but should be sent to a special class for emotionally disturbed children. I started him on niacinamide 1 G bid and ascorbic acid 1 G bid. His spooky dreams vanished in a few weeks, made a sudden burst of improvement, but in April 1971 he suddenly got worse. By June he was almost well. I increased his niacinamide to 1 G tid. Until October 15, 1970 he would get better, than slip again. I increased the niacinamide again to 1 G qid. He again was better but remained depressed. I tried parnate 10 mg but this activated his psychosis, bringing back visual hallucinations which lasted for ten days after it was stopped. By March 31, 1971 he rarely saw visions. I changed him to niacin 1 G tid because of nausea. I increased his niacin to 9 G od, but he could not tolerate this dose and it was decreased to 2 G tid. August 27, 1971 he was normal. His parents did not continue with pyridoxine and in a few days he was much worse. This was restored and once more he was well. This was tried several times with the same results. During 1972 he was getting on well until August when he had infectious hepatitis and was taken off all medication in hospital for two weeks. As his jaundice cleared he began to deteriorate and he was restarted on his vitamins. On July 6, 1973 he was on niacinamide 1 G tid. His jaundice had recurred. There was now a conflict between his pediatrician, who did not seem concerned over his behavior but was worried about his jaundice, and myself. On July 6, 1973 I started him on inositol niacinate 1 G tid, pyridoxine 250 mg bid, and imipramine 25 mg at bed. John Hoffer had found him unimproved, i.e., oooo. By September 28, 1973 he was much better, and according to his mother, was normal. His jaundice did not come back. His hyperactivity score reflected his condition. Before I saw him it was 107. By May 4, 1972 it was 28. On July 6, 1973 it was 119 and on September 28, 1973 it was 37.

(39) Cur.H.: Born June 1967, Cur. H. was first seen in June 1971. Suddenly when he was 4½ years old there was a change in his personality. He became very selfish, jealous of his baby sister, and a speech defect, previously barely noticeable, became worse. When excited, words tumbled out of his mouth and were unintelligible. He had been wetting his bed for the previous year. I started him on niacin 1 G tid, pyridoxine 250 mg bid, ascorbic acid 1 G tid, and the diet. His speech began to improve but the niacin caused nausea and vomiting. He was kept off the niacin until February 14, 1973 without any improvement. Then I resumed the niacin which he could now tolerate. By April he began to get better. He still saw visions and heard voices. On June 1, 1973 he was nearly well, and by September 1973 he was normal, more sociable, concentrated better and wet the bed rarely. His hyperactivity score decreased from 113 on June 14, 1972 to 33 on July 6, 1973.

(40) P.H.: Born February 1969, P.H. was first seen on December 1972. Her mother was very sick during the pregnancy and she was delivered by section. She began to vocalize at 8 months, but at 16 months she abruptly stopped and began to cry excessively until age 2. She was very restless and spent her days sitting in a hall with a blanket over her head rocking. She began to vocalize again at 2½ years old, and when I saw her, had started to babble. She pointed at things she wanted. At play school she was very restless. A special child investigative unit diagnosed her as mentally retarded. I did not agree with this and diagnosed her hyperactive syndrome. She started on niacin 1 G bid, ascorbic acid 1 G tid, thiamin 150 mg tid, and pyridoxine 200 mg tid. One month later she was less active. On January 17, 1973 I increased her niacin to 1 G tid. By April 24, 1973 her mood was much better, she tried to speak more, and could say mama and doll. I increased niacin to 1 G qid. I also added dimethyl glycine, 300 mg od. Dr. Allan Cott had told me he had seen a remarkable acceleration of speech development with this simple natural product. By August 29, 1973 she had started speaking in

sentences. She was more assertive, more self confident, walked better, could color within an outline. I increased the niacin to 2 G tid, and stropped the DMGF because it was expensive. I added a little zinc and manganese. She continued to improve and both parents were pleased with her progress. John Hoffer evaluated her as improved. On January 7, 1974 she was happier, chattered a lot more. She showed more initiative, was less hyperactive, colored well, used her imagination, and could sit quietly. On March 8, 1974 improvement was sustained. She was speaking a lot more, had a large vocabulary, and was socializing well with other children. Her hyperactivity score decreased from 63 on December 14, 1972 to 30 on January 7, 1974. On June 4, 1979 her Principal at the Focus Educational Service wrote, "P.H. is a bright little girl who displays no significant problems in her ability to understand and manipulate academic skills and concepts."

On October 19, 1981 she wrote me as follows: "I am in grade 7 this year but I still have problems that make it necessary for me to spend some time in a specialized program. However, before I can qualify for any of these programs, the school board requires a letter of recommendation from you. Would you please send such a letter to —-. Thank you very much. I hope you are keeping well. On December 1, we are moving to —- Street. It is a very big old house and I am looking forward to having more room and to helping mum decorate as the house needs an awful lot of work done on it." This is certainly not the type of letter a retarded person could have written.

Her mother continued to bring her to see me even after I moved to Victoria. I saw her last on July 29, 1993 and sent the following report back to her referring doctor: "I was very pleased with her continuing improvement when I saw her today with her mother. She reported to me quite happily that she was working at the college in —— as a kitchen helper, working about 6 or 7 months per year, and that this past summer she had been helping her grandmother who needs nursing care, which P.H. does very effectively. I found her speech very much improved, her manner was very good and friendly, and I was really very pleased with her progress. A mental state examination showed there were no changes in perception, she had no thought disorder, her memory was excellent, and her concentration was good. She was cheerful, and slept well. I have suggested that she go back on to ascorbic acid 1 G tid and a B-complex 50s od. This is in striking contrast to the findings on her when she was a baby and was found to have an intelligence quotient of 70 and described as totally non-verbal."

(41) J.H.: Born 1960, J.H. was first seen in May 1971. From birth Joe was a difficult baby. He did not eat well. He began to walk by 20 months and to speak at age 3½ years, but shortly after he was fitted for glasses, he stopped and did not speak again until he was 7. When I saw him, he was confused, read very poorly, words appeared jumbled, and numbers were reversed. He had been diagnosed as perceptually handicapped with mental retardation. He was in a special class for speech and occupational therapy. I started him on niacinamide 1 G tid, ascorbic acid 1 G bid, pyridoxine 250 mg od, and diet. One month later words stopped moving, reading was better, language was better and he enjoyed reading. On December 29, 1971 he was better. He had gotten worse over the summer at camp when he was not given his vitamins. I changed the amide to niacin 1 G qid. His mother then considered him normal. He was in a opportunity class in a regular school. He rarely saw figures reversed. Previous allergies were clearing. On July 19, 1973 he was evaluated by John Hoffer as much improved – i.e., 1011 (3). He was symptom-free, got along well at home and at school, was friendly. He would have been rated 1111 if he had been attending a regular school class. His hyperactivity score decreased from 47 on May 14, 1971 to 31 on July 19, 1971.

His mother wrote an account of his illness and recovery entitled "Bringing Up Joey" which appears in the Foreword to this book.

(42) B.I.: Born October 1963, B.I. was first seen January 1972. In December 1971 B.I.'s mother had consulted me for her depression present for four years. She had not responded to tranquilizers or psychotherapy. She complained of many visual illusions, which she found very frightening, and felt unreal. She was paranoid, blocked, and her ideas ran too quickly through her mind. Memory and concentration were poor. On the ortho-molecular approach she began to improve, and in July 1973 I gave her a series of 7 ECT. By the end of 1973 she was well, but a little tense and restless. She was worried about her son B.I. who was normal away from home but not at home. At home he continually fought with his siblings, cried a lot, complained that everyone was watching him all the time, and had seen visual hallucinations on several occasions. He was started on niaci-

namide 1 G tid and pyridoxine 250 mg od. But he could not swallow any pills and refused to take any. He was seen by John Hoffer on August 14, 1973 and there was no change. He was doing well at school, but his behavior was bad at home. His mother believed that all the difficulty arose out of religious difficulties between her and her husband and made no serious attempt to make him take the vitamins. He was evaluated 0001 (1) – not improved. On September 11, 1973 I saw both parents and they agreed to try to get their son to follow the program. One month later his behavior was much better at home. He was then started on liquid niacinamide 1 G tid. His hyperactivity score decreased from 93 on January 19, 1972 to 59 on November 15, 1973.

(43) R.J.: Born February 1966, R.J. was seen in February 1971. His mother became my patient in March 1969 because of her fear of dying present many years and high anxiety and tension which she had learned to control by excessive consumption of alcohol. She became alcoholic and her behavior became unusual, running around, and one occasion getting ready to leave home and her children for another man when her husband intercepted them. She then joined A.A. and had been abstinent for three weeks. She had experienced visual illusions and hallucinations and auditory hallucination long before she began to drink. She felt unreal, was paranoid and blocked with depression. On megavitamins she began to improve, losing all her symptoms except for depression which remained until she had a series of ECT January 1971. She then was well.

Her son R.J. had become irritable, aggressive, fidgety. His behavior reminded his mother of her own childhood and she was warned he too might become schizophrenic. R.J. described vivid monster nightmares and a few visual illusions. He was started on niacinamide 1 G tid. By May 19, 1971 there was little change. He was seen July 9, 1973 by John Hoffer who found him not improved, i.e., 0001. He did not get on well in school, was erratic in his studies, and his marks were gradually going down. He did not sleep well, was tired in the morning, never laughed or smiled and occasionally went into destructive rages. He was then started on niacinamide capsules 1.5 G tid and pyridoxine 250 mg od. By September 5, 1973 he was slightly better, less fearful, but he was stubborn about not taking pyridoxine as he did not like the taste. On December 12, 1973 he was better and was more cooperative. His behavioral score did not change much, being 79 on September 22, 1970 and 71 on July 9, 1973.

(44) S.J.: Born December 1963, S.J. was first seen in February 1971. Although her mother was worried about her shyness, her slow progress in school, her moodiness and mild hyperactivity, S.J. herself felt normal. I started her on niacinamide 1 G tid. In May 1971 she was better, and when seen in July 9, 1973 by John Hoffer she was normal, 1111 (4). She was taking only 1 G daily. Her hyperactivity score was 63 on September 22, 1970, 67 on February 19, 1971 and 53 on May 19, 1971.

(45) E.J.: Born April 1961, E.J. was first seen in October 1969. By age 2 he had learned 4 words but knew no more when I first saw him. His head was large, suggesting a hydrocephalic problem. He had received a shunt in 1969 and was getting speech therapy. When I saw him he could only say "ay,ay" in response to my questions. According to his mother, he knew 50 words. He made his needs known by pointing. He enjoyed watching T.V. The differential diagnosis included organic brain damage, infantile autism, and childhood schizophrenia. I started him on niacinamide 500 mg tid, ascorbic acid 500 mg tid, and one month later doubled the dose, adding thiamin 100 mg tid and pyridoxine 100 mg tid. There was slight improvement according to the speech therapist and his mother. On March 5, 1971 I could not find any improvement and added dimethyl glycine 100 mg tid. Again his mother saw some additional improvement in a month. He was then evaluated at a childhood retardation center and diagnosed as organic cerebral dysfunction due to arrested hydrocephalus. John Hoffer saw him in August 17, 1973 and found him unimproved 0000 (0). His behavioral scores remained unchanged from May 1970 to August 1973 at around 65.

(46) D.K.: Born November 1958, D.K. was first seen April 1968. Her mother was referred to me after severe mood swings present for seventeen years which were not responsive to the usual treatment for this disorder. But she was not manic depressive. She was schizophrenic with visual illusions, paranoid ideas that everyone was watching her, especially when she was depressed. She would refuse to leave the house. She thought her neighbors and her husband could read her mind. She was also confused, blocked, and

her memory and concentration were very poor. She excreted KP. I started her on treatment which included 6 ECT in August of 1968 and she began to get better. By the end of 1972 she was well after I added pyridoxine to her program.

She was worried about her daughter D.K. who was not doing well at school and was very irritable, very fussy over food and suffered from headaches. I started her on a sugar-free diet, but by February 1970 she was no better. I then added niacinamide 500 mg tid and ascorbic acid 500 mg tid. One month later there was no change. She had been eating large amounts of junk food. I doubled her vitamin intake and added pyridoxine 500 mg od. On August 28, 1972 there was some improvement. On November 6, 1972 her mother reported she had not suffered the usual hay fever and she was better in math and science. In November 1972 she had mononucleosis and was off all vitamins. She quickly relapsed and failed her classes. I started her on niacin 1 G tid. She was then in grade 10. Whenever she stayed on her program, she did well in school, but if she discontinued the program for a few days, she would quickly revert back to her previous state when she was moody, irritable, had many temper tantrums, and used profane language. On November 5, 1973 she was much improved and was well most of the time. John Hoffer found her 1001, (4) − improved, but with a fluctuating course. Her hyperactivity score changed from 79 on June 21, 1972 to 35 on June 19 1973 to 51 on August 3, 1973. Her behavior was remarkably sensitive to whether or not she took her vitamins and followed her diet.

(47) B.K.: Born October 1962, B.K. was first seen in February 1971. Early in 1970 his teacher was very unhappy with his progress. He did not concentrate on or complete his work, and had to be pressed continually to keep at it. He had been on niacinamide 1 G bid for one year with no improvement. When he saw me he described fearful dreams every night of animals and men after him, he was convinced that other children were talking about him and getting him into trouble to hurt him, that no one liked him, and he was often sad. I increased the vitamin to 1 G tid and added ritalin 10 mg od. By April 15, 1971 he slept with no dreams, had a good report from school, and was more cheerful, although still paranoid. On July 14, 1971 he was well. On August 13, 1973 he had been off all his vitamins following

pneumonia in mid-June. His visual illusions were back, his concentration was poor, and he was again sad. His June school report had been the best he had ever had. His mother did not think he had relapsed much, however. He was evaluated 0.5, 1, 0.5, 0 (2) – improved. His hyperactivity score was 57 on February 10, 1971, 38 on April 15, 1971 and 51 on August 13, 1973.

(48) S.K.: Born April 1961, S.K. was first seen in April 1972. He could not remember ever being free of tension and nervousness which caused a marked tremor and made it impossible for him to sit for more than two hours. His mother was worried about his hyperactivity, especially bad in a crowd, and his inappropriate social behavior which she dated from age 5. He occasionally suffered nightmares of monsters, and when he awakened, it took a long time before he realized he was awake. He also heard ugly noises. A loud sound reverberated through his head for a long time and he heard himself think. He was paranoid, had a recurrent fear of being kidnapped with his parents refusing to pay the ransom. Whenever he took a bath, he felt the house was burning down. He was tense, nervous, and often suicidally depressed. I started him on niacinamide 1 G tid and pyridoxine 250 mg bid with his sugar-free diet. One month later he was better, less nervous, no longer heard those noises, was less paranoid, had many more friends, and no longer worried about being kidnapped. On August 23, 1973 he was free of symptoms but his behavior was still bad at school where he was enrolled a special behavioral class. At home he was well. John Hoffer rated him 0001 (1) – unimproved, because of these difficulties at school. I increased his niacinamide to 4 G daily and a few days later there was a marked improvement.

His HOD scores reflected these changes:

Date	Total	Perceptual	Paranoid	Depression
April 13, 1972	47	11	6	6
May 15, 1972	52	9	3	7
August 28, 1972	26	7	0	4
Normal Scores	<30	<3	<3	<3

His hyperactivity scores decreased from 97 on April 13, 1972 to 49 on August 23, 1972.

(49) Ben.K.: Born April 1962, Ben K. was first seen in May 1973. Ben was referred by a child psychiatrist who had diagnosed him obsessive compulsive. He had been started on speech therapy in 1968 with improvement, but in 1970 his compulsive activity became more prominent. Every action was repeated twice – e.g., outside he would walk and then retrace his steps exactly the same way. He wanted every question asked of him to be repeated, and if someone did not do so, he would become very distressed. At first he told me that he could not hear properly but later admitted that he did hear the question. He had to have it repeated anyway. He spoke with a pronounced lisp, repeated words, but was embarrassed if told he had already said the word. Before seeing me, he had experienced voices. He was started in niacinamide 1 G tid and pyridoxine 250 mg bid. One month later his repetitive behavior had eased a little. On August 31, 1973 he was nearly symptom-free and was judged to be well – i.e., 1111 (4). He had never had a behavioral problem and his scores remained low, 43 on May 10, 1973 and 34 on August 31, 1973.

(50) L.L.: Born January 1963, L.L. was first seen in December 1972. During her first year she suffered colic for 9 months and never slept at night. From the beginning she was different from other children and was very hyperactive. She complained her nose was stuffy all the time so she could not concentrate at school. In the dark she saw many visual illusions, monsters and ghosts, and hallucinated her grandmother and her mother in the semi-dark. She could not fall asleep. She also could not concentrate, had a poor memory, and was nervous most of the time. She was not able to take niacin 1 G tid but was able to take 125 mg tid. After one week she was well, but five months later she went off medication and remained well. When seen on July 18, 1973, John Hoffer found her normal – i.e., 1111 (4). Because she was still a little overactive I advised her to start on niacinamide 1 G od. Her hyperactivity score decreased from 77 on December 27, 1972 to 35 on February 19, 1973.

(51) B.L.: Born July 1964, B.L. was first seen in October 1971. After four admissions to University Hospital, B.L.'s father diagnosed himself paranoid schizophrenia. He had set out on his own to read about the disease as he had not been told by any of his psychiatrists what his diagnosis was. He requested a referral to me, and late in 1969 I started him on orthomolecular therapy. This included a brief admission in 1971 for a series of ECT. During that admission, he persuaded his psychiatrist to allow him to continue to take his vitamins. After that he improved slowly and had been well one year when he started his son on a vitamin program. His son B.L. had started telling him he could feel things with his feet under the blanket. He could not read, could not understand the words, and with his eyes closed he saw children, men, and sometimes spiders. In school he cried a lot for no apparent reason. One month after he had been started on niacin 1 G tid he was normal. John Hoffer saw him on July 26, 1973 and found him normal – i.e., 1111 (4).

(52) S.L.: Born December 1965, S.L. was first seen in January 1972. He was B.L.'s brother. He cried a lot in school, lacked confidence and suffered many fears, including a fear of flush toilets, elevators, and doctors. He couldn't play hockey, even though he wanted to, because he was so worried he would not play well enough. He had difficulty reading and enunciating words. His father started him on niacin 1 G tid and I saw him one month later. By then he was nearly well. He played hockey, was cheerful in the mornings, and alert, and could read with no difficulty. When seen by John Hoffer, he was evaluated 0111 (3) – much improved. He still believed children were watching him, still was afraid of elevators, and occasionally heard a voice when he lay in bed at night. Whenever he cheated on his diet and ate sugary foods, his nose would run, his eyes would redden, and his behavior would become bad. His hyperactivity score changed from 79, before he started on the vitamin, to 33 on July 26, 1973.

(53) K.L.: Born October 1969, K.L. was first seen in August 1972. He began to speak at age 2 but knew only 12 words by age 3. He made his wants known by pointing. He was typically overly active, fidgety, unable to stay with any activity very long, clumsy, unpredictable, and wet the bed. I started him on niacinamide 1 G tid and pyridoxine 250 mg bid plus sugarfree diet. A week later he began to talk more and by the end of the year had

made substantial improvement in speech. He still was hyperactive. John Hoffer evaluated him on July 19, 1973 and found him not improved – i.e., oooo (o). He was clinically a little better but not enough to classify him as improved. On January 8, 1974 he was a lot better. His mother discovered coffee relaxed him. His performance at school was normal but he still was getting speech therapy. His behavioral scores decreased from 74 on August 18, 1972 to 50 on July 19, 1973 to 39 on January 8, 1974.

(54) M.L.: Born November 1964, M.L. was first seen in July 1972. He was a very quiet, slow passive baby who began to speak at age 2 without much improvement until age 5. Then he went to a slow learners' class. He had become hyperactive at 2. I found it impossible to talk to him as he did not understand anything and every reply was random and pointless. I started him on niacinamide 1 G tid and pyridoxine 250 mg od plus sugar-free diet. On August 18, 1972 I added ritalin 20 mg. On August 23, 1972 I changed the niacinamide to niacin 1 G tid and increased his ritalin to 30 mg. The first improvement occurred over the next two months. On December 29, 1972 his speech was better and much clearer and he continued to get better at school. I reduced the ritalin to 20 mg. On March 29, 1973 I added liothyronine 5 mcg daily. He continued to improve and some days was very good. He was able to communicate better, began to make friends, rarely wet the bed, and had been promoted to grade one for the following year. John Hoffer evaluated him on July 19, 1993 as not improved – i.e., oooo (o). On July 19. 1974 I started him back on niacinamide. His speech continued to get better and he now enjoyed school. His hyperactivity score changed from 95 on July 26, 1972 to 71 on March 29, 1973 to 67 on July 19, 1973 to 40 at the last evaluation on January 8, 1974.

(55) D.M.: Born March 1960, D.M. was first seen in February 1971. D.M.'s father consulted me in December 1960 complaining about marital difficulties. He was a chronic schizophrenic, which was the main reason he could not get along with his wife. He suffered many illusions, misidentified people, was very paranoid, blocked, often could not find the right word or a word he did not want would pop out, and he was very depressed. On niacin 1 G tid he improved slowly, and on March 5, 1970 he was much improved. The marriage ended in a friendly divorce.

In February 1971 his son D.M. was brought to me by his mother because he had become a severe discipline problem at school. He was loud and noisy in class, was very disturbing and socially inappropriate. He received detentions nearly every week but he did not worry about that. He thought he was normal. At home he was belligerent. He began to fall behind in his work. I started him on niacinamide 1 G tid. By May 17, 1971 he had received very few detentions and his behavior was better. In August 1971 he passed into grade 6. According to his mother, he was normal. When evaluated July 16, 1973 John Hoffer found him well – i.e., 1111 (4). His mother still kept him on the vitamin as a preventive measure as she did not want him to become schizophrenic as she had seen what it done to her husband and recently to a brother of hers. His hyperactivity score changed from 67 on February 18, 1971 to 45 on July 16, 1973.

(56) T.M.: Born July 1964, T.M. was first seen in February 1972. He was a very intelligent boy who was able to describe his difficulties easily. He was very nervous, performance at school was erratic, he fought a lot with other children, and he was paranoid. His behavior became worse in September 1971 when they moved to Saskatoon. His mother described him as very hyperactive. He had the following perceptual symptoms: words moved on the page or became fuzzy, fearful dreams of monsters, dragons, hallucinations of the same objects when awake during the day, voices who introduced themselves by saying "I am the ghost of . . ." These were very frightening. He described his existence as if living in a dream. In thinking he blocked and had no self confidence. His mood was depressed, he had suicide ideas, and once wanted stab himself in the heart. I started him on niacinamide 1 G tid and pyridoxine 250 mg bid. Two months later he was normal. All the symptoms were gone. In July 1973 John Hoffer evaluated him as 1111 (4) – normal. His hyperactivity score descended from 89 on February 29, 1972 to 49 on April 11, 1972 to 35 on July 16, 1973.

(57) R.M.: Born November 1957, R.M. was first seen in March 1970. At age 5 he began to have spells when he would stand and stare for up to one minute, unaware of his surroundings, and often he then urinated. He was extremely restless and almost unmanageable. An EEG showed focal epileptogenic activity in the left frontal area. He had one or two spells each day.

He was examined at a child mental health clinic in 1967. There he told them about his fearful dreams which stuck to him when he awakened, peculiar sensations, for example, of being someone from another planet, and because of his general anxiety and fearfulness, he did very badly at school. He was given medication and psychotherapy for three years which helped him but not his performance at school. In 1970 he started on dilantin 100 mg tid because his father's seizures had been controlled by this anticonvulsant.

When I saw him, he daydreamed a lot at school, often sleepwalked, suffered many visual illusions, heard his mother's voice calling him when he listened to records, felt unreal, was paranoid and hostile and was very rough with his baby brother. I started him on niacin 1 G tid, glutamic acid 1 G bid, and the sugar-free diet while continuing him on his dilantin. On July 6, 1970 he had very few spells and was no longer a behavioral problem. I added pyridoxine 250 mg od. He continued to improve. By August 15, 1973, still on his nutrients, he was unreal very rarely, still had a few spells, and had had one grand mal in April, but continued to improve at school. On August 15, 1973 he was evaluated by John Hoffer who found him 0010 (1) – improved. He denied any perceptual symptoms but scored very high on the perceptual score of the HOD test. He did not have much energy. He found school boring but had passed into grade 10. He had few friends. He was no longer a behavioral problem at home, spent a lot of time reading, and did not mingle with anyone.

Date	HOD Scores				Behavioral Score
	Total	Perceptual	Paranoid	Depression	
March 11-70	91	25	5	7	85
Apr 13-70	99	28	5	9	59
Oct 5-70					55
July 6-70	137	33	6	12	
Aug 30-70	137	30	8	12	
Aug 15-73	70	15	6	8	

(58) J.N.: Born December 1962, J.N. was first seen in February 1969. He began to speak late, was a slow learner, and seemed unaware of his surroundings. He suffered spells lasting two weeks when he was very stubborn, his speech was slurred, and he put strange words together. I started him on niacinamide 1 G od and ascorbic acid 1 G od. After two months he suddenly became normal for a few days. On July 14, 1969 I increased niacinamide to 500 mg tid, in December 3, 1969 to 1 G tid, and in July 15, 1970, as there was no significant improvement, I added niacin 1 G od and ritalin 20 mg od. On August 12, 1971 I stopped the ritalin and niacinamide and added haldol 2 mg od. By March 10, 1971 he was well most of the time and getting on much better in school. I then increased niacin to 4.5 G od, adding pyridoxine 250 mg bid, and stopped the tranquilizer. On May 8, 1972 I increased niacin to 2 G tid. On June 7, 1972 he was nearly normal. I added imipramine 25 mg before bed. He had relapsed by the end of March 1973 and became abusive. John Hoffer evaluated him as 0100 (1) — not improved. But he was still very good at school. On July 18, 1973 I increased his imipramine to 50 mg before bed, and by September 5, 1973 he was normal again. His hyperactivity score descended from 92 on February 27, 1969 to 35 on June 8, 1972, increased to 65 on July 18, 1973 and finally was 27 on September 5, 1973. He was an A student.

(59) D.P.: Born March 1960, D.P. was first seen in April 1969. Six months before I saw him he began to deteriorate. He became slow, inattentive, and often his speech made no sense at home. He called things by the wrong name, began to lie, and to see visions. He described these hallucinations as like watching a movie where he saw a large number of men hurling rocks and sticks at him and heard them shouting to him. When he tried to read, the words blurred. He was diagnosed schizophrenic, as had been his brother. I started him on niacinamide 500 mg tid and ascorbic acid 500 mg tid. One month later his hallucinations were gone and he was able to speak more clearly. Words no longer blurred when he read. By June 23, 1973 he was nearly well. John Hoffer on August 15, 1973 found him well – i.e., 1111 (4). If he missed his vitamins for two days, his symptoms would return. His hyperactivity score on August 15, 1973 was 31.

(60) S.P.: Born December 1969, S.P. was first seen in April 1973. One year after he was adopted, he became very jealous of a baby girl adopted after him, and he became hyperactive. He was tested as part of an experimental group with an I.Q. range of 120 to 140. He was very restless, easily frustrated, very changeable in behavior from angel to devil. His biological mother was subject to episodes of depression and her mother had been in a mental hospital for what appeared to have been schizophrenia. S.P. described nightmares of large monsters. When he walked downstairs, the stair surfaces appeared slippery. I started him on niacin 500 mg tid, pyridoxine 250 mg bid, liothyronine and the sugar-free diet. After 6 weeks he was much better, kinder to his sister. His rash was gone. He saw the monsters rarely and had wet his bed only once. On May 30, 1973 his niacin was increased to 1 g tid. On August 7, 1973 John Hoffer rated him 0101 (2) — improved. His parents reported there was a definite surge of improvement after the dose of niacin had been increased to 1 G tid. His appetite was better, he was more relaxed, he responded better to discipline and communicated better. He slept dry and was socially much better. On September 25 he was normal. Late in November he drank mouthwash and after that began to drink wine whenever he could. He was again restless, had a rich fantasy life involving monsters, guns, shooting. His hyperactivity score decreased from 105 on April 11, 1973 to 33 on September 25, 1973.

(61) L.P.: Born October 1964, L.P. was first seen in June 1973. At 7 years he developed insomnia and slept very few hours. Sedatives made him too dopey during the day. He was depressed and became so awkward he could not hold a spoon or pencil properly. He had just learned to tie his shoes when I saw him. But in school he was very good. He was afraid of the dark, had shadow illusions, was absent-minded. He was started on niacinamide 1 G tid and pyridoxine 250 mg bid plus the diet. On July 26 he was well. He was promoted to a high grade 4 level from the previous low grade 3 level. On July 5, 1973 he was evaluated 1110 (3) – much improved. On November 15, 1973 he began to resent taking pills and became nauseated and would occasionally vomit. He was then given a liquid niacinamide preparation instead which he could tolerate. He remained much improved. His hyperactivity score decreased from 79 on June 5, 1973 to 37 on July 5, 1973.

(62) C.P.: Born June 1962, C.P. was first seen in May 1969. His mother had suffered from schizophrenia for 20 years with alcoholism over the last ten years. But the last two years she was much better. She was then worried about her son because he was so slow in school, wrote backwards even when he did not want to. He became disobedient, did not respond to punishment, did many foolish and hazardous things, wet the bed and was typically hyperactive. Socially he was very inept. She had given him niacinamide 1 G od for a year with no improvement. He had failed to respond to mellaril 30 mg od. I started him on niacin 1 G bid, periactin, and an antidepressant. By March 19, 1970 there had been no change. I then added dexedrine 10 mg and there was a substantial improvement. He stopped bedwetting. On April 20, 1970 I increased niacin to 4 G od. On February 23, 1973 I increased niacin again to 5 G. I had also tried mellaril, tofranil, even going as high as 150 mg of mellaril, but by June 4, 1973 there was no improvement. On July 16 he had passed into grade 3, but he was unimproved – i.e., 0000. His hyperactivity score was 102. He also refused to take any medication, refused to follow his diet, ate a lot of sweets. On November 30, 1973 he was still not improved.

(63) L.A.P.: Born January 1959, L.A.P. was first seen in August 1971. She had such a severe speech defect she could hardly be understood, but she was not aware she had a problem. She was born with spina bifida, which healed by 11 months. She sat by age 8 months, began to talk at age 3, and spoke brief sentences when 5. She was in a special class and making slow progress. Her reading was very poor. Her mother thought she was bright and her memory was good. Because of a peculiar bladder problem, she had to have an in-dwelling catheter attached to a bag. It was hoped this could be removed after puberty. I started her on niacinamide 1 G tid, ascorbic acid 1 G bid, and pyridoxine 250 mg bid. One month later she was more relaxed and less irritable. I increased the niacinamide to 4 G od and the pyridoxine to 500 mg bid. On December 16, 1971 her speech was more distinct, she did not get angry as much, was more inquisitive and helpful. On March 16, 1972 I added DMG 300 mg od. By April 18, 1972 her mother was very pleased with her improvement in speech. She did not stutter as much. I added niacin 1 G tid and ritalin 20 mg od. But the ritalin made her worse. She grew two inches and enjoyed reading. On July 25, 1972 I increased

niacin to 2 G tid. On September 6 she was again much better and had started initiating conversation. I decreased her niacin to 1.5 G tid. On November 28, 1972 her speech was nearly normal but she did not like reading. On February 1973 she ran out of DMG but her improvement was maintained. But on June 28, 1973 her mother reported that her speech defect had later recurred. When the DMG was resumed, her speech became much better again. She later discontinued it once more and this time her speech did not get worse. On September 4, 1973 her behavior was normal but she was still slow in a special class. She was evaluated by John Hoffer as 0001 (1) – improved. Her hyperactivity score decreased from 79, at her worst, to 43 on June 28, 1973.

(64) P.R.: Born July 1963, P.R. was first seen in August 1972. His parents were worried about severe shyness and worsening behavior in school. He admitted he found it hard to concentrate but denied any other symptoms. He was examined by a professor of Child Psychiatry who found him normal, bright, imaginative, and ascribed his poor school performance to lack of teacher attention, believing that P.R. was more intelligent than his teacher. I started him on niacinamide 1 G tid, pyridoxine 250 mg bid, ascorbic acid 1 G od. One month later he was more relaxed, keeping up with his schoolwork for the first time. On June 22, 1973 he had improved steadily. He had many food idiosyncrasies. On July 19, 1973 his brother drowned and he was very upset. He was seen by John Hoffer who evaluated him as 0001 (1) – unimproved. He was restless at school, which he did not like, had few friends, could not relate to his mates, and was disobedient. His parents believed he was better but not well. But his academic performance was very good. His hyperactivity score decreased a little from 75 on August 10, 1972 to 49 on June 22, 1973 and increased to 61 on August 17, 1973.

(65) C.R.: Born July 1960, C.R. was first seen in January 1971. His mother, a recovered schizophrenic on megavitamin therapy, was normal over 3½ years and became worried about her son's slowness in school. He described horrible dreams, saw monstrous faces which went away when he slept. Words moved about on the page and blurred. He had heard footsteps behind him, his hands and feet appeared too small. He was paranoid, thinking no one liked him, that children ganged up on him. He found it hard to

concentrate. I started him on niacinamide 1 G tid. By August 1971 he was better and remained on his vitamins until August 1972. John Hoffer saw him June 1973 and found him well if he took his vitamins – i.e., 1111 (4). His HOD scores were normal except for a slight increase in the perceptual score.

(66)L.R.: Born March 1959, L.R. was first seen in January 1970. She sometimes hallucinated faces, guns and knives at night which vanished when she closed her eyes. She knew they were not real but was still afraid. She was very nervous, often spoke too fast, and had become very irritable. I started her on niacinamide 1 G tid. In August 1971 she was better but still too active. In January 1972 she stopped her vitamins for a month and relapsed. She was advised to go back onto the niacinamide and I added pyridoxine 250 mg od. On August 14, 1973 John Hoffer found her well – i.e., 1111 (4). She had not taken anything for six months.

Date	HOD Scores				Behavioral Score
	Total	Perceptual	Paranoid	Depression	
Jan 4-70	52	13	0	6	
Jan 4-71					67
Aug 6-71	4	0	1	1	55

(67) Ge.R.: Born October 1967, Ge.R. was first seen in March 1973. He was born hyperactive. Special schools were of no help. The situation at home became intolerable, and his father, later diagnosed schizophrenic, moved out. He remained in Regina where he was being treated and Ge.R. and his mother moved to Saskatoon. I started him on niacin 1 G tid, pyridoxine 250 mg bid. On July 30, 1973 he was a little better, but he was evaluated 0000 — unimproved. On December 7, 1973 his father reported he was still taking the vitamins. His hyperactivity score had decreased from 107 to 85 by July 30, 1973.

His father was sufficiently impressed with his son's change that he sought an appointment for himself. He was started on niacin 1 G tid and ascorbic acid 1 G bid. He was nearly normal by December 7, 1973. His father's HOD scores, all high when I first saw him, were by then all normal.

(68) Ga.R.: Born October 1964, Ga.R. was first seen in May 1973. He suffered temper tantrums as a baby. At age 5 he was referred to a mental health clinic and treated for a year. He was then discharged normal, but his mother was diagnosed too anxious. After that he slowly deteriorated and his mother could no longer cope with him. He was easily frustrated, could not be reasoned with, but he was getting along well at school. He complained of frequent stomachaches. In my office he was very fidgety and restless. He was started on niacinamide 1 G tid, ascorbic acid 1 G tid, thiamin 150 mg tid, and pyridoxine 200 mg tid. Two months later he was better, seldom had any pain, was more self-reliant, but still clung a lot to his mother. On July 6, 1973 I changed B-3 to niacin 1 G qid. He was improved by August. On August 30, 1973 he was back on niacinamide but by error had only been taking ¾ God. He remained the same clinically. His hyperactivity score decreased from 77 on May 25, 1973 to 53 on December 12, 1973.

(69) N.R.: Born October 1965, N.R. was first seen in January 1972. Her mother had German measles while pregnant. N.R. was deaf in her left ear and could not localize the source of voices or sounds. She had frequent stomachaches, headaches, and could not sleep at night. She was a little hyperactive, had many temper tantrums, and did not respond to discipline. I started her on niacinamide 2 G tid. After three months she stopped the vitamins because she had nausea. Her parents noted no change. On July 30, 1973 she was rated 0111 (3) – much improved. Occasionally she hallucinated an animal and heard voices. Her behavioral score decreased from 57 on January 31, 1972 to 35 on July 30, 1973.

(70) D.R.: Born October 1961, D.R. was first seen in October 1967. From birth he was uncoordinated, could not learn to read, could not remember words, was easily frustrated, seemed tired all the time, and in the morning appeared to be in a daze. He wet his bed every night. His mother was a recovered schizophrenic and his father also had improved on vitamin B-3. I started him on niacinamide 1 G bid and ascorbic acid 1 G bid. On January

25, 1968 he was much better, wet his bed occasionally, was less tired, and had started reading. I then discontinued the vitamins and started placebo. His eyes became sore, he became overly active, began to whine all the time, became very impatient, and made little progress. He was taken into a special class. On February 8, 1968 I put him back on niacinamide 1 G tid. After five days he began to improve again and was much better, but had not regained his earlier improved condition. On February 26, 1969 he had continued to get better, except over the summer when he began to throw away his pills and by the end of the summer he would not take anything and quickly became much worse. He still had school problems. On October 22, 1969 I tried niacin 1 G tid, and by January 4, 1971 there was some additional improvement. Over the rest of that year I tried deaner and ritalin but they did not help. On April 12, 1973 I added pyridoxine 250 mg od and replaced vitamin B-3 with inositol niacinate 1 G tid. On July 20, 1973 he still had visual illusions, his concentration was poor, he blocked, and was very forgetful. However, his mother considered him nearly normal. He was evaluated 0, 0.5, 1, 0.5 (2) – improved. His hyperactivity score was 47.

(71) W.R.: Born May 1960, W.R. was first seen in April 1969. For 9 months after he was born, he suffered diarrhea, anemia, and malnutrition. After he was started on a proper diet, he developed very quickly but became hyperactive, slept poorly, toilet trained slowly, achieving this by age 20 months. After his sister was born, he regressed and began to soil again. By the time he was in grade 2 he soiled every day. By the time I saw him he soiled only three times each week. He was under severe muscle tension all the time so that he could hardly bend over and skated very stiffly. He was preoccupied with thunder and lightning, of which he was afraid and dreamt about frequently. I started him on niacinamide 500 mg tid and ascorbic acid 1 G tid with mellaril 20 mg od. One month later he was happier, less tense, less disobedient, and soiled less. I doubled his niacinamide. By July 2, 1969 he was a lot better. On August 23, 1973 John Hoffer evaluated him as well – 1111 (4). According to his mother he was on medication for a few months and there was dramatic improvement. But as he found it hard to swallow pills, these were stopped and he had remained well. His mother was watching him very carefully for any evidence of relapse and had seen none.

(72) C.S.: Born August 1964, C.S. was first seen in June 1972. She became very jealous, irritable, and depressed when she was 2½years old. She would not accept any affection. She became very hyperactive, which created problems at school. She told me about her visual and auditory illusions. I started her on niacinamide 1 G tid and pyridoxine 250 mg bid. One month later she was much better and October 18, 1872 she was normal. In July 1973 John Hoffer found her well – 1111 (4). Her hyperactivity score decreased from 85 on June 5, 1972 to 35 by October 18, 1972.

(73) G.S.: Born September 1959, G.S. was first seen in June 1973. He was the brother of C.S. At age 2½ he became very tense and hyperactive. His mother was sick herself and she dealt with his illness by keeping out of his way. He became rebellious, did not respond to discipline, did not make any friends, but got on well at school. Words blurred when he looked at them, he had auditory illusions which frightened him, he heard himself think, felt unreal, and saw his hands get bigger. With his depression he was paranoid, blocked, ideas flashed in and out of his head, and he found it hard to communicate and concentrate. He was tired and disgusted with himself. His mother started him on niacinamide 200 mg od four months before I saw him. I increased his niacinamide to 1 G tid and added pyridoxine 250 mg bid. By October 18, 1972 he was much better. On July 23, 1973 he was almost normal. When he went off medication he became worse. He was evaluated 1110 (3) – much improved. His HOD scores, high in June 1972, were normal by October that year. His hyperactivity score decreased from 99 to 45.

The mother of C.S. and G.S. was the first member of this family to be treated. She had been sick for many years, complaining of many visual illusions, feelings of unreality, paranoid ideas, blocking, and depression. She had been started on niacinamide 300 mg od a year before I saw her and had improved substantially. I increased her niacinamide to 1 G tid and she was well in 4½ months. Her HOD scores, very high before she started taking vitamins, were all normal by May 31, 1972. Two other children were not ill. The recovery of mother and her two children converted a sick family into a normal family. No family therapy was needed.

(74) Gus.S.: Born December 1958, Gus.S. was first seen in April 1973. With a speech defect and a very limited vocabulary, he had great difficulty

expressing himself. He was a slow learner and tested 55 on the I.Q. In addition he was extremely restless and hyperactive. I thought he had childhood schizophrenia. Because he could not be controlled in public school, he had been attending a special school for the mentally retarded for three years where he picked up a number of bad habits from the other children. I started him on niacinamide 1 G tid and pyridoxine 250 mg bid. One month later there was slight improvement. I then added niacin 1 G tid. By August 1973 his speech was distinctly better as was his school performance. He was still a severe behavioral problem. He was evaluated by John Hoffer as 0000 – not improved. By November 1973 I had to stop the niacin because it caused nausea. He was still no better. Nevertheless, his hyperactivity score decreased from 101 on April 2, 1973 to 65 on November 14, 1973.

He had an older brother, retarded since age 2. By age 20 he was a behavioral problem as well. He was a chronic schizophrenic who did not respond to six months of vitamin treatment.

(75) Y.S.: Born June 1955, Y.S. was first seen in June 1969. For one year before she saw me this A student became very nervous and gradually became paranoid about her parents, believing they were watching her and her schoolmates too closely. Most people hated her, she told me. She blocked, her memory and concentration were very poor and she became introverted. Visual hallucinations appeared, words moved up and down on the page, and she would not look directly at people because they could read her mind. She heard herself think and heard voices. I started her on niacinamide 1 G tid, ascorbic acid 1 G tid, and mellaril 30 mg od. One month later she was less paranoid and had fewer suicide ideas. On July 24, 1969 the visual hallucinations were gone, voices were infrequent, she was even less paranoid and therefore more comfortable with people, less tired and not depressed. On October 9, 1969 she was well, as she was when she was seen by John Hoffer on August 9, 1973, who evaluated her 1111 (4). She had stopped taking the vitamins to see if she still needed them and soon became very nervous again, but did not need any tranquilizer for four years. She had been accepted for training as an airline attendant.

Date	HOD Scores			
	Total	Perceptual	Paranoid	Depression
June 3-69	71	17	6	11
June 24-69	37	7	4	6
July 24-69	23	5	4	5
Oct 9-69	2	0	0	0

(76) T.S.: Born January 1955, T.S. was first seen in December 1968. He got on well at school except for outbursts of anger. He could not accept correction, held a grudge for a long time, and blamed his parents irrationally – for example, if he was late he blamed them because he was slow. He was seen at a mental health clinic where his parents were advised never to spank him because it made him insecure. He was placed on tranquilizers which made him too fat. He was clearly schizophrenic. I started him on niacinamide 1 G tid and ascorbic acid, same dose. By the end of December he was much better but had slipped again by mid-January. I added imipramine 30 mg at bed time. By mid-February he no longer wet the bed, was in better spirits, and found school less boring. On June 13, 1969 he had continued to improve. On August 10, 1973 John Hoffer found him not improved. He had stopped all medication in August 1971. He still had many illusions and hallucinations and had some difficulty at school but was no longer a behavioral problem. He was rated 0100 (1) – not improved. He was started back on niacinamide and pyridoxine 250 mg bid was added. On October 10, 1973 he was better again, much improved even though he still had symptoms which did not affect his school performance.

Date	HOD Scores			
	Total	Perceptual	Paranoid	Depression
Dec 4-68	61	18	2	6
Feb 14-69	70	14	2	4
Aug 10-73	88	15	6	11
Oct 10-73	72	16	5	8

(77) E.S.: Born November 1957, E.S. was first seen in September 1971. In 1968 a neighbor had been killed on the block by a milk wagon. Since then E.S. had been very worried, and whenever he saw an accident became very restless and disturbed. Traffic noises were so frightening to him he kept a fan on all night to drown them out. For one year he was seen by a child psychiatrist for psychotherapy with no improvement. His father was a chronic paranoid schizophrenic, impossible to live with, and his parents divorced. I started him on niacinamide 1 G tid and ascorbic acid 1 G tid. Three months later he was no longer worried about accidents but was still afraid of women drivers. He was better at school. I added pyridoxine 250 mg tid. On May 9, 1972 he had shown a lot of additional improvement, and on June 13, 1972 he was nearly normal. His grades had risen to a B average but he was still troubled by street noises. On August 10, 1973 he was well. If he stopped his vitamins he became nervous in a few days. John Hoffer evaluated him as 1111 (4) – normal. His hyperactivity score changed from 41 on September 1971 to 27 on December 15, 1971.

(78) M.A.S.: Born March 1965, M.A.S. was first seen in June 1972. From the time she was adopted as a infant she was allergic to dairy products. She developed well until grade 1 when she was so hyperactive that she could not learn. Milk made her worse and made her wet the bed. She saw words as double, saw animals at dusk, and had nightmares of monsters. She was paranoid, thinking people were making fun of her. Her memory and concentration were poor and she blocked. I started her on niacinamide 1 G tid and pyridoxine 250 mg bid. One month later she was normal. When she stopped medication she quickly relapsed. On July 19, 1973 John Hoffer evaluated her as 0111 (3) – much improved. She occasionally heard a voice say "Go to sleep Mary Ann" and she was still slightly irritable. Her behavioral score decreased from 84 on June 22, 1972 to 39 on July 19, 1973.

(79) R.S.: Born December 1966, R.S. was first seen in June 1971. Soon after he began to walk he was hyperactive with severe tantrums, irritability, and he was unreasonable. His parents were advised by the mental health clinic to give him more love and attention. This they tried with the cooperation of their entire family, but his deterioration was not halted. Later his parents were given a course in behavioral modification. Stimulants made him

worse and mellaril had not helped. He remained very hyperactive, fidgety, and presented with the entire spectrum of hyperactivity, scoring 109 on the hyperactivity scale. I started him on niacinamide 1 G tid, ascorbic acid 1 G tid, and pyridoxine 250 mg bid. Within a few days bedwetting stopped, and he made what appeared a miraculous recovery to his parents. He learned to tie his shoes in a few days. They had never seen him do as well before. On July 8 I changed niacinamide to niacin 1 G tid. On October 19, 1971 he was almost well but did have a few bad days when he was vindictive and mean. I doubled his niacin. He remained improved but was still more active than his parents would like. By February 29, 1972 he was taking niacin 4 G tid. On March 8, 1972 I added lithium carbonate 300 mg tid and imipramine 125 mg at bed. The antidepressant did no good. His parents increased his pyridoxine to 1.5 G od and felt this improved him even more. However, on July 9, 1973 he was seen by John Hoffer who found him 0100 – not improved. His nose was stuffy all the time. He still had mood swings, but they were not as severe as they been before he started lithium. His mother thought his mood swings were precipitated by eating candy which he would do at every opportunity. He was still hyperactive in school but did well scholastically. Later in 1973 he was found to be allergic to several foods which were removed. He also was taken off all medication. Over the next few months there was a major improvement. In February 1974 his parents told me he was in the top of his class in grade 2. He was beginning to become more active again and he was started on back niacin 1 G tid, ascorbic acid 1 G tid, and pyridoxine 250 mg od. His hyperactivity score was 109 on June 3, 1971, 31 on July 8, 1971 and 80 on July 9, 1973.

(80) K.S.: Born October 1955, K.S. was first seen in April 1969. I had seen her older brother first, late in 1968 when he complained of insomnia, difficulty at home and at school. He had experienced visual hallucinations, twice had left his body, heard voices and music, and was nervous and moody. He had become very religious, spent a lot of time reading the Bible, and became introverted. I started him on niacinamide 1 G tid, and in July added pyridoxine 250 mg bid. By then only some residual irritability and depression remained. On September 11, 1972 he was much improved. In May 1973 he married and remained well.

K.S. had resented having been brought to see me and denied everything. According to mother she had been a problem from age 5½, especially at school until a year before I saw her, when her school performance improved. But in its place she began to suffer mood swings. During the interview with me she was immature and hostile. I was not certain she was ill but persuaded her to take niacinamide 1 G tid as a therapeutic trial to see if she was vitamin B-3 dependent. After two months there was no change and she stopped taking vitamins. When seen by John Hoffer on August 10, 1973 she remained the same. She had taken marijuana several times, which made her depressed and made her memory faulty, so she decided not to take it any more. Her mood was good most of the time, but she was irritated by her parents, did not like her mother, and planned on leaving home. Her attitude to school was poor and her grades were mediocre. Her evaluation was much improved – 1, 1, 0.5, 0.5 (3). Her father considered her normal on January 13, 1974.

(81) L.S.: Born April 1966, L.S. was first seen in August 1972. Her mother had come to see me early in 1972 after 12 years of suffering from schizo-phrenia. Her psychiatrist wrote in 1969, "This patient is somewhat out of touch with reality but her mentality is grossly intact. She is a known chronic schizophrenic. She seems to be very unreliable and unpredictable." Before I saw her she had 6 admissions. Early in 1972 she began to attend Schizo-phrenics Anonymous meetings. When I saw her she suffered from voices, unreality feelings, out of the body experiences, paranoia, blocking, and poor memory and concentration with severe depression. In February 1973 she received a series of 9 ECT and after that recovered. She was on niacin 1 G bid, niacinamide 1 G bid, pyridoxine 250 mg tid, and ascorbic acid 1 G tid.

Two years before I saw her daughter L.S., she had developed severe temper outbursts and hyperactivity. She saw words move on the page and collide with each other. She heard voices and footsteps, saw ghosts which were adult size in blue, and saw women. She had seen the faces of a spider monster. They sometimes spoke to her. I started her on niacinamide 1 G tid, pyridoxine 250 mg bid, and ascorbic acid 1 G od. After one month she was free of hallucinations, but the niacinamide dose had to be reduced to 1 G od because it caused nausea. I started her on niacin 1 G bid. Three months late she was more relaxed. On February 19, 1973 she was well. John

Hoffer evaluated her on July 25, 1973 as well – 1111 (4). If she went off her vitamins for two days, her depression would recur. Her hyperactivity score decreased from 91 in August 1972 to 47 on July 25, 1973.

(82) K.S.: Born July 1965, K.S. was first seen in March 1972. She did not sit up until age 27 months. She began to talk but it was not comprehensible for a long time. A pediatric examination found no reason for this. At age 4 she still was not toilet trained. In fall of 1971 she was found to be slow and her mother was blamed for this. Meanwhile she continued to deteriorate. Once, after eating a large amount of sugar, she had a series of convulsions. When I saw her, she told me that words moved about on the page, lines ran together. She was paranoid, believing children were all laughing at her. When anything went wrong, she blamed someone else. I started her on niacinamide 1 G tid and pyridoxine 250 mg bid. One month later she was much better, sleeping dry 3 out of 4 days, her appetite was better, and she was less irritable. Her teacher told her mother she had learned more in three weeks than in the previous year at school. On July 24, 1973 she was evaluated improved – 0011. She could take only 2 G niacinamide daily due to nausea on the higher dose, but on the lower does she was more hyperactive. Words still moved laterally and she had trouble concentrating and remembering. She was then started on inositol niacinate 1 G od to supplement the niacinamide. On January 12, 1974 she was good but still wet her bed every fourth day. The inositol niacinate was increased to 2 G daily. Her hyperactivity score changed from 101 on March 2, 1972 to 39 on April 10, 1972 and was 47 on July 24, 1973.

(83) D.T.: Born 1960, D.T. was first seen in April 1970. He was born 5 weeks premature with jaundice. He began to walk at 8 months and to talk at 2½ years. He suffered a series of infections and colic and became hyperactive. He was started on ritalin, which worked like a miracle. He became normal, completed grade 1 but had difficulty with grade 2. Other problems arose while still on ritalin 40 mg daily and he was referred to a clinic. The drug was stopped and he was given mellaril 10 mg at night. This made him much worse. His appetite became voracious for sweets and his diet was very bad. Two weeks before he saw me he was started on niacinamide 1 G bid and ascorbic acid 1 G bid. Over this period, he became a little better,

less irritable. A five hour glucose tolerance test showed he had very severe relative hypoglycemia. The sugar values at 0, 0.5, 1, 2, 3, 4, and 5 hours were 104, 239, 282, 198, 68, 82 and 90 milligrams per 100 ml of blood. I increased his niacinamide to 1 G tid, ascorbic acid 1 G bid, and kept him on ritalin 45 mg od. Four months later he was better, but his antisocial behavior got worse. He lied, made false reports to the police, and began to steal. His ritalin was slowly reduced to 20 mg. His niacinamide was increased to 2 G tid. On September 4, 1970 he was much better. I changed the vitamin B-3 to niacin 1 G tid. On October 5, 1970 he was normal. In September 1971, after returning from summer camp, he once more began to lie and steal. I increased his niacin to 2 G tid, and on December 3, 1971 he was well again. On December 3, 1972 I decreased his ritalin to 15 mg. He passed into grade 7 with a C average. On June 12, 1973 he was caught stealing twice in school, and was erratic. His parents had divorced and he had not been following his program. On July 27, 1973 he was evaluated 0000 (0) — not improved. He reported visual illusions, bad behavior in school and at home. By December 27, 1973 he had passed forged checks, was caught, appeared in court. But his parents were pleased with his progress. By the end of the year he was almost normal. He was free of symptoms and anti-social behavior. His hyperactivity score decreased from 91 on April 14, 1970 when he was not taking ritalin to 78 on 40 mg ritalin, to 59 when the vitamins were added. On July 27, 1973 it was 67.

(84) P.T.: Born April 1961, P.T. was first seen in April 1972. He could not study and was extremely restless. It started during infancy. At one year he suffered three convulsions. He was then normal until he entered school. Then his learning problems emerged, he suffered many temper tantrums and became a behavioral problem. I started him on niacinamide 1 G tid and pyridoxine 250 mg bid. Two months later he was better. I added ritalin 20 mg to accelerate recovery. This produced a spurt of improvement. School was more fun. On November 29, 1972 his mother told me he had been very good in school but had been stealing all summer. I added imipramine 25 mg before bed. On February 27, 1973 he was getting on well. On July 24, 1973 he was evaluated 1000 – not improved – by John Hoffer. On January 13, 1974 his mother reported she had stopped the ritalin and imipramine the previous October. He was making steady progress, lost his

temper rarely, was easier to get along with. He was evaluated 1111 (4) – well. His hyperactivity score decreased from 93 on April 12, 1972 to 77 on July 24, 1973.

(85) A.U.: Born November 1963, A.U. was first seen in May 1972. For as long as he could remember he was troubled by visual illusions of letter and figure reversal. He also became very fidgety, restless, irritable, easily upset. Words jiggled on the page, collided with each other, figures reversed, a pencil wiggled like a snake. He hallucinated a fish or a whale or other monsters, often heard his parents call him even when they were not around, and felt unreal. In January he was studied by the Institute of Child Guidance and Development and given extensive remedial exercises. He gained seven months of reading skill in two months, and when they had finished, his reading age was 6 years and 10 months (his age was 8 years and 5 months). I started him on niacinamide 1 G tid and pyridoxine 250 mg bid. In two months he was able to read much better, words no longer moved, but figures still reversed. He entered grade 3 and found school more fun. By August 21, 1972 all perceptual symptoms were gone, he was more relaxed and coordinated. On November 20, 1972 he still read slowly and had seen monsters a few times. On June 12, 1973 he was reading normally, but was slow in math and still reversed B and D. He was much improved. On August 23, 1973 John Hoffer found him much improved – 1, 0.5, 1 (3). He still found reading hard and had a few problems relating to other children. Sugar always made him worse. He had advanced into a regular grade 4 class but was one year behind. His hyperactivity score decreased from 45 on May 22, 1972 to 34 on November 20, 1972 and increased a little to 49 on August 23, 1973. These are all normal or near normal scores.

On August 23, 1973 his teacher wrote to his mother, "A.U. has become much more self-assured since the beginning of the year. When something was given to him to do I always got, 'Do I have to do that?' He is now willing to try things and realizes that there are some things he can do well. His printing and reading comprehension have greatly improved. He now likes to read. He also comes up and asks words he doesn't know. Before he would skip them. He had been going to the Reading Clinic half days. This has really been beneficial in bringing about the changes. He has a difficult time concentrating on anything any length of time. He can be reading a story aloud to you and every line or so can lead him into telling you a story of his own. He loves all animals and loves telling about them. He is a quiet pupil and seems to get along quite well with the rest of the class." And on January 13, 1963 his grade 3 teacher wrote, "He has made steady progress." His only residual problem was printing, which he found hard.

(86) R.U.: Born April 1974, R.U. was first seen in October 1971. He had a marked speech defect and it was difficult to understand him. He was irritable, easily angered, and would become violent. A child mental health clinic found him retarded with an I.Q. of 78. I started him on niacinamide 1 G tid and ascorbic acid 1 G tid. In two months he was calmer, his speech was better, and his school reported substantial improvement. I added pyridoxine 250 mg bid, June 1, 1972. He had continued to improve until April. On November 28, 1972 his mother told me he had become jaundiced June 8 to 20, 1972 with high fever. He was taken off his vitamins, even though he clearly had infectious hepatitis, because of the general fear of vitamin B-3 by the medical profession. Off his vitamins he quickly began to deteriorate, his speech became worse. By November 28, 1972 progress was so slow his mother wanted him back on niacinamide. On August 13, 1973 it was still hard to understand him but he no longer heard voices, was not hyperactive, but still suffered from lack of coordination. He was evaluated 0101 (2) – improved. His hyperactivity scores decreased from 59 on October 22, 1971 to 49 on January 13, 1974.

(87) F.U.: Born May 1960, F.U. was first seen in April 1971. At age 12, F.U.'s brother was the first member of this family to consult me in July 1970. He had to repeat grade 5 and he blamed his teacher for this. When he was 5 he fell out of a car going 45 miles per hour. He was close to being unconscious, became delirious, and was in hospital 7 days. Following this, his personality changed markedly. He began to suffer severe temper tantrums, was stubborn, disobedient, had many headaches. When he was 11, he had one grand mal seizure. His father was a paranoid epileptic who refused to take medication. His parents were divorced. His hyperactivity score was 97. I started him on niacinamide 1 G tid. By April 1971 he was well and had been promoted to grade 6. On May 1971 he went to live with his father as his

mother could not cope with 8 children. His father refused to give him any more vitamins, but at the last report July 18, 1972 he was still well.

F.U. complained of pain every Monday. Her mother was worried about her frequent bouts of severe depression lasting up to one day. Otherwise she was cheerful. She was also beginning to have difficulty in school. I started her on niacinamide 1 G tid. One month later she was calmer, better at school, and seldom complained of pain. On April 21, 1972 she was living with her father. Her mother had been ill over the summer and had sent 4 children to him. He did not give F.U. any vitamins. She came home March 1972 very ill and her mother resumed the niacinamide. She began to improve. On October 20, 1972 she was nearly normal. I had added pyridoxine 250 mg bid. On January 19, 1973 she told me she had gone off the vitamins November 15, 1972 as she did not like swallowing pills. On August 1, 1973 her mother reported she had started to get worse during July but she considered her still well. John Hoffer evaluated her as 1111 (4). But when she was on the vitamins she was less irritable and less edgy. On January 13, 1974 she was well.

Her mother came to see me for herself May 1971. She had identified her own behavior as a child with F.U. She had suffered similar fears, stomach-aches, was quiet and kept to herself. For many years she had suffered many visual illusions and hallucinations, heard voices, and felt unreal. She had been paranoid, confused, blocked, depressed, and her memory and concentration were poor. I started her on the megavitamin regimen consisting of niacin 4 G od, ascorbic acid 4 G od, pyridoxine 250 mg bid, and amitriptyline 75 mg od. In January 1973 she was normal.

Date	HOD Scores			
	Total	Perceptual	Paranoid	Depression
May 28-71	76	17	5	13
Aug 10-71	29	1	5	5
Sept 4-73	10	1	1	4

(88) Alb.V.: Born December 1962, Alb.V. was first seen in May 1973. By age 3 his behavior was bizarre. He would throw the cat into the dryer, enjoyed

breaking things. When he started school at 5½ he could not learn to read or print. He wet and defecated into his pants with no concern but refused to shower at the YMCA with other boys without his shorts. He dreamed about skeletons, and when he awakened, the dream would remain with him. He often heard people walking in the basement. He had blocks in his thinking and was depressed. I started him on niacinamide 1 G tid, pyridoxine 200 mg tid, thiamin 150 mg tid, and ascorbic acid 1 G tid. Six weeks later he was better with increased bladder and bowel control. On August 29, 1973 bladder and bowel control were normal, he was free of perceptual symptoms, and had passed into grade 5. He was evaluated as 1001 (2) – improved. On November 5, 1973 he had continued to improve, missed very few days at school, did his homework with no pressure needed from mother. His final rating was 1101 – much improved. His hyperactivity score decreased from 83 on May 22, 1973 to 37 on November 5, 1973.

(89) M.V.: Born March 1959, M.V. was first seen in May 1969. For two years he suffered nightmares in which people were after him. He would then awaken and rush into his parents' room and stay there the rest of the night. Two weeks before he saw me he had been started on a bedtime tranquilizer which eliminated the dreams but not his fear of going to bed. He had told his mother that her face looked old and wrinkled, the sheets looked wrinkled. He would not let her go into the basement where he believed men were running around trying to hurt him. He had started to hear voices and suffered peculiar body image problems. At school he was shy and sensitive. He repeated these perceptual changes during my first examination. I started him on niacinamide 500 mg tid and ascorbic acid 500 mg tid. One month later he was better, free of dreams, free of all perceptual symptoms, but still lost his temper too readily. I increased niacinamide to 1 G bid and added mellaril 10 mg od. On August 29, 1969 he was normal. On February 11, 1969 he was in grade 5 but barely passing. He was independent, clung less to mother, and was considered normal by his family. I started him on placebo to replace the niacinamide. After one month he appeared to start to relapse but did not and remained well. He did, however, hear voices again in his head and the nightmares recurred whenever he was very angry. On August 4, 1970 he had become very restless during July and his mother put him back on mellaril 10 mg. He had become very fidgety, was

irritable. On August 3 his nightmare was so severe he slept with his parents again and cried a lot. His mother felt he had reverted to the situation he was in when I first saw him. I restarted niacinamide 1 G tid and by January 18, 1971 he was normal and slowly improving in school. On April 19, 1971 he was still well. On November 25, 1973 he reported he had passed into grade 5 with a D average. In the fall he was up to a C average in grade 6 and for the first time made an A. On June 5, 1972 he was well. When seen by John Hoffer on August 13, 1973, he was evaluated 1111 (4) — normal. He made a C average out of grade 8, enjoyed high school, athletics and was very popular. In mid-June he had stopped all the vitamins. There was a sudden deterioration in his personality, he developed claustrophobia, and became less friendly. He was restarted on the vitamins and soon was well again. His hyperactivity score decreased from 59 in 1969 to 27 in August 1972.

(90) G.V.: Born April 1956, G.V. was first seen in July 1970. He very shy and sensitive and was described by his mother as an empty child who never gave anything. He was not interested in anything, disliked physical activity and gym because of his stiff back. He had surgery for spina bifida. He was very argumentative and difficult. He was treated at a mental health clinic for a year with no response. They advised his parents that they were too strict with him. He had paranoid ideas which he discussed with me. I started him on niacinamide 1 G tid and ascorbic acid 1 G tid. One month later he was better, less paranoid, and had made a few friends. On January 18, 1971 he was a D student at school, bored with it. He had finally been placed on a good diet. On April 19, 1971 he was the same. He had failed all his exams. It was impossible to keep him away from sweets. I increased niacinamide to 2 G tid. On July 13, 1971 he had passed two classes and would have to repeat the year. I stopped the amide and started him on niacin 1 G tid. On November 25, 1971 he was in grade 9 with a good deal of difficulty. I increased niacin to 2 G tid. On January 4, 1972 he had reached adult height, six feet. School was not as hard and he could concentrate better. On May 10, 1972 I added pyridoxine 500 mg bid. He was normal and a C average student. On August 29, 1972 he was promoted into grade 10 having failed two classes. His mother felt he was well but he still found it hard to concentrate. On February 1, 1973 he decreased his niacin to 2 G od. On April 3, 1973 he was well, found studying much easier. His final evaluation

was 1111 (4). He was not seen by John Hoffer as he was over 14 when he started treatment. His hyperactivity score decreased from 95 on July 9, 1970 to 59 on July 13, 1971.

(91) R.V.: Born October 1963, R.V. was first seen in September 1970. He was the first of three siblings, out of four, to be referred. He had suffered severe nightmares for one year, seeing ghosts and monsters. Sometimes he saw them during the day. He was afraid to be alone in his room and became irritable, disobedient, irrational at times and tended to lose control of his muscles.   He heard voices as well. I started him on niacinamide 500 mg tid and ascorbic acid 500 mg tid. After one month he was less fearful and sleeping better. On January 20, 1971 he felt well but was still overactive. On July 13, 1971 he remained the same. I stopped the amide and started niacin 1 G tid. On January 10, 1972 he appeared no better, was still very irritable, fought a lot, but was free of perceptual symptoms. On niacin 2 G tid he was improved again by February 25, 1972, and by June 5, 1972 was nearly well. At camp he was off all vitamins for one week and did not relapse. On August 28, 1972 he had passed into grade 4. There were no school problems. He was still stubborn and fought with his brothers a lot. On April 3, 1973 his mother had decreased niacin to 2 G od. He was normal. On August 13, 1973 he was started on niacinamide 1 G bid. When seen by John Hoffer he still had nightmares 4 days per week but awakened and went back to sleep. There were some visual illusions and he was often depressed. He was a good student, had many friends, and got on well at home. He did not like taking pills. He was evaluated 0111 (3) – much improved. His hyperactivity score decreased from 101 on September 23, 1970 to 49 on August 13, 1973.

(92) J.V.: Born December 1958, J.V. was first seen in August 1972. He was the second son of the V. family, and his parents were worried about his attitude to school. He had been forced to change schools frequently because his family moved often, and when they did not move, he had a succession of teachers. He was found to have dyslexia by an ophthalmologist and received four months of remedial reading with some improvement. The next year he lost interest in school. His hyperactivity score was 41. I started him on niacinamide 1 G tid and pyridoxine 250 mg bid. Two months later he was more interested and had a slightly better record. On August 13, 1973

he was nearly well in all aspects, except there was little improvement in his attitude to school, especially disliking reading and writing. He was evaluated 1000 (1) – not improved. However, according to his father, he only took half the required vitamin doses.

(93) D.V.: Born August 1964, D.V. was first seen in April 1972. In grade 1, he was slow, could not sound words properly, but was advanced to grade 2. After he was given special attention he began to improve. If he did not get this attention, he would relapse. When I examined him, he reported words moved laterally on the page, he suffered nightmares and monsters which drove him into his parents' room, and sometimes he saw the same monsters in his eye. He was paranoid about children telling secrets about him and he believed everyone hated him. His memory was poor and he blocked. I started him on niacinamide 1 G tid and pyridoxine 250 mg bid. One month later his reading had improved. Words were now quiet on the page, his dreams had gone, his behavior was more purposeful. On June 22, 1972 he was nearly well with marked improvement in school. On August 9, 1973 his mother told me he remained well as long as he took the vitamins. On one occasion he began to deteriorate until his mother discovered he was hiding his pills. John Hoffer found he still had illusions when off medication. He had difficulty in his social relationships at school, was very slow, daydreamed a lot. He was evaluated 1,0.5,0.5,0 (2) — improved. In the fall of 1973 his appetite became poor and medication was stopped. After a few days his appetite returned, but he continued to relapse. He was then given lower doses of both niacinamide and niacin and later niacin 1 G tid. On January 13, 1974 he was well, average at school, but still behind due to his previous years of difficulty. Final evaluation was 1111 (4). His hyperactivity score was 51 on April 14, 1972, 29 on June 22, 1972, and 53 on August 9, 1973.

(94) C.W.: Born January 1959, C.W. was first seen in April 1971. According to his mother, he created minor problems until the fall of 1970 after which he became very nervous. He insisted he was fine. Early in 1972 he left home, leaving a note that no one liked him, that everyone growled at him. He wrote that no one should look for him. Next morning he phoned home and was invited back. A couple of days later he and his cousin stole some money. A week later they discovered he was part of a gang of older boys

who were trying to get him to steal cigarettes for them. Later he became very hostile and angry toward everyone. He was started on niacinamide 1 G tid. One month later he was more alert, brighter, better at school, and appeared nearly normal. On July 23, 1973 he told John Hoffer he had remained on his vitamins only 6 months. His mother thought he had improved because of the increased attention she had given him and not his diet and the supplements. John Hoffer found him very tired. He slept poorly for nearly 18 hours each day. He had gradually become more tired over the previous three months. He was still paranoid, but his mother thought he was well. He was evaluated 0011 (2) – improved. He was started on a multivitamin tablet containing niacinamide 200 mg, thiamin 100 mg, riboflavin 25 mg, pyridoxine 250 mg, and ascorbic acid 500 mg. On January 13, 1974 he was less tired and generally much better. He was then rated 0111 (3) – much improved. His hyperactivity score decreased from 53 on April 22, 1971 to 29 on July 23, 1973.

(95) K.W.: Born June 1964, K.W. was first seen in March 1972. He started walking at 12 months and was hyperactive thereafter. Grades 1 and 2 were very difficult because he could not read and had difficulty expressing himself. I started him on niacinamide 1 G tid and pyridoxine 250 mg bid. One month later words had stopped moving and he could read better. School was more fun and he slept well. I increased his niacinamide to 4 G od. On July 20, 1972 he was much better in school, no mark being less than 75. He enjoyed reading but was still restless. On August 20, 1972 he could not tolerate the bitter taste of niacinamide and I switched the vitamin to niacin 1 G tid. On December 19, 1972 he continued to improve. On April 23, 1973 he was normal. On July 23, 1973 John Hoffer evaluated him 1111 (4) – normal. His parents told John that whenever he got careless about the vitamins his behavior would deteriorate. His hyperactivity score was 51 on March 17, 1972, 45 on April 20, 1972, and 33 on July 23, 1973.

(96) Ca.W.: Born March 1962, Ca.W, was first seen in June 1972. She was very fearful a robber was coming into the house. Her aunt and her two sisters were worried about her paranoid attitude. She believed no one liked her, she was fearful, heard footsteps at night, had night terrors. She gradually became more absent-minded and had started to rock a lot. She told

me about her nighttime illusions when clothes looked like animals. She was sad and felt like killing herself. I started her on niacinamide 1 G tid and pyridoxine 25 mg bid. On March 23, 1973 she was normal. On May 11, 1973 her family reported she could not tolerate either niacinamide or niacin, and I started her on inositol niacinate 1 G tid. She was getting on well but found it hard to fall asleep. On June 21, 1973 she was still easily discouraged, paranoid, felt people were staring at her, was depressed, never laughed and had no friends. I placed her back on niacinamide 1 G bid and decreased the inositol derivative to 1 G od, adding imipramine 25 mg at bed time. On August 23, 1973 she was a lot better, but still shy and fearful. John Hoffer evaluated her 0.5,0.5,0.5,0 (1.5) – improved. She was a lot better but had not quite reached the state called for by the much improved evaluation. On December 4, 1973 she remained about the same. Her hyperactivity score decreased from 71 on June 22, 1972 to 45 on August 2, 1972, then increased to 55 August 23, 1973.

(97) D.W.: Born in December 1953, D.W. was first seen in June 1972. D.W. was Ca.W.'s older sister. She, too, was shy, and had been getting worse. She had been hyperactive and her behavior was identical to that of her sister. She felt people were staring at her, was paranoid, believing people were talking about her. Her memory was poor, she could not concentrate, and she blocked. I started her on vitamin treatment, and December 4, 1973 she was normal.

Date	HOD Scores			
	Total	Perceptual	Paranoid	Depression
June 1972	31	3	4	8
Aug 1972	4	0	0	2
Mar 1973	17	2	4	7

(98) F.W.: Born October 1958, F.W. was first seen in April 1972. She was the third girl from this family. Her aunt was worried about her moodiness and depression present for one year. I did not think she was ill and simply advised her to improve her diet. Two months later she was well. A glucose

tolerance curve done February 1973 showed she had severe relative hypo-glycemia.

(99)   T.W.: Born October 1958, T.W. was first seen in April 1972. For three months he had been very tired. He found it hard to get up in the morning and stayed tired the rest of the morning. His family doctor had started him on niacinamide 1 G bid, which made him more tired. His parents believed, however, that his behavior was better. I increased the niacinamide to 1 G tid and added pyridoxine 250 mg od. By May 1972 he was normal. On July 16, 1973 he had not taken any vitamins for three months but he was still well. His hyperactivity score, 59 at his worst, decreased to 33 when last seen.

(100) M.W.: Born February 1957, M.W. was first seen in December 1970. He was seen at a mental health clinic when he was 8 years because he had poor reading habits and still wet the bed. After several visits enuresis stopped. At age 11, he was seen again because he could not concentrate. Early in 1970 he was started on small doses of niacinamide and showed some improvement. Just before I saw him he had forged two checks to buy drums. The school had decided he could not learn in a regular class and proposed having him go to a special class for emotionally disturbed students. He had a few visual illusions, had some difficulty in concentrating, and was nervous. He was diagnosed schizophrenic by the clinic. His father was a chronic schizophrenic. I increased his niacinamide to 1 G tid, added ascorbic acid 1 G tid, and stelazine 6 mg od. One month later he was better. His school grades went up to a B average. On January 5, 1972 his parents told me his referring physician reduced the niacinamide to 1 G od and he began to relapse. Later in 1971 his parents increased the dose and once more he became well. On April 25, 1972 he was normal and his school performance continued to improve. I added pyridoxine 250 mg bid and decreased the tranquilizer dose. On April 25, 1973 he was normal. June 1973 was not a good month. He was depressed, irritable, could not study, and was worried he would fail. I put him back on stelazine. On June 27, 1973 he was normal most of the time. On September 19, 1973 he was caught stealing money from his parents. On August 15, 1973 he was evaluated 0, 0.5, 0, 1 (1.5) – improved. On December 3, 1972 he was better. He still had visual illusions,

thought too slowly, had some trouble in school, and hoped to go to a special class to complete grade 12. He liked the effect of the vitamins, but did not like the tranquilizer. His hyperactivity score decreased from 75 on December 24, 1970 to 35 on January 5, 1972. On August 15, 1973 his HOD scores were all too high.

(101) L.W.: Born April 1959, L.W. was first seen in May 1971. He told me he was having trouble in school because he was lazy and preferred to daydream. In grade 5 he had been a B student, but in grade 6 he alternated hyperactivity with bouts of severe passivity when he seemed almost dead. Over the years he had become progressively more hyperactive and had developed a marked craving for sugar. His mother thought his symptoms, especially his headaches, fitted the hypoglycemic pattern and had started to curb his excessive intake of sugar with some improvement. I started him on niacinamide 1 G tid, pyridoxine 250 mg od, and ascorbic acid 1 G bid. One month later his mother saw some improvement. He was less tired, easier to live with. I increased his niacinamide to 4 G od. On July 31, 1973 he had passed into grade 9 but still had a short attention span, was restless, moody and bored. During November 1971 his school reported there had been a marked improvement over the previous 2 months. He had remained on the vitamins the whole time but would not keep away from sweets. He had a problem with his schoolmates, had very few friends, and was too aggressive. John Hoffer evaluated him as 1000 (1) – not improved. His hyperactivity score changed from 97 on May 16, 1971 to 51 on September 16, 1971, then increased again to 83 on July 31, 1973. On January 14, 1974 his mother told me he would only take niacinamide 1 G od and pyridoxine 250 mg od, but she considered he was well. He was getting on well in school, was cheerful, but balky at home. There were no major problems. His evaluation was 1111 (4) – normal.

(102) M.W.: Born August 1958, M.W. was first seen in May 1968. She had a problem with math. She had to repeat grade 2 and was slow in grade 3. She did not concentrate, her mind wandered, and often when someone spoke to her she was unaware of them. Her personality had been deteriorating for 2 years and she was depressed. Her sister had chronic schizophrenia. She was started on niacinamide 1 G bid and ascorbic acid 1 G bid. One

month later she was much better, no longer paranoid or fearful. On August 30, 1968 she was normal and enjoyed school. On April 7, 1969 she was more restless and sometimes believed people were watching her. I added chlorpromazine 25 mg before bed. On April 30, 1971 she was well. I increased the niacinamide to 1.5 G tid but this caused nausea. She had to be taken off for ten days and regressed. On September 3, 1971 she was still hyperactive and restless. I changed her to niacin 2 G tid, and by July 24, 1973 she was well, according to her mother. She had finished grade 8 with a B average. John Hoffer evaluated her as 1110 (3) – much improved. On September 4, 1973 she was well. On January 14, 1974 she had made the honor role, was mature and taking on more responsibilities. She remained well.

(103) S.W.: Born December 1955, S.W. was first seen in October 1969. One month before I saw her, she was told she would be expelled from school. She was afraid to go home and wandered about the city for two days. Her girlfriend eventually phoned home and her parents came for her. She was hostile, believing they were too harsh with her. If she came home late they would ground her. She was had a C average in grade 9 but had missed a lot of school because she found it so boring. She thought people were looking at her, heard a man's voice at night calling her, heard herself think, and felt unreal. Reading was difficult because the words moved on the page. She was paranoid, thinking people were talking about her and strangers were laughing at her, and once she was convinced her mother had bugged her room. Group conversation confused her. She had ideas of killing and two years earlier had tried to choke her sister. She was depressed and suicidal. Her mother thought she was becoming gay because of something she had written in her diary and because she was less interested in boys. I started her on niacinamide 1 G tid and the same dose of vitamin C. One month later the perceptual symptoms were gone, school was more fun, and she was less depressed. On December 15, 1969 she was normal. On March 19, 1970 she was well. She enjoyed school, was able to concentrate and remember. She had gained ½ an inch, her hair was growing faster, her nails were better and she no longer had any white areas in them, and her skin, which had been dry and rough, was normal. On August 15, 1973 John Hoffer evaluated her 1111 (4) – normal. She had remained on the vitamins until mid-1971 and after that only when she felt she was not living up to her full

potential. She was completing grade 12. She was active in sports, played baseball and coached basketball in the winter. On February 2, 1974 I ran into her at the airport in Palm Springs on her way home after enjoying a two-week holiday with her mother and two sisters. She was well and enjoying life.

Date	HOD Scores			
	Total	Perceptual	Paranoid	Depression
Oct 15-69	83	19	5	12
Nov 15-69	2	0	0	0

(104) K.Y.: Born October 1964, K.Y. was first seen in November 1970. Although he was intelligent, he fell behind at school and he was harder to manage at home. Three weeks before his mother brought him to see me he had seen an old house and had been told it had snakes in it. He began to dream of snakes and refused to go to bed. His teddy bear looked like a ghost. Often he fled from his bed to spend the rest of the night in his parents' bedroom. When he read, words moved laterally on the page, lines were crooked, faces pulsated. This made him laugh. I started him on niacinamide 1 G bid. Two months later he was much better. Whenever he did not take his vitamins, he would relapse. I added pyridoxine 250 mg bid. On October 6, 1972 he was well. On August 24, 1973 he still had some visual illusion and was sensitive about other children. He did not like taking vitamins and rather than fight with him he was allowed to take them erratically. He was good at school. John Hoffer evaluated him 0111 (3) – much improved. His hyperactivity score was 59 on November 2, 1970, 49 on February 12, 1971, and 43 on August 24, 1973. His mother, a chronic schizophrenic, was under treatment with vitamins since November 1970. She was much improved, except she still was jealous of her husband without reason.

(105) E.Y.: Born April 1961, E.Y. was first seen in August 1968. Two months before I saw him, he began to cry a lot for no reason, became stubborn, complained of stomach and head aches, became sleepless, and had bad thoughts. At school he became childish. He had monster nightmares and

saw ghosts. He would awaken in terror and run to his mother. He would fall asleep if she stayed with him. He hallucinated the same objects in the daytime when awake. He also heard the ghosts talk to him. He was convinced they were real and that someone was putting poison into his food. I started him on niacinamide 500 mg tid and ascorbic acid 500 mg od. Two months later he did not hear voices but still had visual hallucinations. His fears were gone as were his temper tantrums. On July 3, 1969 he had been normal since the beginning of the year. I then stopped the niacinamide and gave him placebo. In two weeks he began to relapse, became irritable, began to pick fights, and could not fall asleep. The niacinamide was resumed. He was well in a few days. On March 24, 1970 he reported he was again fearful of spiders and wolves under his bed. I increased the niacinamide to 1 G bid and later to 1 G tid. On February 19. 1971 he was in hospital for investigation for his stomach pain. He was found to have hypoglycemia. Off all medication for the one week in hospital he began to hallucinate again. After discharge, back on niacinamide, he recovered. On August 19, 1973 John Hoffer found him normal – 1111 (4). He was a high B student, friendly, had no fears, was free of all symptoms, and was considered normal by his mother. Last seen on December 14, 1973, he was normal.

(106) V.Y.: Born 1965, V.Y. was first seen in February 1973. He was the third child of the Y. family to be seen. In the fall of 1972 he began to see visual illusions. Objects appeared first too large, then too small. When he closed his eyes, he felt he floated off the bed. He was afraid to go to school and became hyperactive. By mid-January he was well again. Apparently he had flu. His mother was worried he might become sick like his brothers. He was started on niacinamide 1 G od with pyridoxine 250 mg od. When seen on December 14, 1973, he was normal.

(107) R.Y.: Born May 1960, R.Y. was first seen in March 1968. He was the first of four sons seen. In the summer of 1967 he became a behavioral problem, disobedient at home, and jealous of his younger brothers. He could not learn and was afraid to go to sleep without the lights on. He had frightening monster nightmares. He was nervous, lost his temper frequently. I started him on niacinamide 1 G od and ascorbic acid 1 G od. After four months he was better. His behavior had stated to normalize, his marks in

school went up, and he was promoted to grade 3 with 2 As. He was more restless. I added chlorpromazine 75 mg at bed time and increased his niacinamide to 1.5 G od. Three months later he was normal, according to his parents and his teachers. On March 26, 1969 his school average continued to improve but he was more disobedient. Niacinamide was increased to 1 G tid, chlorpromazine was stopped, and he was given imipramine 20 mg at bed time. On October 17, 1969 he was free of perceptual symptoms but still had a problem with other children. His constipation, present since birth, was completely cleared. On March 24, 1970 the antidepressant was stopped. On October 27, 1970 he was irritable. On August 17, 1973 John Hoffer evaluated him 1111 (4) – normal. He had passed into grade 8 and got on well at home and at school. His hyperactivity score was 43 on August 14, 1973 and 55 on December 14, 1973.

(108) S.V.: Born October 1965, S.V. was first seen in December 1970. He did not sit until 1 year old, began to walk at 1½ years and to speak by age 3. Seen at a mental health clinic he was found hyperactive and fearful. He was started on a tranquilizer. In December 1969 he had a grand mal convulsion, and after three more, in July 1970 he was given anticonvulsant medication. He remained seizure-free but ill. He tired easily, perspired a lot, was physically awkward, and could not run properly. His mother told me he described to her being bitten by a little girl, he was very sensitive to noise, and when he heard or saw trains he screamed, cried and ran away. He was very shy and it was hard to get him to speak. He was hyperactive in my office. He still was not toilet trained. I started him on niacinamide 1 G tid, ascorbic acid 1 G bid, and continued mysoline 250 mg od. Two months later his coordination was better, and his speech was clearer. I increased niacinamide to 2 G tid and added ritalin 10 mg od. He was placed in a special home to train him in bladder and bowel control. He could not take the higher dose of vitamin and vomited. On May 21, 1971 his mother discontinued his mysoline. On May 25 he was admitted to hospital convulsing, and mysoline was reinstated. He left the special home toilet trained and was more alert and physically better on niacinamide 1 G tid. A professor of pediatrics advised his mother never to given him any more "junk" vitamins and never to take him back to see me. This elicited a minor explosion from his mother who had always considered mysoline junk and considered

vitamins important. On July 22, 1971 I added pyridoxine 100 mg tid and DMG 300 mg od. On August 19, 1971 he was better. His mother found that contrary to the opinion of the special home he had not been toilet trained but he was much better. His color was normal, his enunciation was better, and he learned to count. He had no more temper tantrums. On January 13, 1972 he was toilet trained. By October 28 he had moved into the city so he could attend special classes. His landlady did not believe in vitamins and discontinued his program without consulting his mother. His pediatrician stopped the mysoline. On June 7, 1972 I increased pyridoxine to 250 mg bid. He had continued to improve but had one convulsion June 7. He had one seizure in July and five in September. He had not shown any additional improvement and appeared to be in a trance. He was given dilantin 150 mg and phenobarbital 20 mg od. His speech began to improve again, but he was still hyperactive and he still averaged two seizures per month. He was speaking more clearly. On May 24, 1973 he continued to improve, except for his convulsions. On July 26, 1973 I replaced niacinamide by inositol niacinate 1 G tid. On January 18, 1974 his mother discovered that when he did not take pyridoxine he had no convulsions. He was more independent, began to do things for himself, and his speech was much clearer. His hyperactivity score changed from 73 on December 17, 1970 to 49 on May 21, 1971. He was evaluated improved.

(109) R.W.: Born June 1962, R.W. was first seen in January 1968. His mother was a chronic schizophrenic from 1954. While sick, she had married, later divorced, and was left alone to care for 4 children. In 1968 she was started on orthomolecular treatment and followed the program faithfully. She became much improved. She was worried about R.W. because often his speech would become incomprehensible. He was very quiet and shy, was becoming a behavioral problem, and fought a lot with his twin sister. He was positive for KP. I started him on niacinamide 500 mg tid and ascorbic acid 500 mg tid. One month later he had stopped stuttering, stopped playing with dolls, spoke more clearly, stopped running around in circles, and was more active. On October 10, 1968 his mother reported that in the spring he had not followed the program and had begun to stutter once more. He began to wet the bed in the fall. I increased the niacinamide to 1 G tid. In March 1969 he was sleeping dry, had continued to improve slowly,

but remained behind his sister. I increased the niacinamide to 4 G od. On March 31 he was speaking more distinctly. I added dexedrine 5 mg and pyridoxine 100 mg od. On March 2, 1971 his mother considered him normal. He spoke to me much more freely, was making better grades in school, but was still shy. On July 30, 1973 he was doing well. John Hoffer evaluated him 0111. He still had a few visual illusions. When he closed his eyes, he saw holes in a graveyard passing by him. His hyperactivity score was 37.

(110) C.W.: Born June 1962, C.W. was first seen in January 1968. She was R.W.'s twin and was normal. Her mother was worried she might also become ill. She excreted KP in her urine. I started her on niacinamide 1 G od and ascorbic acid 1 G od. On July 22, 1969 she had started to show behavioral problems and had started to baby talk. She had not taken any vitamins for 7 days. I increased her niacinamide to 1 G qid, adding mellaril 50 mg od. On March 31, 1970 she was much improved. I decreased the niacinamide to 1 G bid, stopped mellaril, and added dexedrine 5 mg. On July 27, 1970 she had passed into grade 2, cried a lot, and disliked being touched. I added niacin 12 G od. On December 30, 1970 she was better but now refused to take any vitamins. On March 2, 1971 she needed glasses but refused to wear them. She was getting on well at school. On July 30, 1973 there was no change. She refused medication, was passing in school, but was clearly behind her brother. John Hoffer found her 1000 – not improved. She was slow, paranoid, irritable, and depressed. When she could be persuaded to take her vitamins, she would become well. Her hyperactivity score was 75.

An older sister was started on vitamins at age 6 and was normal by October 1970. She refused further treatment. In November 1973 she was admitted to hospital after a suicide attempt. She had been living with her father and her behavior had been gradually getting worse.

CONCLUSION

New Case Histories

The therapeutic program that was so effective twenty years ago remains effective today, perhaps even more so because of the increased awareness of the role played by food allergies. But to establish the fact that the 1970 results were not due to a peculiar, unreproducible series of events present then and not now I will describe just a few of my recent cases. Since 1976 when I started to practice in Victoria, British Columbia, I have seen well over 500 children. These children have been referred to me by their family physicians who have seen the results of the treatment. They were very skeptical at first and only yielded to the pressure from the families before making the referral. After a while they began to make the referrals on their own.

Here I will only include children who have failed to respond to orthodox treatment. They are a special group of failures. Children seen without a history of previous treatment respond much more quickly to treatment. I am not critical of the professional skills of the psychiatrists who failed to help these children because they are at fault only because they have not adopted the new and better treatment. If they use the orthomolecular program, they will be just as successful and they can treat much larger numbers of patients since they will not have to spend as much time with their child patients.

(1) W.E.: Born 1967, W.E. was first seen in June 1982. W.E. did not think there was anything wrong. His parents were very worried about the deterioration in his behavior and by his excessive craving for sweets, present since infancy. He had started running away from home. On the ninth runaway the police were called. In addition, his grades had deteriorated in school in spite of his intelligence. He did not want to study. He scored 75 on the hyperactivity scale. I started him on a sugar-free/junk food Saturday program: he would not have any sugar whatever until Saturday when he could eat as much as he liked. I added niacinamide 500 mg tid, ascorbic acid 500 g bid, pyridoxine 250 mg od, and zinc sulfate 220 mg od. One month later he was a little better, more relaxed. He decided not to do the Junk Saturday any more. On June 27, 1995 his mother came to see me about a problem of her own. She told me her son was well. He is in a relationship with a woman who is becoming a nurse; he is a hard worker, fully employed. His present scores are 1111 (4) – well.

(2) C.M.: C.M. came to the office with her mother on May 17, 1994 who described her as destructive, foul-mouthed, non-compliant, and suffering from severe temper tantrums. This behavior was so bad her mother was considering giving her up. She had been well until age 3. It was then noted she could not get along with other children. After that she became worse. She was treated by a child psychiatrist for two years with the usual psychiatric treatment used by child psychiatrists, including tegretal, but there had been no improvement. On March 24, 1994 her psychiatrist reported to her general practitioner that earlier improvement had not been sustained, that she remained negative and opposed. He continued to meet with a group of professional workers involved in her care. The school wanted her medicated. But she had not responded to medication. She still presented a behavioral disturbance, he wrote, but not clearly attention deficit disorder.

   In my office she was atrocious. She was crude, difficult, just on the verge of violence, ready to throw my furniture about. She resented any conversation, kept telling me she hated me, and stated that she would never cooperate with any treatment. Her eyes flashed with rage as she stared at me; if she had had a gun in her little hand, I believe she would have used it. She had not wanted to come and resented me before she even knew me. Her mother stated she behaved this way all the time. Tegretal created visual difficulties and the dose had to be reduced. She had been suspended from school twice because of her foul language and for a while was hyperactive. She loved sweets, and when she could get them, her behavior would soon become much worse. She had white areas on her finger nails indicating a deficiency of pyridoxine and zinc.

After awhile she told me she had nightmares, could not sleep without a night light. She had told her mother she had been seeing things in her room. She had a reading problem and was receiving tutoring. She was very irritable and hostile. On the hyperactivity scale, she scored 99. I started her on a dairy-free, sugar-free program with niacinamide 500 mg tid, ascorbic acid 500 mg tid, pyridoxine 100 mg od, and zinc sulfate drops.

On June 21 there was no improvement. She had been suspended from school for five days. She was still very hostile, threw two chairs over in my office. I added imipramine 25 mg at bedtime. On September 20, 1994 she was slightly more relaxed but was still very angry, and her behavior was so bad in my office I could hardly bear to have her there. I added thioridazine 25 mg hs. On October 26 her mother came alone. Her daughter had been suspended again but was not able to go to school without crying. In December I doubled her imipramine. There had been substantial improvement. On March 9, 1995 she was reasoning better, performed better at school, had only a few minor incidents but was still easily upset. She was more friendly to me and showed me her pogs. On June 23, her mother called. She had sores in the corner of her mouth. I added riboflavin and increased the pyridoxine to 500 mg od. On July 13, 1995 she was normal. She was in grade 5, getting good grades. She enjoyed school. That day the school was having a western party. She was dressed as a cowgirl and happily showed her costume to me and to Fran, my secretary. Her mother stated she was well, she stated she felt well, and I agreed with both of them. Her hyperactivity score was normal – 43. By eliminating sugar and dairy products, adding the correct vitamins and using tiny amounts of a tranquilizer and a low dose antidepressant, this little girl was transformed from a child monster to a friendly, likable, attractive girl who enjoyed school, had many friends, and made good grades. The life of her whole family was transformed by this change. She had failed to respond to the large amount of care her behavior had previously elicited. Had she been started on this progam when she was three all that trouble would not have occurred and the province would have had a much lower medical care bill. She was transformed from a Miss Hyde to a Dr Jekyll. Within a year or two I expect to have her off her two drugs and on vitamins and good nutrition only.

(3) R.G.: Born December 22, 1992, R.G. was first seen on January 25, 1995. Her parents were concerned over her global developmental delay. She was breastfed for only 4 months and fully weaned by 8 months. She was very slow to move, to roll over, but they did not really become worried until September 1994 when following a cold which lasted one month, development stopped. She also began to hyperventilate and once was taken to the Emergency department of the local hospital. Later investigation at the Children's Hospital, Vancouver revealed no reason for her condition. When I saw her, she was just beginning to walk from chair to chair but was very awkward. Within her limitations of movement, she appeared to be hyperactive. She could feed herself but was very messy. She appreciated attention but when held was very restless and tended to scratch and pull on things. She could say "mama," did respond to play, and laughed when her father acted in a certain way. She had a chronic runny nose, which improved when dairy products had been decreased. She had been drinking a lot of milk. Apple juice caused stomachache. When it touched her skin, it turned red. She had evidence of zinc pyridoxine deficiency, with white areas on her nails. I placed her on a dairy-free diet, ascorbic acid 1 G od, zinc chelate 15 mg od, and a vitamin mineral preparation specially designed for children. On May 15, she could stand alone and walk by herself but was still unsteady. She vocalized more, was growing faster. Her parents described her condition as if she were waking up. They were very pleased with her progress. On July 17, 1995 her nose no longer ran. She was found allergic to bananas and to oats. Her comprehension was better, her response to her parents normal. For 20 minutes she lay quietly in her father's arms, something she could not have done before. I had started niacinamide 100 mg tid on May 15 with dimethyl glycine 50 mg bit. In July I increased the niacinamide to 500 mg tid and the DMG to 50 mg tid. A

few days before she came to see me, she was seen by a pediatric geneticist with expertise in Retts syndrome. He classified her as a good example of this condition. Whatever she has, there is no doubt she has shown a major improvement with the nutritional approach and probably will continue to improve substantially over the years.

(4) J. D.: Born September 1980, J.D. was first seen on September 15, 1987. He had been diagnosed as suffering infantile autism at the Pearkes Center. Birth was difficult and he was in an incubator for five days. He was breast-fed until 15 months but had been started on milk before that. At age 13 months he began to speak, saying "mama," but three months later speech stopped. By age 18 months his parents were concerned at his failure to develop. He was unresponsive. At age 2 he had a very high fever. At age 2½ he was found normal on physical examination by his physician and pediatrician. In pre-school his teachers found him to be different, and when he was 7 he was diagnosed autistic followed by treatment.

When I saw him he was able to talk but was easily confused, and one had to speak very slowly and distinctly. He could only grasp one concept at a time. He had been on mellaril 25 mg hs, which calmed him. It was impossible to obtain a mental state. He did report hearing things at night like a humming. I advised his parents to place him on sugar-free and milk-free program and to add niacinamide 500 mg tid, ascorbic acid 500 mg tid, pyridoxine 250 mg od, and zinc 15 mg with calcium magnesium to prevent any adverse effect from the B-6. On February 9, 1988 he was calmer, took direction better, and his speech was improving. He was able to sleep through the night. On May 9, 1988 he was much better, his emotional reactions were more appropriate, communicated easier. On August 1, 1988 he had completed grade 1, did math at a grade 2 level. One month later he was more restless at school. I had added imipramine 25 mg before bed. On March 21, 1989 his mother was pleased with his progress. She had taken him off the program two months before. On April 6, 1989 it was necessary to place him back again because he had slipped. One year later he was normal and still improving, in Grade 3 in the normal school. On January 3, 1995 he was in Grade 8, with As and Bs. He liked school, got on well with his mates, but felt lonely. At home he was making more friends. He was still on the vitamin program, and his parents were content with his continuing progress.

(5) T.A.: Born October 1985, T.A. was first seen on November 5, 1987. When she was 2½ months old she was given pertussis vaccine. Soon she developed seizures, arched her back and screamed for ten days. Following a grand mal seizure, she was admitted to hospital for four days where she continued to have convulsions. After being placed on medication, dilantin 50 mg bid, tegretal 300 mg od, clobazam 20 mg, chloral 300 to 500 mg at bed time, halcion or nembutal as needed, and ativan SL as needed she continued to have two seizures each day when I saw her, usually in her sleep. She was now mentally handicapped, could not walk properly even with a walker, wore a helmet, but was hyperactive within the limits of her physical disability. She had started to walk at 7½ months. She was not toilet trained. I started her on a sugar and dairy-free diet adding a vitamin-mineral mixture from Bronsons, three tablets od, ascorbic acid 500 mg bid, cod liver oil 1 teaspoon od, pyridoxine 100 mg od, and folic acid 1 mg od.

Six weeks later she was much better, could walk without her walker and did not need her helmet. She had started baby talk, was less hyperactive, and had fewer seizures. By January 5, 1988 she had been seizure free for four weeks. Her parents had started to take her off the tegretol. She could sleep without any sedatives. On October 31, 1988 her parents told me she had been getting along very well. In April 1989 she was placed on depakene and by June was in status epilepticus. The depakene level was twice normal. It was suddenly discontinued, the seizures worsened, and it was resumed and slowly decreased. The doctor at the Children's Hospital accused her parents of mistreating her and lying about her seizures. The family fired her neurologist and soon after the social worker seized this child and made her a ward. She was admitted to hospital. There they would not allow her to take any vitamins. The last I heard they had retained a lawyer to get her released. They were very worried that what she had gained in a few months would vanish in the hospital. It is not rare for children to develop seizure after vaccination. It would become even rarer if each child were getting ample amounts of vitamin C before the vaccination. I do not consider her a success because I have no follow up. Her treatment was interrupted by physicians who were hostile to any nutritional approach. But after a fantastic amount of medication had failed to stop the seizuring, a simple vitamin program did.

(6) H.M.: Born October 1982, H.M. was first seen on November 9, 1983. By age 5 months it was clear she was not developing normally. She was very flaccid and did not move around much. At age 7 months she was diagnosed infantile spasms by the Pearkes Clinic and was started on prednisone and ACTH. She received vaccination at age 3 and age 6 and after each one became much worse. Her EEG was abnormal and she continued to have seizures. Eventually the ACTH was stopped and the prednisone reduced. When I saw her, she slept all the time, except when she fed. Still, she was growing. She was able to move her arms and legs, but could not turn over. I started her on a vitamin-mineral mixture and dimethyl glycine 12.5 mg tid. On December 22 she was much better until she got the flu. By February 8, 1984 she was vocalizing a lot more, had been free of seizures. On May 3, 1984 she was able to sit up alone, was aware, could understand, obey her mother, could hold her bottle, and smiled. She was taken off DMG but was to go back on if she relapsed. On July 5, 1984 she was seizure-free, stable, stronger, walking in her jumper. She was vocalizing well and her parents were pleased with her progress.

(7) C.A.: Born January 1987, he was first seen June 1994. At 8 months it was found his left hand was not working properly. This was worse at one year. With this exception he had developed normally. At age 3½ he was diagnosed to have infantile autism and cerebral palsy. It was concluded he had had a stroke in utero. He began to suffer convulsions every November beginning in the left hand, then into his eyes. On tegretol 900 mg he still had seizures. I started him on niacin 100 tid, ascorbic acid 500 mg tid, pyridoxine 250 mg, magnesium oxide 420 mg od, and zinc 15 mg od. By February 1995 he was better and had been making steady improvement.

(8) J.T.: Born January 1984, J.T. was first seen in May 1989. He was referred as a behavioral and language development problem. As an infant he suffered repeated ear infections. He walked by age 10 months. After each of four vaccinations he had relapsed. When age 17 months, he had his first seizure and was placed on dilantin and phenobarbital. He had severe side effects and was switched to depakene and later tegretol 100 mg bid. He had his last seizure January 1989, 4 months before I saw him. When I saw him, he was irritable, cranky, sullen, aggressive, depressed, and cried a lot. He

still suffered frequent colds, his face was pale, and he had allergy shiners. I started him on a dairy-free diet and decreased sugar intake, adding pyridoxine 100 mg od, ascorbic acid 500 mg bid, and a liquid B complex preparation. Four days after he was on this program he was much better, and by June 22, 1989 was normal. In July 1995 he was still well.

(9) A.I.: Born January 1984, A.I. was first seen on March 1, 1995. Breastfed until age 6 months, he was then started on cows' milk and became very constipated. He walked by age 10 months. At age 4 years his behavior had become very bad. He was silly, giddy, raced around, would not obey his parents. But he was very bright, and at age 4 was discussing the merits of free trade. He was started on ritalin 30 mg od, which reduced his hyperactivity. When I saw him, he had typical pink cheeks and red ears of the allergic child and was very restless. He had been to the Emergency of the hospital 27 times over the years because of his behavior and accidents. His mother had taken him off dairy products with no improvement, but off sugar he was much better. I started him on the vitamin regimen. On April 4, 1995 he had new glasses which improved his behavior. On June 20, he was better but had not taken his vitamins regularly. On July 20, 1995 his mother was pleased with his improvement. He no longer ran away from home, was more responsive, calmer, and had graduated into grade 6 with a B average. He was still on ritalin, but I planned that on the full dose of niacinamide 1 G tid I would start to decrease the amount of ritalin.

Orthomolecular or nutritional treatment is clearly the best treatment available for children with learning or behavioral disorders as my clinical experiences continue to prove since 1960 when I first began to treat these children. Over the past 40 years I have seen at least 1,500 children ages 14 or less. The results of treatment remain good – most of these children recover and go on to lead normal and productive lives. This means that they are getting on pretty well with their families and the community, that they are free of the disease which first brought them to me, and that they are able to play a productive role in our society.

This treatment can be provided by any physician trained in these methods. No special skill is required, and for most patients, psychiatric treatment is not indicated. In fact, I think these children would be better off never to see a psychiatrist if the psychiatrist is going to use the same old approach which inevitably leads the child to be labeled with one of fifty useless diagnostic terms so loved by the American Psychiatric Association and to be treated with the same old treatment, the stimulant ritalin.

Parents will have difficulty finding physicians willing to use this approach, however. It is so difficult to overcome decades of bias and prejudice, decades of blaming someone, either parents or society. Parents with these children should read as much as they can, and consult their family doctor. If their doctors are not interested in orthomolecular treatment, they should shop around until they find one who is. Once the doctor's interest is aroused, it does not take long before they become enthusiastic therapists because the results are so positive. Parents and physicians will in many cases need to be very patient since treatment with nutrients does not produce overnight results but the slow, steady recoveries which are much more exciting than the rapid responses to drugs which in the end lead nowhere. Drugs should be used as needed very sparingly and removed as soon as the child has shown an adequate response to diet and nutrient supplements. The good health of our children must be placed above the financial interests of physicians and pharmaceutical companies.

THE NUTRIENT CONTENT
OF COMMON FOODS

I t is always best to acquire all of the daily allotment of nutrients you need from the nutritional quality of foods eaten. The following list of the vitamin and mineral content of many foods will help you tailor your eating to your specific dietary needs. Use the listing to identify foods that are good sources for the particular vitamin or mineral you are interested in.

While the values given in these lists can be useful in comparing nutritional content in foods, the absolute values for food nutrients will vary, depending on such factors as the condition of the soil where the food was grown (or what type of nutrition an animal received), the amount of processing or refining, and the method of preparation.

The serving size of each food in the lists has been standardized to 100 grams. This was done to provide a more appropriate comparison between the relative amounts of nutrients in foods and allows them to be ranked from highest to lowest. Remember, however, not all foods are consumed in 100-gram quantities, especially if they are highly concentrated, like kelp, dulse, wheat germ, and brewer's yeast. Such foods often appear at the top of the list, indicating that they are concentrated nutritional sources. To get an idea of what 100 grams of a food represents, it may be helpful to consider what it is equivalent to in common measurements. A 100-gram serving size is approximately equal to any one of the following:

- about ⅜ cup fluid measure
- about ¼ cup dry measure
- 3¼ ounces of milk or yogurt
- slightly more than 1 cup leafy vegetable
- ¾ cup root vegetable
- 5½ ounces nuts, seeds
- ⅔ cup of sliced fruit
- ½ cup cereal grain, uncooked
- 7 tablespoons cooking oil
- 5 tablespoons honey, molasses

The following lists indicate the amounts of important nutrients available in 100-gram portions of various foods.

Bad Food

The following foods contain large amounts of sodium chloride, added during processing, and should generally be avoided.

Canned or frozen vegetables
Cured, smoked,
or canned meats
Commercial peanut butter
Potato chips, corn chips, etc.
Processed cheeses
Luncheon meats
Salted nuts

Packaged spice mixes
Bouillon cubes
Canned fish
Salted crackers
Canned or packaged soups
Commercial salad dressings
Meat tenderizers

Vitamins

Vitamin A (Carotene)

I.U. per 100-gram (3.5 oz) portion		I.U. per 100-gram (3.5 oz) portion	
50,500	Lamb liver	43,900	Beef liver
22,500	Calf liver	21,600	Peppers, red chili
14,000	Dandelion greens	12,100	Chicken liver
11,000	Carrots	10,900	Apricots, dried
9,300	Collard leaves	8,900	Kale
8,800	Sweet potatoes	8,500	Parsley
8,100	Spinach	7,600	Turnip greens
7,000	Mustard greens	6,500	Swiss chard
6,100	Beet greens	5,800	Chives
5,700	Butternut squash	4,900	Watercress
4,800	Mangos	4,450	Peppers, sweet red
4,300	Hubbard squash	3,400	Cantaloupe
3,300	Endive	2,700	Apricots
2,500	Broccoli spears	2,260	Whitefish
2,000	Green onions	1,900	Romaine lettuce
1,750	Papayas	1,650	Nectarines
1,600	Prunes	1,600	Pumpkin
1,580	Swordfish	1,540	Whipping cream
1,330	Peaches	1,200	Acorn squash
1,180	Eggs	1,080	Chicken
1,000	Cherries, sour red	970	Butterhead lettuce
900	Asparagus	900	Tomatoes, ripe
770	Peppers, green chili	690	Kidneys
640	Peas	600	Green beans
600	Elderberries	590	Watermelon
580	Rutabagas	550	Brussels sprouts
520	Okra	510	Yellow cornmeal
460	Yellow squash		

Vitamin A from animal source foods occurs mostly as active, preformed vitamin A (retinol), while that from vegetable source foods occurs as pro-vitamin A (beta-carotene and other carotenoids) that must be converted to active vitamin A by the body to be utilized. The efficiency of conversion varies among individuals; however, beta-carotene is converted more efficiently than other carotenoids. Green and deep-yellow vegetables, as well as deep-yellow fruits, are highest in beta-carotene.

Vitamin B-1 (Thiamin)

I.U. per 100-gram (3.5 oz) portion		I.U. per 100-gram (3.5 oz) portion	
15.61	Brewer's yeast	14.01	Torula yeast
2.01	Wheat germ	1.96	Sunflower seeds
1.84	Rice polishings	1.28	Pine nuts
1.14	Peanuts, with skins	1.10	Soybeans, dry
1.05	Cowpeas, dry	.98	Peanuts, without skins
.96	Brazil nuts	.93	Pork, lean
.86	Pecans	.85	Soybean flour
.84	Beans, pinto and red	.74	Split peas
.73	Millet	.72	Wheat bran
.67	Pistachio nuts	.65	Navy beans
.63	Veal heart	.60	Buckwheat
.60	Oatmeal	.55	Whole wheat flour
.55	Whole wheat	.51	Lamb kidneys
.31	Garbanzos	.48	Lima beans, dry
.46	Hazelnuts	.45	Lamb heart
.45	Wild rice	.43	Cashews
.43	Rye, whole grain	.40	Lamb liver
.40	Lobster	.38	Mung beans
.38	Cornmeal, whole	.37	Lentils
.36	Beef kidneys	.35	Green peas
.34	Brown rice	.33	Walnuts
.30	Pork liver	.25	Garlic, cloves

.25	Beef liver	.24	Almonds, ground
.24	Lima beans, fresh	.24	Pumpkin and squash seeds
.23	Brains, all kinds	.23	Soybean sprouts
.22	Peppers, red chili		

Vitamin B-2 (Riboflavin)

I.U. per 100-gram (3.5 oz) portion		I.U. per 100-gram (3.5 oz) portion	
5.06	Torula yeast	4.28	Brewer's yeast
3.28	Lamb liver	3.26	Beef liver
3.03	Pork liver	2.72	Calf liver
2.55	Beef kidneys	2.49	Chicken liver
2.42	Lamb kidneys	1.36	Chicken giblets
1.05	Veal heart	.92	Almonds
.88	Beef heart	.74	Lamb heart
.68	Wheat germ	.63	Wild rice
.46	Mushrooms	.44	Egg yolks
.38	Millet	.36	Peppers, hot red
.35	Soy flour	.35	Wheat bran
.33	Mackerel	.31	Collards
.31	Soybeans, dry	.30	Eggs
.29	Split peas	.29	Beef tongue
.29	Brains, all kinds	.26	Kale
.26	Parsley	.25	Cashews
.25	Rice bran	.25	Veal
.24	Lamb, lean	.23	Broccoli
.23	Chicken, meat and skin	.23	Pine nuts
.23	Salmon	.23	Sunflower seeds
.22	Rye, whole grain	.22	Navy beans
.22	Beet and mustard greens	.21	Beans, pinto and red
.22	Lentils	.22	Pork, lean
.22	Prunes	.21	Mung beans
.21	Blackeyed peas	.21	Okra
.13	Sesame seeds, hulled		

Vitamin B-3 (Niacin)

I.U. per 100-gram (3½ oz) portion		I.U. per 100-gram (3½ oz) portion	
44.4	Torula yeast	37.9	Brewer's yeast
29.8	Rice bran	28.2	Rice polishings
21.0	Wheat bran	17.2	Peanuts, with skins
16.9	Lamb liver	16.4	Pork liver
15.8	Peanuts, without skins	13.6	Beef liver
11.4	Calf liver	11.3	Turkey, light meat
10.8	Chicken liver	10.7	Chicken, light meat
8.4	Trout	8.3	Halibut
8.2	Mackerel	8.1	Veal heart
8.0	Chicken, meat only	8.0	Swordfish
8.0	Turkey, meat only	7.7	Goose, meat only
7.5	Beef heart	7.2	Salmon
6.4	Veal	6.4	Beef kidneys
6.2	Wild rice	6.1	Chicken giblets
5.7	Lamb, lean	5.6	Chicken, meat and skin
5.4	Sesame seeds	5.4	Sunflower seeds
5.1	Beef, lean	5.0	Pork, lean
4.7	Brown rice	4.5	Pine nuts
4.4	Buckwheat, whole grain	4.4	Peppers, red chili
4.4	Whole wheat grain	4.3	Whole wheat flour
4.2	Mushrooms	4.2	Wheat germ
3.7	Barley	3.6	Herring
3.5	Almonds	3.5	Shrimp
3.0	Haddock	3.0	Split peas

Pantothenic Acid (a B vitamin)

I.U. per 100-gram (3.5 oz) portion		I.U. per 100-gram (3.5 oz) portion	
12.0	Brewer's yeast	11.0	Torula yeast
8.0	Calf liver	6.0	Chicken liver

3.9	Beef kidneys	2.8	Peanuts
2.6	Brains, all kinds	2.6	Heart
2.2	Mushrooms	2.0	Soybean flour
2.0	Split peas	2.0	Beef tongue
1.9	Perch	1.8	Blue cheese
1.7	Pecans	1.7	Soybeans
1.6	Eggs	1.5	Lobster
1.5	Oatmeal, dry	1.4	Buckwheat flour
1.4	Sunflower seeds	1.4	Lentils
1.3	Rye flour, whole	1.3	Cashews
1.3	Salmon	1.2	Camembert cheese
1.2	Garbanzos	1.2	Wheat germ, toasted
1.2	Broccoli	1.1	Hazelnuts
1.1	Turkey, dark meat	1.1	Brown rice
1.1	Wheat flour, whole	1.1	Sardines
1.1	Peppers, red chili	1.1	Avocados
1.1	Veal, lean	1.0	Blackeyed peas, dry
1.0	Wild rice	1.0	Cauliflower
1.0	Chicken, dark meat	1.0	Kale

Vitamin B-6 (Pyridoxine)

I.U. per 100-gram (3.5 oz) portion		I.U. per 100-gram (3.5 oz) portion	
3.00	Torula yeast	2.50	Brewer's yeast
1.25	Sunflower seeds	1.15	Wheat germ, toasted
.90	Tuna	.84	Beef liver
.81	Soybeans, dry	.75	Chicken liver
.73	Walnuts	.70	Salmon
.69	Trout	.67	Calf liver
.66	Mackerel	.65	Pork liver
.63	Soybean flour	.60	Lentils, dry
.58	Buckwheat flour	.58	Lima beans, dry
.56	Blackeyed peas, dry	.56	Navy beans, dry
.55	Brown rice	.54	Garbanzos, dry
.53	Pinto beans, dry	.51	Bananas

.45	Pork, lean	.44	Albacore
.43	Beef, lean	.43	Halibut
.43	Beef kidneys	.42	Avocados
.41	Veal kidneys	.34	Whole wheat flour
.33	Chestnuts, fresh	.30	Egg yolks
.30	Kale	.30	Rye flour
.28	Spinach	.26	Turnip greens
.25	Beef heart	.26	Peppers, sweet
.25	Potatoes	.24	Prunes
.24	Raisins	.24	Sardines
.24	Brussels sprouts	.23	Elderberries
.23	Perch	.22	Cod
.22	Barley	.22	Camembert cheese
.22	Sweet potatoes	.21	Cauliflower
.20	Popcorn, popped	.20	Red cabbage
.20	Leeks	.20	Molasses

Folic Acid (a B vitamin)

I.U. per 100-gram (3.5oz) portion		I.U. per 100-gram (3.5oz) portion	
2022	Brewer's yeast	440	Blackeyed peas
430	Rice germ	425	Soy flour
305	Wheat germ	295	Beef liver
275	Lamb liver	225	Soybeans
220	Pork liver	195	Bran
180	Kidney beans	145	Mung beans
130	Lima beans	125	Navy beans
125	Garbanzos	110	Asparagus
105	Lentils	77	Walnuts
75	Spinach, fresh	70	Kale
65	Filbert nuts	60	Beet and mustard greens
57	Textured vegetable protein	56	Peanuts, roasted
		56	Peanut butter

53	Broccoli		50	Barley
50	Split peas		49	Whole wheat cereal
49	Brussels sprouts		45	Almonds
38	Whole wheat flour		33	Oatmeal
32	Dried figs		30	Avocado
28	Green beans		28	Corn
28	Coconut, fresh		27	Pecans
25	Mushrooms		25	Dates
14	Blackberries		7	Ground beef
5	Oranges			

Vitamin B12 (Cobalamin)

I.U. per 100-gram (3.5 oz) portion

I.U. per 100-gram (3.5 oz) portion

104	Lamb liver		98	Clams
80	Beef liver		63	Lamb kidneys
60	Calf liver		31	Beef kidneys
25	Chicken liver		18	Oysters
17	Sardines		11	Beef heart
6	Egg yolks		5.2	Lamb heart
5.0	Trout		4.0	Brains, all kinds
4.0	Salmon		3.0	Tuna
2.1	Lamb		2.1	Sweetbreads
2.0	Eggs		2.0	Whey, dried
1.8	Beef, lean		1.8	Edam cheese
1.8	Swiss cheese		1.6	Brie cheese
1.6	Gruyere cheese		1.4	Blue cheese
1.3	Haddock		1.2	Flounder
1.2	Scallops		1.0	Cheddar cheese
1.0	Cottage cheese		1.0	Mozzarella cheese
1.0	Halibut		1.0	Perch, fillets
1.0	Swordfish			

Biotin (a B vitamin)

I.U. per 100-gram (3.5 oz) portion		I.U. per 100-gram (3.5 oz) portion	
200	Brewer's yeast	127	Lamb liver
100	Pork liver	96	Beef liver
70	Soy flour	61	Soybeans
60	Rice bran	58	Rice germ
57	Rice polishings	52	Egg yolk
39	Peanut butter	37	Walnuts
34	Peanuts, roasted	31	Barley
27	Pecans	24	Oatmeal
24	Sardines, canned	22	Eggs
21	Blackeyed peas	18	Split peas
18	Almonds	17	Cauliflower
16	Mushrooms	16	Whole wheat cereal
15	Salmon, canned	15	Textured vegetable protein
14	Bran	13	Lentils
12	Brown rice	10	Chicken

Choline (a B vitamin)

I.U. per 100-gram (3.5 oz) portion		I.U. per 100-gram (3.5 oz) portion	
2200	Lecithin	1490	Egg yolk
550	Liver	504	Whole eggs
406	Wheat germ	340	Soybeans
300	Rice germ	257	Blackeyed peas
245	Garbanzo beans	240	Brewer's yeast
223	Lentils	201	Split peas
170	Rice bran	162	Peanuts, roasted
156	Oatmeal	145	Peanut butter
143	Bran	139	Barley
122	Ham	112	Brown rice

104	Veal	102	Rice polishings
94	Whole wheat cereal	86	Molasses
77	Pork	75	Beef
75	Green peas	48	Cheddar cheese
66	Sweet potatoes	42	Green beans
29	Potatoes	23	Cabbage
22	Spinach	20.5	Textured vegetable protein
15	Milk	12	Orange juice
5	Butter		

Inositol (a B vitamin)

I.U. per 100-gram (3½ oz) portion		I.U. per 100-gram (3½ oz) portion	
2220	Lecithin	770	Wheat germ
500	Navy beans	460	Rice bran
454	Rice polishings	390	Barley, cooked
370	Rice germ	370	Whole wheat
270	Brewer's yeast	270	Oatmeal
240	Blackeyed peas	240	Garbanzo beans
210	Oranges	205	Soy flour
200	Soybeans	180	Peanuts, roasted
180	Peanut butter	170	Lima beans
162	Green peas	150	Molasses
150	Grapefruit	150	Split peas
130	Lentils	120	Raisins
120	Cantaloupe	119	Brown rice
117	Orange juice	110	Whole wheat flour
96	Peaches	95	Cabbage
95	Cauliflower	88	Onions
67	Whole wheat bread	66	Sweet potatoes
64	Watermelon	60	Strawberries
55	Lettuce	51	Beef liver
46	Tomatoes	33	Eggs
13	Milk	11	Beef, round

Vitamin B17 (Amygdalin)

For certain nutrients, there are few foods sources that contain appreciable quantities. In these cases we list those foods that are best sources, rather than relative nutrient amounts.

Foods containing more than 500 milligrams per 100-gram portion:

Wild blackberries	Apple seeds	Cherry seeds
Elderberries	Apricot seeds	Nectarine seeds
Peach seeds	Fava beans	Bamboo sprouts
Pear seeds	Mung beans	Alfalfa leaves
Plum seeds	Bitter almonds	
Prune seeds	Macadamia nuts	

Foods containing between 100 and 500 milligrams per 100-gram portion:

Boysenberries	Raspberries	Garbanzo beans
Currants	Alfalfa sprouts	Blackeyed peas
Gooseberries	Buckwheat	Kidney beans
Huckleberries	Flax seed	Lentils
Loganberries	Millet	Lima beans
Mulberries	Squash seed	
Quince	Mung bean sprouts	

Foods containing below 100 milligrams per 100-gram portion:

Commercial blackberries	Peas	Cashews
Cranberries	Lima beans	Beet tops
Black beans	Sweet potatoes, yams	

Para-Aminobenzoic Acid (paba)
(a B vitamin)

Good sources include:

Mushrooms	Sunflower seeds	Whole milk
Liver	Wheat germ	Eggs
Bran	Oats	
Cabbage	Spinach	

Pangamic Acid (Vitamin B15)

Good sources include:

Apricot kernels	Corn grits	Oat grits
Yeast	Wheat germ	Sunflower seeds
Liver	Wheat bran	Pumpkin seeds
Rice bran		

Vitamin C (Ascorbic Acid)

I.U. per 100-gram (3.5 oz) portion		I.U. per 100-gram (3.5 oz) portion	
1300	Acerola	369	Peppers, red chili
242	Guavas	204	Peppers, red sweet
186	Kale leaves	172	Parsley
152	Collard leaves	139	Turnip greens
128	Peppers, green sweet	113	Broccoli
102	Brussels sprouts	97	Mustard greens
79	Watercress	78	Cauliflower
66	Persimmons	61	Cabbage, red
59	Strawberries	56	Papayas
51	Spinach	50	Oranges and juice
47	Cabbage	46	Lemon juice
38	Grapefruit and juice	36	Elderberries

36	Calf liver	36	Turnips
35	Mangoes	33	Asparagus
33	Cantaloupes	32	Swiss chard
32	Green onions	31	Beef liver
31	Okra	31	Tangerines
30	New Zealand spinach	30	Oysters
29	Lima beans, young	29	Blackeyed beans
29	Soybeans	27	Green peas
26	Radishes	25	Raspberries
25	Chinese cabbage	25	Yellow summer squash
24	Loganberries	23	Honeydew melon
23	Tomatoes	23	Pork liver

Vitamin D

I.U. per 100-gram (3.5 oz) portion		I.U. per 100-gram (3.5 oz) portion	
500	Sardines, canned	350	Salmon
250	Tuna	150	Shrimp
90	Sunflower seeds	90	Butter
50	Liver	50	Eggs
40	Milk, fortified	40	Mushrooms
30	Natural cheeses		

Vitamin E (Tocopherol)

I.U. per 100-gram (3.5 oz) portion		I.U. per 100-gram (3.5 oz) portion	
216	Wheat germ oil	90	Sunflower seeds
88	Sunflower seed oil	72	Safflower oil
48	Almonds	45	Sesame oil
34	Peanut oil	29	Corn oil
22	Wheat germ	18	Olive oil
18	Peanuts	14	Soybean oil

13	Peanuts, roasted	11	Peanut butter
3.0	Bran	3.6	Butter
3.2	Spinach	3.0	Oatmeal
2.9	Asparagus	2.5	Salmon
2.5	Brown rice	2.3	Rye, whole
2.2	Rye bread, dark	1.9	Pecans
1.9	Wheat germ	1.9	Rye and wheat crackers
1.4	Whole wheat bread	1.0	Carrots
0.99	Peas	0.92	Walnuts
0.88	Bananas	0.83	Eggs
0.72	Tomatoes	0.29	Lamb

Vitamin K

I.U. per 100-gram (3.5 oz) portion		I.U. per 100-gram (3.5 oz) portion	
650	Turnip greens	200	Broccoli
129	Lettuce	125	Cabbage
92	Beef liver	89	Spinach
57	Watercress	57	Asparagus
35	Cheese	30	Butter
25	Pork liver	20	Oats
19	Green peas	17	Whole wheat
14	Green beans	11	Pork
11	Eggs	10	Corn oil
8	Peaches	7	Beef
7	Chicken liver	6	Raisins
5	Tomatoes	3	Milk
3	Potatoes		

Bioflavonoids (Vitamin P)

Goods sources include:

Grapes	Black currants	Peppers
Rose hips	Plums	Papaya

Prunes   Parsley   Cantaloupe
Oranges   Grapefruit   Tomatoes
Lemon juice   Cabbage   Cherries
Apricots

Minerals

Calcium

I.U. per 100-gram (3.5 oz) portion		I.U. per 100-gram (3.5 oz) portion	
1093	Kelp	925	Swiss cheese
750	Cheddar cheese	352	Carob flour
296	Dulse	250	Collard leaves
246	Turnip greens	245	Barbados molasses
234	Almonds	210	Brewer's yeast
203	Parsley	200	Corn tortillas (lime added)
187	Dandelion greens	186	Brazil nuts
151	Watercress	129	Goat's milk
128	Tofu	126	Dried figs
121	Buttermilk	120	Sunflower seeds
120	Yogurt	119	Beet greens
119	Wheat bran	118	Whole milk
114	Buckwheat, raw	110	Sesame seeds, hulled
106	Ripe olives	103	Broccoli
99	English walnut	94	Cottage cheese
93	Spinach	73	Soybeans, cooked
73	Pecans	72	Wheat germ
69	Peanuts	68	Miso
68	Romaine lettuce	67	Dried apricots
66	Rutabaga	62	Raisins
60	Black currants	59	Dates
56	Green snap beans	51	Globe artichokes
51	Dried prunes	51	Pumpkin and squash

50	Cooked dry beans		seeds
49	Common cabbage	48	Soybean sprouts
46	Hard winter wheat	41	Oranges
39	Celery	38	Cashews
38	Rye grain	37	Carrots
34	Barley	32	Sweet potatoes
32	Brown rice	29	Garlic
28	Summer squash	27	Onions
26	Lemons	26	Fresh green peas
25	Cauliflower	25	Lentils, cooked
22	Sweet cherries	22	Asparagus
22	Winter squash	21	Strawberry
20	Millet	19	Mung bean sprouts
17	Pineapple	16	Grapes
16	Beets	14	Cantaloupe
14	Jerusalem artichokes	13	Tomatoes
12	Eggplant	12	Chicken
11	Orange juice	10	Avocado
10	Beef	8	Bananas
7	Apples	3	Sweet corn

Magnesium

I.U. per
100-gram (3.5 oz) portion

I.U. per
100-gram (3.5 oz) portion

760	Kelp	490	Wheat bran
336	Wheat germ	270	Almonds
267	Cashews	258	Blackstrap molasses
231	Brewer's yeast	229	Buckwheat
225	Brazil nuts	220	Dulse
184	Filberts	175	Peanuts
162	Millet	160	Wheat grain
142	Pecan	131	English walnut
115	Rye	111	Tofu
106	Beet greens	90	Coconut meat, dry

88	Soybeans, cooked	88	Spinach
88	Brown rice	71	Dried figs
65	Swiss chard	62	Apricots, dried
58	Dates	57	Collard leaves
51	Shrimp	48	Sweet corn
45	Cheddar cheese	41	Parsley
40	Prunes, dried	38	Sunflower seeds
37	Common beans, cooked	37	Barley
36	Dandelion greens	36	Garlic
36	Raisins	35	Fresh green peas
34	Potatoes with skin	34	Crab
33	Bananas	33	Sweet potatoes
30	Blackberries	25	Beets
25	Broccoli	24	Cauliflower
23	Carrots	22	Celery
21	Beef	20	Asparagus
19	Chicken	18	Pepper, green
17	Winter squash	16	Cantaloupe
16	Eggplant	14	Tomato
13	Cabbage	13	Grapes
13	Milk	13	Pineapple
13	Mushrooms	12	Onions
11	Oranges	11	Iceberg lettuce
9	Plums		

Phosphorus

I.U. per 100-gram (3.5 oz) portion		I.U. per 100-gram (3.5 oz) portion	
1753	Brewer's yeast	1276	Wheat bran
1144	Pumpkin and squash seeds	1118	Wheat germ
		837	Sunflower seeds
693	Brazil nuts	592	Sesame seeds, hulled
554	Soybeans, dried	504	Almonds
478	Cheddar cheese	457	Pinto beans, dried

409	Peanuts	400	Wheat
380	English walnuts	376	Rye grain
373	Cashews	352	Beef liver
338	Scallops	311	Millet
290	Barley, pearled	289	Pecans
267	Dulse	240	Kelp
239	Chicken	221	Brown rice
202	Garlic	175	Crab
152	Cottage cheese	150	Beef or lamb
119	Lentils, cooked	116	Mushrooms
116	Fresh peas	111	Sweet corn
101	Raisins	93	Milk
88	Globe artichoke	87	Yogurt
80	Brussels sprouts	79	Prunes, dried
78	Broccoli	77	Figs, dried
69	Yams	67	Soybean sprouts
64	Mung bean sprouts	63	Dates
63	Parsley	62	Asparagus
59	Bamboo shoots	56	Cauliflower
53	Potato, with skin	44	Green beans
44	Pumpkin	42	Avocado
40	Beet greens	39	Swiss chard
38	Winter squash	36	Carrots
36	Onions	35	Red cabbage
51	Spinach	33	Beets
31	Radishes	29	Summer squash
28	Celery	27	Cucumber
27	Tomatoes	26	Bananas
26	Persimmon	26	Eggplant
26	Lettuce	24	Nectarines
22	Raspberries	20	Grapes
20	Oranges	205	Eggs
17	Olives	16	Cantaloupe
10	Apples	8	Pineapple

Sodium

I.U. per 100-gram (3.5 oz) portion		I.U. per 100-gram (3.5 oz) portion	
3007	Kelp	2400	Green olives
2132	Salt (1 teaspoon)	1428	Dill pickles
1319	Soy sauce (1 tablespoon)	828	Ripe olives
747	Sauerkraut	700	Cheddar cheese
265	Scallops	229	Cottage cheese
210	Lobster	147	Swiss chard
130	Beet greens	130	Buttermilk
126	Celery	122	Eggs
110	Cod	71	Spinach
70	Lamb	65	Pork
64	Chicken	60	Beef
60	Beets	60	Sesame seeds
52	Watercress	50	Whole milk
49	Turnips	47	Carrots
47	Yogurt	45	Parsley
43	Artichoke	34	Dried figs
30	Lentils, dried	30	Sunflower seeds
27	Raisins	26	Red cabbage
19	Garlic	19	White beans
15	Broccoli	15	Mushrooms
13	Cauliflower	10	Onions
10	Sweet Potatoes	9	Brown rice
9	Lettuce	6	Cucumber
5	Peanuts	4	Avocado
3	Tomatoes	2	Eggplant

Potassium

I.U. per 100-gram (3.5 oz) portion		I.U. per 100-gram (3.5 oz) portion	
8060	Dulse	5273	Kelp
920	Sunflower seeds	827	Wheat germ
773	Almonds	763	Raisins
727	Parsley	715	Brazil nuts
674	Peanuts	648	Dates
640	Figs, dried	604	Avocado
603	Pecans	600	Yams
550	Swiss chard	540	Soybeans, cooked
529	Garlic	470	Spinach
450	English walnuts	430	Millet
416	Beans, cooked	414	Mushrooms
407	Potatoes, with skin	382	Broccoli
370	Bananas	370	Meats
369	Winter squash	366	Chicken
341	Carrots	341	Celery
322	Radishes	295	Cauliflower
282	Watercress	278	Asparagus
268	Red cabbage	264	Lettuce
251	Cantaloupe	249	Lentils, cooked
244	Tomatoes	243	Sweet potatoes
234	Papaya	214	Eggplant
213	Peppers, green	208	Beets
202	Peaches	202	Summer squash
200	Oranges	199	Raspberries
191	Cherries	164	Strawberries
162	Grapefruit juice	158	Grapes
157	Onions	146	Pineapple
144	Milk	141	Lemon juice
130	Pears	129	Eggs
110	Apples	100	Watermelon
70	Brown rice, cooked		

Iron

I.U. per 100-gram (3.5 oz) portion		I.U. per 100-gram (3.5 oz) portion	
100.3	Kelp	17.3	Brewer's yeast
16.1	Blackstrap molasses	14.9	Wheat bran
11.2	Pumpkin and squash seeds	9.4	Wheat germ
		8.8	Beef liver
7.1	Sunflower seeds	6.8	Millet
6.2	Parsley	6.1	Clam
4.7	Almond	3.9	Dried prunes
3.8	Cashews	3.7	Beef, lean
3.5	Raisins	3.4	Jerusalem artichokes
3.4	Brazil nuts	3.3	Beet greens
3.2	Swiss chard	3.1	Dandelion greens
3.1	English walnuts	3.0	Dates
2.9	Pork	2.7	Cooked dry beans
2.4	Sesame seeds, hulled	2.4	Pecans
2.3	Eggs	2.1	Lentils
2.1	Peanuts	1.9	Lamb
1.9	Tofu	1.8	Green peas
1.6	Brown rice	1.6	Ripe olives
1.5	Chicken	1.3	Mung bean sprouts
1.2	Salmon	1.1	Broccoli
1.1	Currants	1.1	Whole wheat bread
1.1	Cauliflower	1.0	Cheddar cheese
1.0	Strawberries	1.0	Asparagus
0.9	Blackberries	0.8	Red cabbage
0.8	Pumpkin	0.8	Mushroom
0.7	Bananas	0.7	Beets
0.7	Carrots	0.7	Eggplant
0.7	Sweet potatoes	0.6	Avocado
0.6	Figs	0.6	Potatoes
0.6	Corn	0.5	Pineapple

0.5	Nectarines	0.5	Winter squash
0.5	Brown rice, cooked	0.5	Tomatoes
0.4	Oranges	0.4	Cherries
0.4	Summer squash	0.3	Papaya
0.3	Celery	0.3	Cottage Cheese
0.3	Apples		

Copper

I.U. per 100-gram (3.5 oz) portion		I.U. per 100-gram (3.5 oz) portion	
13.7	Oysters	2.3	Brazil nuts
2.1	Soy lecithin	1.4	Almonds
1.3	Hazelnuts	1.3	Walnuts
1.3	Pecans	1.2	Split peas, dry
1.1	Beef liver	0.8	Buckwheat
0.8	Peanuts	0.7	Cod liver oil
0.7	Lamb chops	0.5	Sunflower oil
0.4	Butter	0.4	Rye grain
0.4	Pork loin	0.4	Barley
0.4	Gelatin	0.3	Shrimp
0.3	Olive oil	0.3	Clams
0.3	Carrots	0.3	Coconut
0.3	Garlic	0.2	Millet
0.2	Whole wheat	0.2	Chicken
0.2	Eggs	0.2	Corn oil
0.2	Ginger root	0.2	Molasses
0.2	Turnips	0.1	Green peas
0.1	Papaya	0.1	Apples

Black pepper, thyme, paprika, bay leaves, and active dry yeast are also high in copper.

Manganese

I.U. per 100-gram (3.5 oz) portion		I.U. per 100-gram (3.5 oz) portion	
3.5	Pecans	2.8	Brazil nuts
2.5	Almonds	1.8	Barley
1.3	Rye	1.3	Buckwheat
1.3	Split peas, dry	1.1	Whole wheat
0.16	Carrots	0.15	Broccoli
0.14	Brown rice	0.14	Whole wheat bread
0.13	Swiss cheese	0.13	Corn
0.11	Cabbage	0.10	Peaches
0.8	Walnuts	0.8	Fresh spinach
0.7	Peanuts	0.6	Oats
0.5	Raisins	0.5	Turnip greens
0.5	Rhubarb	0.4	Beet greens
0.3	Brussels sprouts	0.3	Oatmeal
0.2	Cornmeal	0.2	Millet
0.19	Gorgonzola cheese	0.09	Butter
0.06	Tangerines	0.06	Peas
0.05	Eggs	0.04	Beets
0.04	Coconut	0.03	Apples
0.03	Oranges	0.03	Pears
0.03	Lamb chops	0.03	Pork chops
0.03	Cantaloupe	0.03	Tomatoes
0.02	Milk	0.02	Chicken breasts
0.02	Green beans	0.02	Apricots
0.01	Beef liver	0.01	Scallops
0.01	Halibut	0.01	Cucumbers

Cloves, ginger, thyme, bay leaves, and tea are also high in manganese.

Zinc

I.U. per 100-gram (3.5 oz) portion		I.U. per 100-gram (3.5 oz) portion	
148.7	Fresh oysters	6.8	Ginger root
5.6	Ground round steak	5.3	Lamb chops
4.5	Pecans	4.2	Split peas, dry
4.2	Brazil nuts	3.9	Beef liver
3.5	Nonfat dry milk	3.5	Egg yolk
3.2	Whole wheat	3.2	Rye
3.2	Oats	3.2	Peanuts
3.1	Lima beans	3.1	Soy lecithin
3.1	Almonds	3.0	Walnuts
2.9	Sardines	2.6	Chicken
2.5	Buckwheat	2.4	Hazelnuts
1.9	Clams	1.7	Anchovies
1.7	Tuna	1.7	Haddock
1.6	Green peas	1.5	Shrimp
1.2	Turnips	0.9	Parsley
0.9	Potatoes	0.6	Garlic
0.5	Carrots	0.5	Whole wheat bread
0.4	Black beans	0.4	Raw milk
0.4	Pork chops	0.4	Corn
0.3	Grape juice	0.3	Olive oil
0.3	Cauliflower	0.2	Spinach
0.2	Cabbage	0.2	Lentils
0.2	Butter	0.2	Lettuce
0.1	Cucumber	0.1	Yams
0.1	Tangerines	0.1	String beans

Chromium

The values listed below show the total chromium content of these foods, and do not indicate the amount that may be biologically active as the Glucose Tolerance Factor (GTF). Those foods marked with an * are high in GTF.

I.U. per 100-gram (3.5 oz) portion		I.U. per 100-gram (3.5 oz) portion	
112	Brewer's yeast*	57	Beef round
55	Calf liver*	42	Whole wheat bread*
38	Wheat bran	30	Rye bread
30	Fresh chili	26	Oysters
24	Potatoes	23	Wheat germ
19	Peppers, green	16	Hen's eggs
15	Chicken	14	Apples
13	Butter	13	Parsnips
12	Cornmeal	12	Lamb chop
11	Scallops	11	Swiss cheese
10	Bananas	10	Spinach
10	Pork chop	9	Carrots
8	Navy beans, dry	7	Shrimp
7	Lettuce	5	Oranges
5	Lobster tails	5	Blueberries
4	Green beans	4	Cabbage
4	Mushrooms	3	Beer
3	Strawberries	1	Milk

Selenium

I.U. per 100-gram (3.5 oz) portion		I.U. per 100-gram (3.5 oz) portion	
144	Butter	141	Smoked herring
123	Smelts	111	Wheat germ

103	Brazil nuts	89	Apple cider vinegar
77	Scallops	66	Barley
66	Whole wheat bread	65	Lobster
63	Bran	59	Shrimps
57	Red swiss chard	56	Oats
55	Clams	51	King crab
49	Oysters	48	Milk
43	Cod	39	Brown rice
34	Top round steak	30	Lamb
27	Turnips	26	Molasses
25	Garlic	24	Barley
19	Orange juice	19	Gelatin
19	Beer	18	Beef liver
18	Lamb chop	18	Egg yolk
12	Mushrooms	12	Chicken
10	Swiss cheese	5	Cottage cheese
5	Wine	4	Radishes
4	Grape juice	3	Pecans
2	Hazelnuts	2	Almonds
2	Green beans	2	Kidney beans
2	Onions	2	Carrots
2	Cabbage	1	Oranges

Iodine

I.U. per 100-gram (3.5 oz) portion		I.U. per 100-gram (3.5 oz) portion	
90	Clams	65	Shrimp
62	Haddock	56	Halibut
50	Oysters	50	Salmon
37	Sardines, canned	19	Beef liver
16	Pineapple	16	Tuna, canned
14	Eggs	11	Peanuts
11	Whole wheat bread	11	Cheddar cheese
10	Pork	10	Lettuce

9	Spinach		9	Green peppers
9	Butter		7	Milk
6	Cream		6	Cottage cheese
6	Beef		3	Lamb
3	Raisins			

Nickel

I.U. per 100-gram (3.5 oz) portion			I.U. per 100-gram (3.5 oz) portion	
700	Soybeans, dry		500	Beans, dry
410	Soy flour		310	Lentils
250	Split peas		175	Green peas
153	Green beans		150	Oats
132	Walnuts		122	Hazelnuts
100	Buckwheat		90	Barley
90	Corn		90	Parsley
38	Whole wheat		35	Spinach
30	Fish		27	Cucumbers
26	Liver		25	Rye bread
25	Pork		25	Carrots
24	Eggs		22	Cabbage
20	Tomatoes		20	Onions
16	Potatoes		16	Beef
16	Apricots		16	Oranges
15	Cheese		15	Watermelon
14	Lettuce		13	Apples
12	Whole wheat bread		12	Beets
12	Pears		8	Grapes
8	Radishes		6	Pine nuts
6	Lamb		3	Milk

Molybdenum

I.U. per 100-gram (3.5 oz) portion		I.U. per 100-gram (3.5 oz) portion	
155	Lentils	135	Beef liver
130	Split peas	120	Cauliflower
110	Green peas	109	Brewer's yeast
100	Spinach	100	Wheat germ
77	Beef kidney	75	Brown rice
70	Garlic	60	Oats
53	Eggs	50	Rye bread
45	Corn	42	Barley
40	Fish	36	Whole wheat
32	Whole wheat bread	32	Chicken
31	Cottage cheese	30	Beef
30	Potatoes	25	Onions
25	Peanuts	25	Coconut
25	Pork	24	Lamb
21	Green beans	19	Crab
19	Molasses	16	Cantaloupe
14	Apricots	10	Raisins
10	Butter	7	Strawberries
5	Carrots	5	Cabbage
3	Whole milk	1	Goat's milk

Vanadium

I.U. per 100-gram (3.5 oz) portion		I.U. per 100-gram (3.5 oz) portion	
100	Buckwheat	80	Parsley
70	Soybeans	64	Safflower oil
42	Eggs	41	Sunflower seed oil
35	Oats	30	Olive oil
15	Sunflower seeds	15	Corn

14	Green beans	11	Peanut oil
10	Carrots	10	Cabbage
10	Garlic	6	Tomatoes
5	Radishes	5	Onions
5	Whole wheat	4	Lobster
4	Beets	3	Apples
2	Plums	2	Lettuce
2	Millet		

REFERENCES

While writing this book, I have consulted the following list of publications. Some of the authors are named in the book as the sources of my information. Health care professionals and parents may find this bibliography useful for reading more about children's nutrition.

Aaronson, A. "Hypnosis, time perception and personality." Schizophrenia, 2: 11-14, 1968.

Altschul. R., Hoffer, A., and Stephen, J.D. "Influence of nicotinic acid on serum cholesterol in man." Archives of Biochemistry and Biophysics, 54: 558-559,1955.

Altschul, R. and Hoffer, A. "Effects of salts of nicotinic acid on serum cholesterol." British Medical Journal, 2: 713-714, 1958.

Alvarez, W.D. "Ways of discovering foods that are causing distress." Proceedings of Staff Meetings Mayo Clinic, 7: 443- , 1932.

Anderson, P. "Clozapine comes with money-back offer." The Medical Post, May 16, 1995.

Anderson, W.W. "The hyperkinetic child: A neurological appraisal." Neurology, 13: 968- , 1963.

Anonymous. "Molecules and Minds." The Lancet, 343: 681-682, 1994.

Anonymous. "Hyper children may be tamed by the right diet." The Medical Post, July 20, 1993.

Barnes, B.B. and Galton, L. Hypothyroidism : The Unsuspected Illness. New York, NY: Thomas Y. Crowell Company, 1976.

Bateson, G. Percival's Narrative: A Patient's Account of His Psychosis. Stanford,CA: Stanford University Press, 1961.

Bender, L. "Childhood schizophrenia." American Journal Orthopsychiatry, 26: 499-506, 1955.

Bender, L. and Helme, W.H. "A quantitative test of theory and diagnostic indicators of childhood schizophrenia." Archives Neurology & Psychiatry,70: 413-453, 1953.

Benton, D. and Roberts, G. "Effect of vitamin and mineral supplementation on intelligence of a sample of school children." The Lancet, 1: 140-143, 1988.

Benton, D. "Dietary sugar, hyperactivity and cognitive functioning: A methodological review." Journal of Applied Nutrition, 41: 13-0, 1989.

Benton, D. and Buts, J.P. "Vitamin/mineral supplementation and intelligence." The Lancet, 1: 1158-1160, 1990.

Benton, D. and Cook, R. "Vitamin and mineral supplements improve the intelligence scores and concentration of six-year-old children." Personality and Individual Differences, 12: 1151-1158, 1991.

Benton, D., Haller, J., and Fordy, J. "Vitamin supplementation for one year improves mood." Neuropsychobiology, 32: 98-105, 1995.

Birkmayer, W. and Birkmayer, G.J.D. "Nicotinamide adenine dinucleotide (NADH): the new approach in the therapy of Parkinson's disease." Annals of Clinical and Laboratory Science, 19: 38-43, 1989.

Birkmayer, J.G.D. and Birkmayer, W. "The coenzyme nicotinamide adenine dinucleotide (NADH) as biological antidepressive agent: Experience with 205 Patients." New Trends in Clinical Neuropharmacology, 5: 19-25, 1991.

Birkmayer, J.G.D., Vrecko. C., Volc, D., and Birkmayer, W. "Nicotinamide adenine dinucleotide (NADH) – a new therapeutic approach to Parkinson's disease. Acta Neurologica Scandanvica, 87, Supp 146: 32-35, 1993.

Birkmayer, J.G.D. "Nicotinamide adenine dinucleotide (NADH): the new therapeutic approach for improving dementia of the Alzheimer's type." Forschungs und Lehreinrichtung des Birkmayer Instituts fur Parkinsontherapie. Vienna, Austria. (Available from Menuco Corp., 350 Fifth Ave., Suite 7509, New York, NY 10118.)

Blackburn, M. "Use of efamol (oil of evening primrose) for depression andhyperactivity in children." In Omega-6 Essential Fatty Acids: Pathophysiology and Roles in Clinical Medicine. Ed. Horrobin, D.F. New York, NY: Liss, 1990.

Bray, G.W. "Enuresis of allergic origin." Archives of Disabled Children, 6: 251, 1931.

Breneman, J.C. "Nocturnal enuresis, a treatment regimen for general use." Annals of Allergy, 24: 185- , 1965.

Canner, P.L., Berge, K.G., Wenger, N.K., Stamler, J., Friedman, L., Prineas, R.J., and Freidewald, W. "Fifteen year mortality coronary drug project: Patients' long term benefit with niacin." American College of Cardiology, 8: 1245-1255, 1986.

Caplan, Paula J. They Say You're Crazy. New York, NY: Addison-Wesley, 1995.

Carroll, H.C.M. "A psychometric critique of Nelson et al's 1990 paper: Nutrient intakes, vitamin-mineral supplementation and intelligence in British school children." Personality and Individual Differences, 18: 669-675, 1995.

Cheraskin, E., Ringsdorf, W.M., and Sisley, E.L. The Vitamin C Collection. New York, NY: Harper and Row, 1983.

Cleave, T.L., Campbell, G.D., and Painter, N.S. Diabetes, Coronary Thrombosis and the Saccharine Disease. Bristol, UK: John Wright and Sons, 1969.

Cleave, T.L. The Saccharine Disease. New Canaan, CT: Keats Publishing, 1975.

Colgan, M. and Colgan, L. "Do nutrient supplements and dietary changes affect learning and emotional reactions of children with learning difficulties? A controlled series of 16 cases." Nutrition and Health, 3: 69-77, 1984.

Colquhoun, I. and Buondy, S. "A lack of essential fatty acids as a possible cause of hyperactivity in children." Medical Hypothesis, 7: 673-679, 1981.Compendium of Pharmaceuticals and Specialties. 30th ed. Ottawa, ON: Canadian Pharmaceutical Association, 1995.

Cott, A. "Treatment of ambulant schizophrenics with vitamin B-6 and relative hypoglycemic diet." Journal of Schizophrenia, 2: 189-196, 1967.

Cott, A. "Treatment of schizophrenic children." Schizophrenia, 1: 44- , 1969.

Cott, A. "Orthomolecular approach to the treatment of learning disabilities." Schizophrenia, 3: 95-105, 1971.

Cott, A. "Treatment of learning disabilities." Journal of Orthomolecular Psychiatry, 3: 343-355, 1974.

Cott, A., Agel, J., and Boe, E. Dr. Cott's Help for Your Learning Disabled Child: The Orthomolecular Treatment. New York, NY: Times Books, 1985.

Crawford, M. and Marsh, D. Nutrition and Evolution. New Cannan, CT: Keats Publishing, 1995. (First published in 1989 as The Driving Force).

Crook, W.G. The Allergic Tension-Fatigue Syndrome in Allergy of the Nervous System. Ed. F. Speer. Springfield, IL: C.C. Thomas, 1970.

Crook, W.G. and Stevens, L. Solving the Puzzle of Your Hard to Raise Child. Jackson, TN: Professional Books, 1987.

Davis, D.R. "The Harrell study and seven follow-up studies: A brief review." Journal of Orthomolecular Medicine, 2: 11-115, 1987.

Davison, H.M. "Allergy of the nervous system." Quarterly Review of Allergy, 6: 157- , 1952.

Egger, J., Wilson, J., Carter, C.M., Turner, M.W., and Southill, J.F. "Is migraine food allergy? A double blind controlled trial of oligoantigenic diet treatment." The Lancet, 2: 865-868, 1983.

Egger, J., Carter, C.M., Graham, P.J., Gumley, D., and Soothill, J.F. "A controlled trial of aligoantigenic diet treatment in the hyperkinetic syndrome." The Lancet 1: 940-945, 1985.

Egger, J., Stolla, A., and McEwen, L.M. "Controlled trial of hyposensitization in children with food induced hyperkinetic syndrome." The Lancet, 339: 1150-1153, 1992.

Esperenca, M. and Gerrard, J.W. "Nocturnal enuresis studies in bladder function in normals and enuretics." Canadian Medical Association Journal, 101: 269- , 1969.

Esperenca, M. and Gerrard, J.W. "Nocturnal enuresis comparison of the effect of imipramine and dietary restrictions on bladder capacity." Canadian Medical Association Journal, 191: 721- , 1969.

Feingold, S.F. Introduction to Clinical Allergy. Springfield, IL: C.C. Thomas, 1973.

Fogel, S. and Hoffer, A. "Perceptual changes induced by hypnotic suggestions for the post hypnotic state." Journal of Clinical Experimental Psychopathology 23: 24-35, 1962.

Gerrard, J.W., MacKenzie, J.W.A., Goluboff, N., Gardson, J., and Manangas, C.S. "Cows' milk allergy: prevalence and manifestations in an unselected series of newborns." Acta Pediatrica Scandanavica, Supp. 234, 1- , 1973.

Gerrard, J.W. Understanding Allergies. Springfield, IL: C.C. Thomas, 1973.

Gillberg, C. and Coleman, M. The Biology of the Autistic Syndromes. 2nd ed. New York, NY: MacKeith Press and Oxford Blackwell Scientific, 1992.

Goldman, B. "Pertussis vaccine: Why do some parents say no?" Canadian Medical Association Journal, 139: 1174-1177, 1988.

Gottschalk, L.A., Rebello, T., Buchsbaum, M.S., Tucker, H.G., and Hodges, E.L. "Abnormalities in hair trace elements as indicators of aberrant behavior." Comprehensive Psychiatry, 32: 229-237, 1991.

Green, R.G. "Subclinical pellagra: its diagnosis and treatment." Schizophrenia, 2: 70-79, 1970.

Green, G. "Learning disability." Canadian Medical Association Journal, 110: 617- , 1974.

Green, R.G. "Subclinical pellagra – a CNS allergy. Journal of Orthomolecular Psychiatry, 3: 312-318, 1974.

Green, R.G. "To be or not to be sublinical pellagra." Journal of Orthomolecular Psychiatry, 6: 186-193, 1977.

Green, R.G. "Hyperactivity and the learning disabled child." Journal of Orthomolecular Psychiatry, 9: 93-104, 1980.

Hallaway, N. and Strauts, Z. Turning Lead into Gold: How Heavy Metal Poisoning Can Affect Your Child and How to Prevent and Treat It. Vancouver, BC: New Star Books, 1995.

Harrell, R.F., Capp, R.H., Davis, D.R., Peerless, J., and Ravitz, L.R. "Can nutritional supplements help mentally retarded children? An exploratory study." Proceedings of the National Academy of Sciences. 78: 574-578, 1981.

Hattersley, J.G. "The answer to crib death." Journal of Orthomolecular Medicine, 8: 229-245, 1993.

Hauser, P., Zametkin, A.J., Martinez, P., Vitiello, B., Matochik, J.A., Mixson, A.J., and Weintraub, B.D. "Attention deficit-hyperactivity disorder in people with generalized resistance to thyroid hormone." New England Journal of Medicine, 328: 997-1001, 1993.

Hemila, H. "Is there a biochemical basis for 'nutrient need'?" Trends in Food Science and Technology, 73: 1991.

Heseker, H., Kubler, W., Pudel, V., and Westenhoffer, J. "Psychological disorders as early symptoms of a mild-to-moderate vitamin deficiency." In Beyond Deficiency. Ed. H.E. Sauberlich and L.J. Machlin. Annals of the New York Academy of Sciences, 669: 352-357, 1992.

Hoffer, A., Osmond, H., and Smythies, J. "Schizophrenia: a new approach. II. Results of a year's research." Journal of Mental Science, 100: 29-45, 1954.

Hoffer, A. "Adrenochrome and adrenolutin and their relationship to mental disease." In Psychotropic Drugs. Eds. S. Garattini and V. Ghetti. London, UK: Elsevier Press, 1957.

Hoffer, A., Osmond, H., Callbeck, M.I., and Kahan, I. "Treatment of schizophrenia with nicotinic acid and nicotinamide." Clinical Experimental Psychopathology, 18: 131-158, 1957.

Hoffer, A. and Osmond, H. "The adrenochrome model and schizophrenia." Journal of Nervous and Mental Disorders, 128: 18-35, 1959.

Osmond, H. and Hoffer, A. "Schizophrenia: a new approach. III." Journal of Mental Science, 105: 653-673, 1959.

Hoffer, A. and Osmond, H. The Chemical Basis of Clinical Psychiatry. Springfield, IL: C.C. Thomas, 1960.

Hoffer, A. and Osmond, H. "A card sorting test helpful in making psychiatric diagnosis." Journal of Neuropsychiatry, 2: 306-330, 1961.

Hoffer A. and Osmond, H. "A card sorting test helpful in establishing prognosis." American Journal of Psychiatry, 118: 840-841, 1962.

Hoffer, A. Niacin Therapy in Psychiatry. Springfield, IL: C.C. Thomas, 1962.

Hoffer, A. "The effect of adrenochrome and adrenolutin on the behavior of animals and the psychology of man." International Review of Neurobiology, 4: 307-371, 1962.

Hoffer, A. and Osmond, H. "Malvaria: a new psychiatric disease." Acta Psychiatrica Scandanavica, 39: 335-366, 1963.

Hoffer, A. "The presence of malvaria in some mentally retarded children." American Journal of Mental Deficiency, 67: 730-732, 1963.

Osmond, H. and Hoffer, A. "Massive niacin treatment in schizophrenia: Review of a nine-year study." The Lancet, 1: 316-320, 1963.

Hoffer, A. and Osmond, H. "Treatment of schizophrenia with nicotinic acid – a ten year follow-up." Acta Psychiatrica Scandanavica, 40: 171-189, 1964.

Hoffer, A. "D-lysergic acid diethylamide (LSD): a review of its present status." Clinical Pharmacology and Therapeutics, 6: 183-255, 1965.

Hoffer, A. "A comparison of psychiatric inpatients and outpatients and malvaria." International Journal of Neuropsychiatry, 1: 430- 432, 1965.

Hoffer, A. "Malvaria, schizophrenia and the HOD test." International Journal of Neuropsychiatry, 2: 175-177, 1965.

Hoffer, A. "Malvaria and the law." Psychosomatics, 7: 303-310, 1966.

Hoffer, A. "Quantification of malvaria." International Journal of Neuropsychiatry, 2: 559-561, 1966.

Hoffer, A. and Osmond, H. "Nicotinamide adenine dinucleotide (NAD) as a treatment for schizophrenia." Psychopharmacology, 1: 79-95, 1966.

Hoffer, A. "Use of nicotinic acid and/or nicotinamide in high doses to treat schizophrenia." Canadian Journal of Psychiatric Nursing, 76: 5-6, 1966.

Hoffer, A. "Enzymology of Hallucinogens." In Enzymes in Mental Health. Eds. J.G. Martin and B. Kisch. New York, NY: J.B. Lippincott Co., 1966.

Hoffer, A. and Osmond, H. How To Live With Schizophrenia. New York, NY: University Books and London, UK: Johnson, 1966. New and Revised Ed; New York, NY: Citadel Press, 1992; Kingston, ON: Quarry Press, 1999.

Hoffer, A. "Families of malvarians." Schizophrenia, 1: 77-89, 1967.

Hoffer, A. "Treatment of schizophrenia with a therapeutic program based upon nicotinic acid as the main variable." In Molecular Basis of Some Aspects of Mental Activity, Vol II. Ed. o. Walaas. New York, NY: Academic Press, 1967.

Hoffer, A. and Osmond, H. The Hallucinogens. New York, NY: Academic Press, 1967.

Hoffer, A. "A program for the treatment of alcoholism: LSD, malvaria and nicotinic acid." In The Use of LSD in Psychotherapy and Alcoholism. Ed. H.A. Abramson. New York, NY: Bobbs-Merril, 1967.

Hoffer, A. and Osmond, H. "Nicotinamide adenine dinucleotide." Psychopharmacology, 1: 79-95, 1967.

Hoffer, A. "Safety, side effects and relative lack of toxicity of nicotinic acid and nicotinamide." Schizophrenia, 1: 78-87, 1969.

Hoffer, A. "Childhood schizophrenia: a case treated with nicotinic acid and nicotinamide." Schizophrenia, 2: 43-53, 1970.

Hoffer, A. "Vitamin B-3 dependent child." Schizophrenia, 3: 107-113, 1971.

Hoffer, A. "A vitamin B-3 dependent family." Schizophrenia, 3: 41-46, 1971.

Hoffer, A. "Treatment of hyperkinetic children with nicotinamide and pyridoxine." Canadian Medical Association Journal, 107: 111-112, 1972.

Hoffer, A. "Mechanism of action of nicotinic acid and nicotinamide in the treatment of schizophrenia." In Orthomolecular Psychiatry. Eds. D.R. Hawkins and Linus Pauling. San Francisco, CA: W.H. Freeman and Co., 1973.

Hoffer, A. "Hallucinogens." Encyclopedia Britannica, 15th ed. 557-560, 1974.

Hoffer, A., Kelm, H., and Osmond, H. The Hoffer-Osmond Diagnostic Test. Huntington, NY: R.E. Krieger, 1975.

Hoffer, A. "Children with learning and behavioral disorders." Journal of Orthomolecular Psychiatry, 5: 228-230, 1976.

Hoffer, A. and Osmond, H. In Reply to The American Psychiatric Association Task Force Report on Megavitamin and Orthomolecular Therapy in Psychiatry. Toronto, ON: Canadian Schizophrenia Foundation, 1976.

Hoffer, A. and Walker, M. Orthomolecular Nutrition. New Cannan, CT: Keats Publishing Inc, 1978. Rev. ed. Putting It All Together: The New Orthomolecular Nutrition, 1996.

Hoffer, A. "The adrenochrome hypothesis of schizophrenia revisited." Journal of Orthomolecular Psychiatry, 10: 98-118, 1981.

Hoffer, A. "Orthomolecular nutrition at the zoo." Journal of Orthomolecular Psychiatry, 12: 116-128, 1983.

Hoffer, A. Vitamin B-3 (Niacin). New Canaan, CT: Keats Publishing, 1984.

Hoffer, A. "Dopamine, noradrenalin and adrenalin metabolism to methylated or chrome indole derivatives: two pathways or one?" Journal of Orthomolecular Psychiatry, 14: 262-272, 1985.

Hoffer, A. Common Questions on Schizophrenia and Their Answers. New Canaan, CT: Keats Publishing, 1988. Rpt. Kingston, ON: Quarry Press, 1999.

Hoffer, A. and Osmond, H. "The adrenochrome hypothesis and psychiatry." Journal of Orthomolecular Medicine, 5: 32-45, 1990.

Hoffer, A. Vitamin B-3 (Niacin) Update. New Roles For a Key Nutrient in Diabetes, Cancer, Heart Disease and Other Major Health Problems. New Canaan, CT: Keats Publishing, 1990.

Hoffer, A. "Chronic schizophrenic patients treated ten years or more." Journal of Orthomolecular Medicine, 9: 7-37, 1994.

Hoffer, A. Hoffer's Laws of Natural Nutrition: Eating Well for Pure Health. Kingston, ON: Quarry Press, 1996.

Hoffer, A. Vitamin B-3 & Schizophrenia: Discovery, Recovery, Controversy. Kingston, ON: Quarry Press, 1998.

Hoffer, A. Vitamin C & Cancer: Discovery, Recovery, Controversy. Kingston, ON: Quarry Press, 1999.

Hoffer, L.J. "Beyond deficiency: the therapeutic actions of nutrients." Personal communication. July, 1995.

Hoobler, B.R. "Some early symptoms suggesting protein sensitization in infancy." American Journal of Disabled Children, 12: 129- , 1916.

Horrobin, D.F. "Essential fatty acids, psychiatric disorders and neuropathis." In Omega-6 Essential Fatty Acids: Pathophysiology Indoles in Clinical Medicine. Ed. D.F. Horrobin. New York, NY: Wiley-Liss, 1990.

Kaplan, B.J., McNicol, J., Conte, R.A., and Moghadam, H.K. "Dietary replacement in preschool-aged hyperactive boys." Pediatrics, 83: 7-17, 1989.

Jones, B., Gerrard, J.W., Shokeir, M.K., and Houston, C.S. "Recurrent urinary infections in girls: relation to enuresis." Canadian Medical Association Journal, 106: 127- , 1972.

Kahan, F.H. "Schizophrenia, mass murder and the law." Journal of Orthomolecular Psychiatry, 2: 127-146, 1973.

Kahan, F.H. "A strange case." Journal of Orthomolecular Psychiatry, 3: 111-132, 1974.

Kahn, I.S. "Pollen toxemia." Journal of the American Medical Association, 82: 241- , 1927.

Kalokerinos, A. Every Second Child. New Canaan, CT: Keats Publishing, 1981.

Kaufman, W. "Niacinamide: A most neglected vitamin." In New Dimensions in Preventive Medicine. New Dimensions in Health. Ed. L.R. Pomeroy. International Academy of Preventive Medicine, 8: 5-25, 1983.

Kaufman, W. The Common Forms of Niacinamide Deficiency Disease: Aniacinamidosis. Bridgeport, CN: Yale University Press, 1943.

Kaufman, W. The Common Form of Joint Dysfunction: Its Incidence and Treatment. Brattleboro, VT: E.L. Hildreth & Co, 1949.

Kelm, H., Hoffer, A., and Hall, R.W. "Reliability of the Hoffer-Osmond Diagnostic test." Journal of Clinical Psychology, 23: 380-382, 1967.

Kelm, H. and Hoffer, A. "Age and the Hoffer-Osmond Diagnostic test." International Journal of Neuropsychiatry, 3: 406-407, 1967.

Krilanovich, N.B. No Sugar Added or Redesigning our Children's Future. Santa Barbara, CA: November Books, 1982.

Langer, S.E. and Scheer, J.F. Solved: The Riddle of Illness. New Canaan, CT: Keats Publishing, 1995.

Lucas, A., Morley, R., Cole, T.J., Lister, G., and Leeson-Payne, C. "Breast milk and subsequent intelligence quotient in children born preterm." The Lancet, 339: 261-264, 1992.

Mandell, M. and Rose, G.J. "May emotional reactions be precipitated by allergens?" Connecticut Medicine, 32: 300- , 1968.

Mandell, M. "Central nervous system hypersensitivity to housedust, molds, and foods: Provocation of acute cerebral reactions in an asthmatic child: The case report of a cerebral respiratory syndrome and a motion picture film record of test-induced reactions." Review of Allergy, April 24, 1970.

Marlowe, M. and Bliss, L.B. "Hair element concentrations and young children's classroom and home behavior." Journal of Orthomolecular Medicine, 8: 79-88, 1993.

Marlowe, M. "The violation of childhood: Toxic metals and developmental disabilities." Journal of Orthomolecular Medicine, 10: 79-86, 1995.

Marlowe, M. and Palmer, L. "Hair trace element status of Appalachian Head Start children." Journal of Orthomolecular Medicine, 11: 15-22 1996.

Meiers, R. "Personal communication," 1972.

Miller, J.B. "Sweets can cause hyperactivity!" Latitudes, 2: 4-5, 1995.

Minskoff, J.G. "Differential approaches to prevalence estimates of learning disabilities." In Minimal Brain Dysfunction. Eds. F.F. de la Cruz, B.H.Fox, and R.H. Roberts. Annals of the New York Academy of Sciences, 205: 139-XX, 1973.

Mullenix, P.J., Denbesten, P.K., Schunior, A., and Kernan, W.J. "Neurotoxicity of sodium fluoride in rats." Neurotoxicology and Teratology, 17: 169-177, 1995.

Needleman, H.L. and Landrigan, P. "Toxic de-ja vu all over again." Letter, February 1996, from Red Hodges.

Nelson, P., Naismith, D.J., Burley, J., Gatenby, S., and Geddes, N. "Nutrient intake

vitamin/mineral supplementation and intelligence in British school children."
British Journal of Nutrition, 64: 13-22, 1989.

Nesse, R.M. and Williams, G.C. Why We Get Sick. New York, NY: Random
House, 1994.

Newbold, H.L., Philpott, W.H., and Mandell, M. "Psychiatric syndromes produced by allergies: Ecological mental illness." Orthomolecular Psychiatry, 2:
84- , 1973.

Newbold, H.L. The Psychiatric Programming of People. Elmsford, NY:
Pergamon Press, 1972.

Olney, J.W. "Excitotoxins in foods." Neurotoxicology, 15: 535-544, 1994.

Parsons, W.B. "Cholesterol Control Without Diet." In The Niacin Solution.
Scottsdale, AR: Lilac Press, 1998.

Pauling. L. "Orthomolecular Psychiatry." Science, 160: 265-271, 1968.

Pauling, L. Vitamin C and the Common Cold. New York, NY: Bantam Books, 1971.

Pauling, L. How To Live Longer and Feel Better. New York, NY: W.H. Freeman
and Co., 1986.

Pfeiffer, C.C., Ward, J., El-Meligi, M., and Cott, A. The Schizophrenias: Yours and
Mine. New York: Pyramid Books, 1970.

Pfeiffer, C.C. and Iliev, V. "A study of zinc deficiency and copper excess in the
schizophrenias." International Review of Neurobiology, Supp 1, 141, 1972.

Pfeiffer, C.C., Iliev, V., and Goldstein, L. "Blood histamine, basophil counts and
trace elements in the schizophrenias." Orthomolecular Psychiatry. Ed. D.R.
Hawkins and L. Pauling. San Francisco, CA: W.H. Freeman, 1973.

Pfeiffer, C.C. Sohler, A., Jenney, M.S., and Iliev, V. "Treatment of pyrroluric
schizophrenia (malvaria) with large doses of pyridoxine and a dietary
supplement of zinc." Journal of Applied Nutrition, 26: 21-28, 1974.

Pfeiffer, C.C. Zinc and Other Micronutrients. New Cannan, CT: Keats
Publishing, 1978.

Pfeiffer, C.C. Mental Illness and Schizophrenia: The Nutrition Connection.
Wellingborough, Northamptonshire, UK and Rochester, VT: Thorsons
Publishing, 1987.

Pfeiffer, C.C., Mailloux, R., and Forsythe, L. The Schizophrenias: Ours To
Conquer. Wichita, KS: Biocommunications Press, 1988.

Philpott, W.H. "Food and chemical hypersensitivity as an aspect of molecular
disease and stress decompensation" and "The significance of adreno-cortical
pituitary normalization and detoxification as a preparation for behavioral
desensitization practice." International Academy of Metabology, New York,
March 23, 1973.

Philpott, W.H. "Methods of relief of acute and chronic symptoms of deficiency -
allergy - addiction maladaptive reactions to foods and chemicals." Seventh
Advanced Seminar in Clinical Ecology, Ft Lauderdale, January 9, 1974.

Powell, N.B., Boggs, P.B., and McGovern, J.P. "Allergy of the lower urinary tract." Annals of Allergy, 28: 252, 1970.

Powell, N.B., Powell, E.B., Thomas, O.C., Queng, J.T., and McGovern, J.P. "Allergy of the lower urinary tract." Journal of Urology, 107: 631- , 1972.

Randolph, T.G. "Ecological mental illness – Levels of central system reactions." The Third World Congress of Psychiatry, Montreal, 1: 379, 1961.

Randolph, T.G. "Clinical ecology as it affects the psychiatric patient." International Journal of Social Psychiatry, 12: 245- , 1966.

Randolph, T.G. "Domiciliary chemical air pollution in the etiology of ecologic mental illness." International Journal of Social Psychiatry, 16: 243- , 1970.

Rapp, Doris J. with Bamberg, D. The Impossible Child. Buffalo, NY: Practical Allergy Research Foundation, 1986.

Rees, E.L. "Clinical observations on the treatment of schizophrenic and hyperactive children with megavitamins." Orthomolecular Psychiatry, 2:93- , 1973.

Rimland, B. Infantile Autism: The Syndrome and Its Implications for a Neural Theory of Behavior. New York, NY: Appleton-Century Crofts, 1964.

Rimland, B. "High dosage levels of certain vitamins in the treatment of children with severe mental disorders." In Orthomolecular Psychiatry. Edited by David Hawkins and Linus Pauling. San Francisco, CA: W.H. Freeman, 1973.

Rimland, B. "An orthomolecular study of psychotic children." Orthomolecular Psychiatry, 4: 371-377, 1974.

Rimland, B., Callaway, E., and Dreyfus, P. "The effect of high doses of vitamin B-6 on autistic children: A double blind crossover study." American Journal of Psychiatry, 135: 472-475, 1978.

Rimland, B. "Recent research in infantile autism." Journal of Operational Psychiatry, 3: 35, 1972; and Autism Research Review International, 7: No. 2, 1993.

Rimland, B. "Address to California State Senate." Autism Research Review International, 9: 3, 1995.

Rimland, B. "Nutritional treatment for autism: The history." Latitudes, 1: 5- 13, 1995.

Rinkle, H.J., "The technique and clinical application of individual food tests." Annals of Allergy, 2: 504- , 1944.

Robertson, W.O. "Does iron prevent effects of lead exposure?" Canadian Medical Association Journal, 154: 146 & 148, 1996.

Rossi, A.D. "Psychoneurologically impaired child." New York State Journal of Medicine. 67: 902- , 1967.

Rowe, A.H. "Allergic toxemia and migraine due to food allergy." California West Medical Journal, 33: 785- , 1930.

Rudin, D.O. "The major psychoses and neuroses as Omega-3 essential fatty acid deficiency syndrome: substrate pellagra." Biological Psychiatry, 16: 837-850, 1981.

Rudin, D.O. "The three pellagras." Journal of Orthomolecular Psychiatry, 12: 91-110, 1983.

Rudin, D.O. and Felix, C. with Schrader, C. The Omega-3 Phenomenon. New York, NY: Rawson Associates, 1987.

Schoenthaler, S.J. "The impact of a low food additive and sucrose diet on academic performance in 803 New York City Public Schools." International Journal of Biosocial Research, 8: 185-195, 1986.

Schoenthaler, S.J., Doraz, W.E., and Wakefield, J.A. "The testing of various hypotheses as explanations for the gains in a national standardized academic test scores in the 1978-1983 New York City Nutrition policy modification project." International Journal of Biosocial Research, 8: 196-203, 1986.

Schulz, J.B., Henshaw, D.R., Matthews, R.T., and Beal, M.F. "Coenzyme Q_{10} and nicotinamide and a free radical spin trap protect against MPTP neurotoxicity." Experimental Neurology, 132: 279-83, 1995.

Schroeder, H.A. The Trace Elements and Man. Old Greenwich, CN: Devin Adair Co., 1973.

Shannon, W.R. "Neuropathic manifestations in infants and children as a result of anaphylactic reactions to food contained in their diet." American Journal of Disabled Children, 24: 89- , 1922.

Silverman, L.J. and Metz, A.S. "Numbers of pupils with specific learning disabilities in local public schools in the United States: Spring 1970." In Minimal Brain Dysfunction, Ed. F.F. de la Cruz, B.H. Fox, and R.H. Roberts. Annals of the New York Academy of Sciences, 205: 146- , 1973.

Silverman, L. "Orthomolecular treatment in disturbances involving brain function." Journal of Orthomolecular Psychiatry, 4: 71-84, 1975.

Simons, F.E.R., Chad, Z.H., and Collins, S.M. "Food allergy and intolerance: New directions." Annals of the Royal College Physicians and Surgeons, Canada, 26: 29-32, 1993.

Spies, T.D., Aring, C.D., Gelperin, J., and Bean, W.B. "The mental symptoms of pellagra: their relief with nicotinic acid." American Journal Medical Science, 196: 461- , 1938.

Soothill, J. "Food intolerance." The Practitioner, 233: 596-598, 1989.

Stevens, L.J., Zentall, S.S., Deck, J.L., Abate, M.L., Watkins, B.A., Lipp, S.R., and Burgess, J.R. "Essential fatty acid metabolism in boys with attention deficit hyperactivity disorder." American Journal of Clinical Nutrition, 62: 761-768, 1995.

Stewart, M.A. "Hyperactive children." Scientific American, 222: 94-98, 1970.

Stewart, M., Ferris, A., Pitts, N., and Craig, A.G. "The hyperactive child syndrome." American Journal of Orthopsychiatry, 36: 861- , 1966.

Stipp, D. "The way we were – Our prehistoric past casts new light, some scientists say." Wall Street Journal, May 24, 1995.

Stone, I. The Healing Factor: Vitamin C Against Disease. New York, NY: Grosset and Dunlap, 1970.

Towbin, A. "Mental retardation due to germinal matrix infections." Science, 164: 156- , 1969.

Towbin, A. "Organic causes of minimal brain dysfunction." Journal of the American Medical Association. 217: 1207- , 1971.

Trent, J.W. Jr. "Suffering fools." The Sciences, 35: 18-22, 1995.

Tuormaa, T.E. "The adverse effects of food additives on health with a special emphasis on childhood hyperactivity: A review of the literature." Journal of Orthomolecular Medicine, 9: 225-243, 1994.

Turkel, H. and I. Nussbaum. Medical Treatment of Down Syndrome and Genetic Diseases. Southfield, MI: Ubiotica, 1986.

Wald, G. and Jackson, B. "Activity and nutritional deprivation." Proceedings of the National Academy of Science, 30: 255-263, 1944.

Walker, S. A Dose of Sanity: Mind, Medicine and Misdiagnosis. New York, NY: John Wiley and Sons, 1996.

Warden, N., Duncan, M., and Sommars, E. "Nutritional changes heighten children's achievement: A five year study." International Journal of Biosocial Research, 3: 72-74, 1982.

Weiss, J.M. and Kaufman, H.S. "A subtle organic component in some cases of mental illness." Archives of General Psychiatry, 25: 74- , 1971.

Westad, K. "Descent into Madness." Times Colonist (Victoria, BC), June 8, 1995.

Wilson, E.D. Wilson's Syndrome. Orlando, FL: Cornerstone Publishing, 1993.

Winneke, G. "Zinc to prevent lead poisoning." Canadian Medical Association Journal, 154: 1622-1623, 1996.

Zaleski, A., Shokier, M.K., and Gerrard, J.W. "Enuresis: Familial incidence and relationship to allergic disorders." Canadian Medical Association Journal, 106: 30- , 1972.

Zametkin, A.J. "Attention deficit disorder: Born to be hyperactive?" Journal of the American Medical Association, 273: June 21, 1995.